Influenza: Diagnosis, Prevention and Management

Influenza: Diagnosis, Prevention and Management

Editor: Edwin Simpson

MURPHY & MOORE
www.murphy-moorepublishing.com

www.murphy-moorepublishing.com

MURPHY & MOORE

Cataloging-in-Publication Data

Influenza : diagnosis, prevention and management / edited by Edwin Simpson.
p. cm.
Includes bibliographical references and index.
ISBN 978-1-63987-322-7
1. Influenza. 2. Influenza--Diagnosis. 3. Influenza--Prevention. 4. Influenza--Treatment.
5. Virus diseases. 6. Respiratory infections. I. Simpson, Edwin.
RC150 .I54 2022
616.203--dc23

Murphy & Moore Publishing,
1 Rockefeller Plaza,
New York City, NY 10020, USA

ISBN 978-1-63987-322-7 (Hardback)

Contents

Preface

This book aims to highlight the current researches and provides a platform to further the scope of innovations in this area. This book is a product of the combined efforts of many researchers and scientists, after going through thorough studies and analysis from different parts of the world. The objective of this book is to provide the readers with the latest information of the field.

The infectious diseases caused by influenza viruses are termed as influenza. Symptoms of influenza generally begin after 1-4 days of exposure to the virus and last for 2-8 days. They include runny nose, sore throat, fever, headache, muscle pain, fatigue and coughing. In children, diarrhea and vomiting may also occur. The progression of influenza may cause pneumonia. It can be caused by a primary viral infection or a secondary bacterial infection. Other complications of influenza are worsening of pre-existing health problems such as asthma and cardiovascular diseases, and diseases such as meningitis, acute respiratory distress syndrome and encephalitis. Influenza viruses are classified into 4 types, namely, influenza virus A, B, C, and D. This book unfolds the different aspects of the diagnosis and management of influenza. It unravels the recent studies in this field. The extensive content of this book provides the readers with a thorough understanding of the subject.

I would like to express my sincere thanks to the authors for their dedicated efforts in the completion of this book. I acknowledge the efforts of the publisher for providing constant support. Lastly, I would like to thank my family for their support in all academic endeavors.

Editor

1

The Efficacy of Immunoadjuvant-Containing Influenza Vaccines in Pregnancy

Kostinov Mikhail Petrovich,
Cherdantsev Alexander Petrovich,
Shmitko Anna Dmitrievna,
Akhmatova Nelly Kimovna,
Kostinova Aristitsa Mikhailovna,
Praulova Darya Alexandrovna,
Polyschuk Valentina Borisovna,
Protasov Andrey Dmitrievich,
Zhestkov Alexander Victorovich and
Tezikov Yuriy Vladimirovich

Abstract

The aim of the work was to determine the clinical safety and immunogenicity of immunoadjuvant vaccines against influenza (MonoGripol Plus and Grippol® Plus) in 182 pregnant women in the II and III trimesters of gestation , and further assessment of fetal conditions and infants of the first 6 months of life. Results: It was shown that immunoadjuvant vaccines do not have a negative effect on the physiological course of pregnancy and the functional state of the fetoplacental complex. In the early postpartum period, the rates of physical and neuro-psychological development and the nature of feeding of children did not differ from the control group. In pregnant women vaccinated with Grippol® plus, the levels of seroprotection to strains of A/H1N1/v are 82.0%, A/H3N2/—88.0%, B—88.3% that measure the CPMP criteria and last more than a year . After birth, transplacental antibodies in children in protective values were observed in 52.3–68.9% of cases, did not differ from the control group, and disappear after 6 months. Respiratory infections during the first 6 months of life of infants born from mothers vaccinated against influenza registered in 1.8 times less frequently.

Keywords: pregnant women, vaccine against influenza, post-vaccination immunity.

1. Introduction

The reports of Strategic Advisory Group of Experts (SAGE) on Immunization underscore that between 7 and 10% of all hospitalized patients with severe influenza are women in the second and third trimester of pregnancy. The requirements of pregnant women with influenza infection for providing medical care in an intensive care unit are 10 times that of other population groups diagnosed with influenza [1–4].

Vaccination of pregnant women using the subunit and split influenza vaccines is routinely performed in a number of countries of Europe and America for over 20 years, and the vaccine efficacy reaches 70–85% [5, 6]. Clinical studies have shown that vaccination of pregnant women using modern inactivated influenza vaccines neither affect the course of pregnancy and fetal growth nor cause undesirable post-vaccination effects. It was found that vaccination of pregnant women using inactivated influenza vaccines leads to 50–63% reduction of flu-related morbidity among infants up to 6 months of age [7, 8].

The WHO Global Advisory Committee on Vaccine Safety indicates that influenza vaccination is a non-alternative approach to safe and effective prevention of influenza in pregnancy [1, 9, 10]. In Russia, the indications for vaccination of pregnant women using modern vaccines are defined within the National Immunization Program Schedule of Russian Federation (RF) (order of Ministry of Healthcare of Russian Federation №125n of 21 March 2014). Federal clinical guidelines "Influenza vaccination of pregnant women" and manuals for physicians have been published which establish the main vaccination requirements for the primary health care in Russia [11–13].

The unfavorable epidemiological situation with influenza that occurred in 2009 has accelerated the development and implementation in healthcare practices of adjuvant-containing pandemic influenza vaccines such as Fluad (containing squalene) and Arepanrix™H1N1 (containing AS03—squalene + α-Tocopherol acetate) which confer enhanced immunogenicity [1, 14]. Adjuvants accelerate, change the dynamics of development of the immunity, and increase its level and the duration of persistence of post-vaccination antibodies. With the help of an adjuvant, durable and solid immunity is achieved by administering small doses of antigen and a less number of injections.

In Russia, two adjuvant-containing subunit influenza vaccines have been developed (monovalent (pandemic) and trivalent preparations). These drugs, in contrast to non-adjuvant subunit vaccines against influenza (e.g., Agrippal S1 containing 15 μg strains of influenza viruses type A and B), have 5 μg of both strains of the influenza virus and an adjuvant-immunomodulator polyoxidonium. In clinical trials, immunoadjuvant vaccines demonstrated high efficacy and safety in children aged 6 months and older and in adults. The trivalent adjuvant-based influenza vaccine is used in clinical practice for more than 20 years [15–24]. In experimental studies, these vaccines showed no teratogenic effect on the developing fetus. Despite extensive use of these vaccines for specific prevention of influenza in Russia, studies on their safety in pregnancy have not been conducted until recently. The information on the effects of adjuvant-containing vaccines on the fetus and post-natal development was missing. The information on vaccine immunogenicity for pregnant women at different gestational age, as well as vaccine ability to confer an adequate passive immunity to a fetus, was insufficient.

The study aimed at determining clinical safety and immunogenicity of "MonoGrippol Plus" and "Grippol® Plus" vaccines in pregnant women in the second and third trimesters of pregnancy with assessment of fetal condition and condition of infants during the first 6 months of life.

2. Materials and methods

2.1. Legal basis of the research

The study was carried out according to the protocol which met the National standard of Russian Federation—GOST P 52379-2005 "Good Clinical Practice" and the international GCP (good clinical practice) standards. Vaccination of pregnant women was carried out with adherence to the ethical norms and guidelines of the WHO and Ministry of Health care of RF.

Women to be vaccinated and followed up were selected strictly in accordance with a case report form that was examined and approved by the Ethics Committee of the Ulyanovsk State University (protocol №35 of 14.01.2010).

The observation of pregnant women before and after vaccination was carried out jointly with an obstetrician-gynecologist in accordance with requirements of the Order of Ministry of Health care and Social Development of RF of 02.10.2009 N 808n "On the approval of the Order of providing obstetric and gynecologic care." Before vaccination, women underwent laboratory testing after they have given the informed consent to participate in the study (**Figure 1**).

During observation and examination of infants, we also adhered to the ethical requirements applicable to biomedical studies. Development of the order and scope of studied parameters was based on provisions listed in the Order № 370 of Ministry of Healthcare of RF of 28.04.2007.

2.2. Randomization

The study was a randomized, placebo-controlled, single-blind, comparative, parallel-group study conducted on pregnant women and infants.

All candidates for study program underwent a preliminary assessment of whether they met the protocol inclusion and exclusion criteria (in accordance with the GMP standards).

Eligibility criteria:

1. Healthy pregnant women aged 20–40.
2. Volunteers capable of fulfilling the protocol requirements (i.e., able to fill in the self-observation diary and turn up for the scheduled visits).
3. Written informed consent of the volunteers to participate in the clinical study.

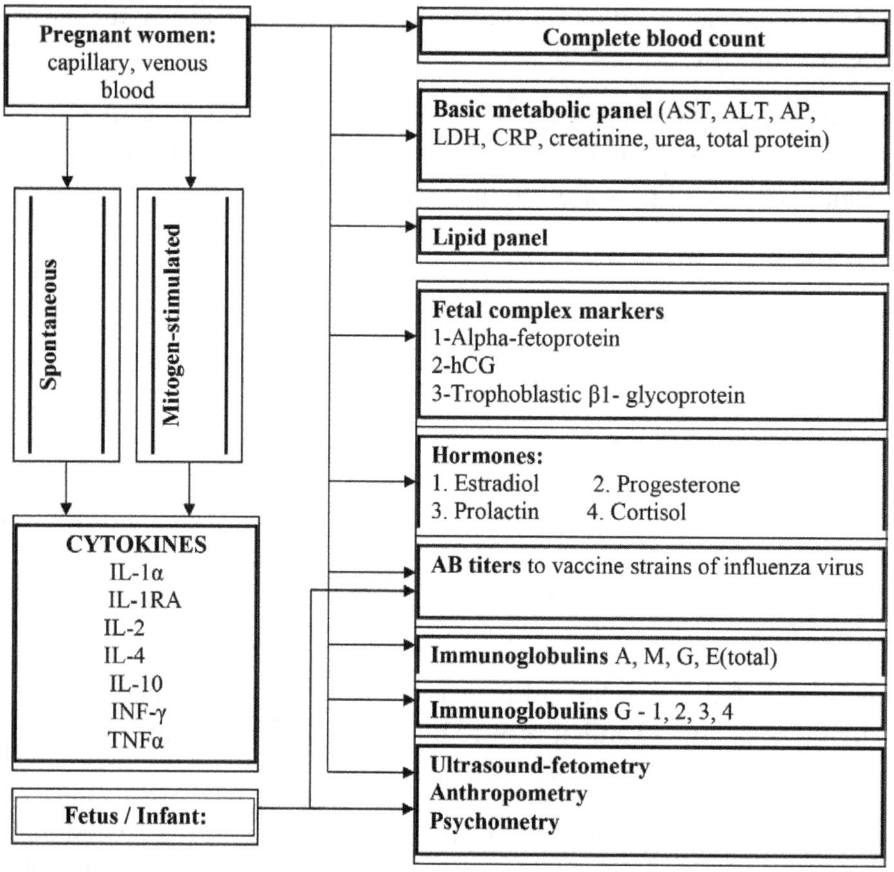

Figure 1. An algorithm of laboratory, physical and instrumental investigation.

Exclusion criteria:

1. History of leukemia, oncologic conditions or positive tests for HIV, hepatitis B and C.
2. Volunteers who had received the immunoglobulin preparations or blood transfusions within the last three months prior to the study.
3. Long-term (more than 14 days) administration of immunodepressants or other immunomodulating drugs within the last six months prior to the study.
4. Any confirmed or suspected immunosuppressive or immunodeficiency disorder.
5. History of chronic alcohol abuse and/or substance abuse.
6. Presence of respiratory or cardiovascular insufficiency, hepatic or renal impairment revealed during physical examination or by laboratory tests at visit 1.
7. Severe congenital defects or serious chronic diseases including any clinically significant diseases of lungs, kidneys, cardiovascular system, nervous system, psychiatric diseases or metabolic disorders confirmed by anamnestic data or objective clinical examination.

8. Presence of acute infectious and/or non-infectious diseases at the time of enrollment in the study.
9. Pregnancy via IVF procedure.

2.3. Duration of observation

A total number of pregnant women vaccinated against influenza during the epidemic seasons of 2009–2010, 2010–2011, and 2011–2012 were 345 subjects. Of those, the number of women and their children participated in an in-depth examination and their assignment to groups and subgroups is presented in **Table 1**.

The frequency of clinical examination and blood collection for laboratory testing in the post-vaccination period was based on the gestational age at the start of observation. Women vaccinated in the second and third trimesters underwent 7 and 6 examinations, respectively.

2.4. Assessment of fetal conditions

Fetometric measurements were carried out using the ultrasound (US) examination during pregnancy weeks 21–22 and 33–35 and included determination and calculation of biparietal diameter (BPD), fronto-occipital size (FOS), head circumference (HC), abdominal circumference (AC), estimated fetal weight (FW) and the femur length/abdominal circumference (FL/AC) ratio. The generally accepted guidelines were followed to evaluate the parameters obtained.

2.5. Assessment of infant conditions

Infant observation started from the first hours and days of life (day 2–3) and was conducted jointly with a neonatologist at maternity home. The basic signs of functional and morphological maturity of the newborn (Apgar score), blood work parameters/biochemical profile and antibody levels to influenza virus strains have been analyzed. All newborns at maternity home underwent neurosonography and cardiac sonography. Basic anthropometric measurements included body weight (BW), body length (BL), head circumference (HC), chest circumference (CC), and height-weight index (Ketle 1).

At the age of 3 and 6 months, the main parameters of physical and neuropsychological development and feeding pattern have been recorded.

2.6. Hormonal status in pregnant women

Hormone concentration in pregnant women was measured using the licensed immunoenzyme test-systems (IETS) such as "Estradiol-EIA" (LLC "Chema," Germany), "EIA-Progesterone,"

	Group I Pregnant women vaccinated with "MonoGrippol Plus"		Group II Pregnant women vaccinated with "Grippol® Plus"		Group III Pregnant women vaccinated with "Agrippal S1"		Group IV Pregnant women who had received "Placebo"		Group V Non-pregnant women, who had received	
	Trimesters of pregnancy								MonoGrippol Plus	Grippol Plus
	II	III	II	III	II	III	II	III		
Number of women participated in study program	28	15	27	23	27	21	22	19	30	19
Total:	43		50		48		41		49	
Average age (years)	25.1 ± 0.7		23.3 ± 0.4		27.8 ± 0.6		24.1 ± 0.3		23.1 ± 0.4	
Number of children born to women vaccinated during pregnancy	24	14	27	21	23	19	18	17		
Total:	38		48		42		35			

Table 1. Study participants' assignment to observation groups.

"EIA-Prolactin," "EIA-Cortisol" (LLC "Alcor Bio Company, Russia"). Fetoplacental complex markers, such as serum alpha-fetoprotein (AFP), human chorionic gonadotropin (hCG) and trophoblastic β1-glycoprotein (TBG), were tested using the IETS from CJSC "Vector-Best," Russia.

2.7. Cytokine profile

Serum cytokines were measured to determine levels of interleukin-1α (IL-1α), interleukin-2 (IL-2), interleukin-4 (IL-4), interferon-γ (IFN-γ), tumor necrosis factor α (TNFα), interleukin-1α receptor antagonist (IL-1RA), and interleukin-10 (IL-10). We used a dual cytokine assay to measure spontaneous and mitogen-induced cytokine production using a system of sample preparation from "Cytokine-Stimul-Best" (CJSC "Vector-Best", Russia). As the test systems, we used standard EIA kits (CJSC "Vector-Best" and LLC "Cytokine", Russia).

2.8. Humoral immune response to vaccination

Concentration of serum immunoglobulins A, M, G, E and IgG subclasses was determined using the appropriate IETS from CJSC "Vector-Best," Russia. Titers of antibodies to influenza virus strains A and B were measured in the hemagglutination inhibition test (HAI) as recommended by the WHO for this kind of studies. As viral antigens, we used the A/California/7/2009/H1N1/v-like, A/H3N2/(Victoria)-like and B (Brisbane)-like strains provided by the laboratory of artificial antigens (FSFI "State Research Center at the Institute of Immunology" of FMBA, Russia).

Vaccine immunogenicity was determined based on criteria established by the Committee for Proprietary Medicinal Products (CPMP) according to the protocol CPMP/BWP/214/96:

1. *Seroprotection level* (>70%).
2. *Seroconversion level* or *vaccine immunologic activity* (>40%).
3. *Seroconversion factor* or *geometric mean fold rise* (>2.5).

2.9. Vaccines

All vaccines used in the study were subunit inactivated preparations. Development of "MonoGrippol Plus" and "Grippol® Plus" vaccines (LLC "NPO Petrovax Pharm," Russia) is based on a special technology of coupling of highly purified protective influenza virus antigens with a polymeric, water-soluble, high-molecular weight adjuvant polyoxidonium. This technology enables a threefold reduction of hemagglutinin (HA) of each viral strain (down to 5 μg) in the vaccine compared to the analog subunit, adjuvant-free vaccine "Agrippal S1" ("Novartis Vaccines and Diagnostics," Italy).

"MonoGrippol Plus" contains antigens of only one influenza virus strain, namely A/California/7/2009/H1N1/v and belongs to the monovalent pandemic influenza vaccines, whereas

"Grippol Plus" and "Agrippal S1" additionally contain antigens of other strains, that is, A/H3N2/(Victoria)-like and B/Brisbane-like (trivalent vaccines).

2.10. Placebo

As a placebo, we used phosphate buffer saline ("GlaxoSmithKline Biologicals") which is used as a diluent for lyophilized vaccines.

2.11. Vaccination

Vaccination of pregnant women was performed in the vaccination room with adherence to sanitary and hygiene regulations, with emergency care available at once. Vaccine preparations were injected intramuscularly as a single-dose of 0.5 mL in the upper third of the arm (deltoid muscle).

2.12. Evaluation of vaccination safety

After an injection, the woman was observed for 40 min for the adverse reaction(s), which were scored to categorize reactions as described in **Table 2**.

Local reactions	
0—absent	Absence of symptoms
1—mild	Hyperemia up to 50 mm in diameter or infiltrate up to 25 mm in diameter
2—moderate	Hyperemia over 50 mm in diameter or infiltrate 26–50 mm in diameter
3—severe	Infiltrate over 50 mm in diameter
Systemic reactions	
0—absent	Absence of symptoms
1—mild	Presence of mild symptoms
2—moderate	Symptoms which markedly impair normal daily activity
3—severe	Symptoms which interfere with normal daily activity
Fever	
0—absent	≤37°C
1—mild	>37°C to ≤37.5°C
2—moderate	>37.6°C to ≤38.5°C
3—severe	>38.6°C

Table 2. Assessment of undesirable post-vaccination reactions.

All possible changes in the well-being and health state were recorded in the case report form (CRF) and self-observation diary (SOD) which the women continued to fill in on a daily basis throughout the first month of the follow-up.

2.13. Statistical analysis

Statistical analysis of samples which did not follow a normally distributed pattern was carried out using the non-parametric tools or parametric methods when the samples followed a normal distribution. We used the applied software package "Microsoft Excel" with the "AtteStat" application (version 10.10.2.). The differences were considered significant at $p < 0.05$.

3. Results and discussion

3.1. Particulars of the course of pregnancy in women vaccinated with "Grippol® Plus"

Although many pregnant women had a history of somatic diseases before they entered the study, as a rule, no exacerbation of pre-existing disease has been observed. The most commonly encountered illness was a mild hypochromic anemia (60.5, 70.0, 61.3, and 60.9% of pregnant women in group I–IV, respectively). Markers of chronic urogenital infection were detected fairly often (44.2% in group I, 46.0% in group II, 59.1% in group III, and 41.5% in group IV). Also, the syndrome of vegetative dystonia (20.9% in group I, 38.0% in group II, 20.5% in group III, and 29.3% in group IV) and altered allergic response (16.3% in group I, 20.0% in group II, 18.2% in group III, and 19.5% in group IV) had been observed. All women had approximately the same frequency of cases of threatened miscarriage in the past (53.5% in group I, 48.0% in group II, 47.7% in group III, and 51.2% in group IV). Therefore, clinical condition of pregnant women was comparable among the groups [25].

3.1.1. Clinical course of the post-vaccination period

Evaluation of the clinical course of the post-vaccination period has shown that it was asymptomatic in 58.1% of women from group I, 60.0% from group II, 54.5% from group III, and 60.9% from group IV ($p > 0.05$). It came under notice that in groups I, II, and III, women vaccinated in the third trimester of pregnancy developed the post-vaccination local and systemic undesirable effects significantly less often than women vaccinated in the second trimester ($p < 0.05$ to $p < 0.01$). The local symptoms occurred in the first few days after vaccination included pain, hyperemia, and infiltration at the site of injection. Such reactions occurred more often in pregnant women immunized with trivalent vaccines (group II—8.0%, group III—10.4%) than in women from placebo group (4.9%), ($p < 0.05$). It was noted that pregnant women from group I developed no or minimal systemic adverse reactions (nausea, fatigability, dizziness or myalgia) where intensity was significantly lower compared to that in women vaccinated with trivalent vaccine, namely group I—6.9% ($p < 0.05$ versus group II), group II—12.0%, group III—10.4%, and group IV—10.2% [26, 27].

3.1.2. Clinical blood analysis

In the late (8–30 days) post-vaccination period, no local post-injection reactions have been reported in either group. Systemic reactions included frequent complaints on increased fatigability and headaches in women from group III ($p < 0.05$). With regard to other symptoms, the groups did not differ significantly between each other and the placebo group (group I—9.3%, group II—14.0%, group III—12.5%, and group IV—12.2%). All symptoms were of a transient nature and required no medication management [26, 27].

Analysis of complete blood count has shown that for the majority of formed elements, cell counts did not differ from normal values in both pre-vaccination and post-vaccination periods. Occasional differences were mostly related to the particulars of the pregnancy period. Analysis of basic metabolic panel performed in dynamics on day 7 and day 30 of the post-vaccination period in each group also did not reveal significant abnormalities which could reflect changes in the metabolic homeostasis ($p > 0.05$). Small changes in creatinine level (minimal value in group III at day 30 post-vaccination—58.04 ± 1.57 μmol/L) and alkaline phosphatase (AP) (maximum value in group III at day 30 post-vaccination—86.23 ± 7.84 IU/L) are not remarkable and fall within the average normal values, attesting to normal variability of this parameter [28, 29].

3.1.3. Lipid metabolism

Analysis of lipid panel obtained 30 days post-vaccination has shown that in all groups, the parameters of lipid/cholesterol metabolism are not significantly altered, and remain within physiological variations [12, 13].

3.1.4. Hormonal profile

Analysis of hormonal profile among vaccinated women has revealed only the intra-group changes in hormone levels which are not so much related to vaccination but rather are due to the gestational age.

Significant differences in prolactin, progesterone, estradiol, and cortisol serum levels were observed in women of different gestational age regardless of whether they received monovalent or trivalent influenza vaccine or placebo ($p < 0.05$). Therefore, it can be affirmed that, despite certain differences in the composition of influenza vaccines used in the study, there are no hormonal changes which could have influenced the state of the fetoplacental unit [12, 13].

3.1.5. Humoral immunity

Serum levels of immunoglobulins measured immediately after vaccination and on day 7 post-vaccination were comparable in pregnant women immunized with different influenza vaccines. At day 30, post-vaccination pregnant women who had received the monovalent influenza vaccine demonstrated higher IgA levels (2.56 ± 0.27 mg/mL) compared to women vaccinated with trivalent preparations (1.61 ± 0.09 mg/mL in group II, 1.34 ± 0.11 mg/mL in group III, and 1.14 ± 0.14 mg/mL in group IV) ($p < 0.01$ to $p < 0.001$). Despite the above differences, the antibody levels reflect normal serum IgA variations. Despite the established difference, the IgA content in all comparison groups was recorded within the physiological norm. Levels of IgM and IgG antibodies did not differ significantly between the groups.

Some variations in the IgG subclasses (1, 2, 3, 4) in the early and late post-vaccination periods were found. However, these variations remained within the acceptable range. In pregnant women with a history of allergic diseases, vaccination against influenza had no subsequent effect on serum total IgE levels.

3.1.6. Cytokine profile

It was noted that all pregnant women vaccinated with different vaccine preparations had elevated levels of mitogen-stimulated IL-1α at day 7 post-vaccination. By day 30, concentration of IL-1α remained elevated as compared to placebo control ($p < 0.05$) although was significantly lower than in vaccinated non-pregnant women ($p < 0.01$). No changes in the IL-2 and TNFα levels have been observed in vaccinated pregnant women although were also significantly higher than in non-pregnant women ($p < 0.01$). The IL-1RA values in a spontaneous cytokine production assay were significantly elevated only after vaccination with trivalent preparations by day 7 (group II) and by day 30 (groups II and III) post-vaccination ($p < 0.01$). At the same time, following mitogen stimulation, no significant changes in the IL-2 concentration have been found in any group. All pregnant women demonstrated significant increase in the IL-IRA and IL-10 following mitogen stimulation regardless of the type of vaccine that reflected the mechanism of physiological control of immune activation.

The IL-4 levels were most stable, with no significant dynamic changes among the groups. The only exception was a subgroup of women immunized with a non-adjuvanted trivalent vaccine in different trimesters of pregnancy. It was noted that by day 7 post-vaccination, a higher level of stimulated IL-4 was found in vaccinated women in the third trimester of pregnancy (6.85 ± 0.11 pg/mL in group III) as compared to pregnant women who had received the adjuvant-containing vaccine during the same period (2.95 ± 0.09 pg/mL in group II) ($p < 0.05$). Subsequently (on day 30 post-vaccination), such differences between the groups could not be found.

Pregnant women had lower IFNγ levels in the mitogen-stimulated cytokine production assay (881.86 ± 92.93 pg/mL in group I, 784.17 ± 65.03 pg/mL in group II, 854.89 ± 68.71 pg/mL in group III, and 790.30 ± 45.55 pg/mL in group IV) than the non-pregnant women (1419.60 ± 69.45 pg/mL in group V) which reflected a natural background level of physiological immune response ($p < 0.05$). At the same time during the first 7 days, post-vaccination elevated IFNγ was detected only in pregnant women who had received the polymer-subunit vaccines (6.47 ± 1.68 pg/mL in group I and 5.89 ± 1.08 pg/mL in group II) as compared to group III (3.03 ± 0.39 pg/mL) ($p < 0.05$). These differences were short-lived, and by day 30, post-vaccination was undetectable [30].

Therefore, the overall picture of cytokine profile in pregnant women had a trend characteristic of physiologic immunosuppression in pregnancy, that is, moderately elevated IL-IRA and

IL-10 and the absence in the post-vaccination period of significantly elevated anti-inflammatory cytokines in the mitogen-stimulation cytokine production assay. Nonetheless, the adjuvanted subunit vaccines had certain differences in their ability to influence cytokine secretion and short-term elevation of IFNγ which is most prominent in women in the second trimester of pregnancy that may reflect active involvement of the Th_1-mediated mechanisms of post-vaccination immunity. Use of non-adjuvanted vaccines leads to immune processes in the early post-vaccination period which are accompanied by increased IL-4 synthesis by blood leukocytes (a sign of Th_2-mediated activation) especially in women vaccinated in late pregnancy. The indirect evidence in favor of this suggestion is the absence of significance changes in the IFNγ levels in the early and late post-vaccination periods. All found changes of parameters recorded in different groups of vaccinated women remained within an acceptable range of variation. Also, no changes pertaining to destabilization of regulation and functioning of immune system due to influenza vaccination of pregnant women have been found [31].

3.2. Effect of vaccination of pregnant women using "Grippol® Plus" influenza vaccine on the antenatal fetal development

3.2.1. *Fetoplacental complex*

Monitoring of fetal development was carried out using a complex of measures, which included analysis of markers of fetoplacental complex and ultrasound fetometry. In all groups of women in the early and late post-vaccination period, no changes in the basic parameters of embryo/fetogenesis (AFP, hCG, TBG) have been found (**Table 3**). Changes in the above parameters did not depend on the type of influenza vaccine used and corresponded to the gestational age (second and third trimesters of pregnancy). Thus, for example, the TBG level in all

Parameter		**Group I "MonoGrippol Plus" (n = 43)**	**Group II "Grippol® Plus" (n = 50)**	**Group III "Agrippal S1" (n = 48)**	**Group IV "Placebo" (n = 41)**
In 7 days	TBG Ng/mL	97.93 ± 20.97	72.69 ± 11.89	88.04 ± 15.46	92.69 ± 20.88
	AFP IU/mL	60.05 ± 13.39	69.59 ± 7.62	81.09 ± 17.88	75.41 ± 10.36
	hCG IU/mL	36.51 ± 4.62	39.74 ± 8.22	40.43 ± 3.10	36.15 ± 2.48
In 30 days	TBG Ng/mL	124.85 ± 14.43	109.17 ± 10.81	118.21 ± 13.99	110.35 ± 13.12
	AFP IU/mL	98.65 ± 8.33	100.43 ± 11.01	110.84 ± 11.19	115.29 ± 9.92
	hCG IU/mL	29.52 ± 3.62	33.84 ± 7.55	29.24 ± 5.20	28.95 ± 1.88

Note: $p > 0.05$ for differences between groups.

Table 3. Fetal complex markers in pregnant women vaccinated against influenza (M ± m).

groups (including placebo control) of women vaccinated in the second trimester of pregnancy was significantly lower than in the third trimester ($p < 0.05$ to $p < 0.01$). A direct relationship was found between the TBG and AFP concentrations ($r = 0.60$; $p < 0.05$) with TBG levels rising as pregnancy progresses ($p < 0.001$). The hCG levels were dropping during the follow-up and inversely correlated with the TBG levels ($r = -0.50$; $p < 0.01$). All serum markers had no deviations from the reference values and reflected physiological changes in pregnancy [32].

3.2.2. Fetometry

Fetometry performed in the second (21–22 weeks) and third (33–35 `) trimester of pregnancy failed to reveal differences among the groups of pregnant women (**Table 4**).

Therefore, study results indicate that vaccination of pregnant women using the adjuvant-containing influenza vaccines "MonoGrippol Plus" and "Grippol® Plus" has no effect on the intrauterine fetal development. Changes of the basic parameters of fetoplacental unit are comparable between the groups and reflect physiological changes during fetal growth.

3.3. Pregnancy outcomes in women vaccinated with "MonoGrippol Plus" and "Grippol® Plus" influenza vaccines

In the majority of cases (85.4–90.7%), pregnancy resulted in physiologic birth (**Table 5**). In a fraction of women, their pregnancy terminated prematurely with the birth of preterm babies (between 2.0 and 8.3%) which corresponds to the preterm birth rate in the Ulyanovsk region of Russia (3.7–5.8%) where the study was taking place. Such outcome was due to the obstetric pathology which was unrelated to prior vaccination. Also, cases of birth of babies with perinatally acquired neurological impairment were mostly associated with gestational immaturity (7.3–10.4%). A fraction of babies had the intrauterine infection-like syndrome (2.0–6.3%) and developmental abnormalities and defects in 2.0–4.9% of cases (3.8–5.9% across the Ulyanovsk region) [33]. Owing to the above abnormalities, such babies were excluded from further study.

3.4. Particulars of development of up to 6 month old infants born to mothers vaccinated during pregnancy with "MonoGrippol Plus" and "Grippol® Plus" influenza vaccines

3.4.1. Apgar scale

The early neonatal period of infants born to mothers vaccinated during pregnancy had a comparable dynamics between the groups. It was shown that, immediately after birth, the number of babies with Apgar score of 8–9 points was similar between the groups (group I—92.1%, group II—87.5%, group III—80.9%, and group IV—94.3%) which attests to the overall good functional maturity. The period of adaptation in newborns passed without complications [34, 35].

3.4.2. Feeding

The feeding of infants born to mothers vaccinated with different influenza vaccines did not differ significantly between the groups. The highest number of nursing mothers (100%) during the neonatal period was observed in groups I and IV and was somewhat lower in groups

Clinical groups	Gestational age	Parameter					
		BPD (mm)	FOS (mm)	HC (mm)	AC (mm)	Fetal weight (g)	$\frac{FL}{AC} \times 100$ (%)
Group I "MonoGrippol Plus" (n = 43)	21–22 weeks	53.18 ± 3.20	73.87 ± 8.11	188.12 ± 13.72	162.81 ± 17.08	527.10 ± 92.31	21.54 ± 0.57
	33–35 weeks	87.81 ± 5.52	111.67 ± 12.9	313.01 ± 24.18	311.60 ± 18.57	2539.40 ± 437.10	22.04 ± 0.44
Group II "Grippol® Plus" (n = 50)	21–22 weeks	54.04 ± 2.70	70.07 ± 7.42	183.90 ± 11.86	170.11 ± 15.98	504.70 ± 96.01	19.49 ± 0.86
	33–35 weeks	89.11 ± 5.31	109.80 ± 14.20	304.21 ± 38.73	295.90 ± 21.07	2489.70 ± 367.30	23.13 ± 0.78
Group III "Agrippal S1" (n = 48)	21–22 weeks	52.56 ± 2.62	68.55 ± 8.12	180.87 ± 18.66	175.44 ± 16.08	489.50 ± 110.10	20.26 ± 0.93
	33–35 weeks	81.49 ± 6.53	106.12 ± 11.40	301.01 ± 21.74	298.30 ± 33.15	2595.2 ± 455.1	22.96 ± 1.04
Group IV "Placebo" (n = 41)	21–22 weeks	52.01 ± 3.9	67.22 ± 9.02	181.01 ± 15.31	178.79 ± 13.9	497.72 ± 138.03	20.99 ± 1.02
	33–35 weeks	82.77 ± 7.71	103.07 ± 8.33	299.82 ± 28.53	301.02 ± 29.34	2607.7 ± 631.0	22.73 ± 1.38

Note: $p > 0.05$ for differences between groups.

Table 4. Ultrasound-fetometry data in pregnant women vaccinated against influenza (M ± m).

Parameter		Group I "MonoGrippol Plus" (n = 43)	Group II "Grippol® Plus" (n = 50)	Group III "Agrippal S1" (n = 48)	Group IV "Placebo" (n = 41)
Women	Physiological birth	39 (90.7%)	48 (96.0%)	43 (89.5%)	35 (85.4%)
	Miscarriage	0	1 (2.0%)	1 (2.1%)	1 (2.4%)
	Premature birth	4 (9.3%)	1 (2.0%)	4 (8.3%)	3 (7.3%)
Infants	Without pathology	38 (88.4%)	46 (92.0%)	42 (87.5%)	33 (85.4%)
	Birth of babies with abnormalities or developmental defects	1 (2.3%)	1 (2.0%)	2 (4.2%)	2 (4.9%)
	Perinatal CNS lesions	4 (9.3%)	3 (6.0%)	5 (10.4%)	3 (7.3%)
	Intrauterine infection-like syndrome	2 (4.6%)	1 (2.0%)	4 (6.3%)	2 (4.9%)

Note: $p > 0.05$ for differences between groups.

Table 5. Outcomes of pregnancy and birth in women vaccinated against influenza.

II and III (85.4 and 92.9%, respectively) ($p > 0.05$). Further onwards, the number of infants receiving only breast milk gradually diminished (92.1% at 3 months and 65.8% at 6 months in group I; 85.4% at 3 months and 72.9% at 6 months in group II; 83.3% at 3 months and 69.0% at 6 months in group III; and 88.6% at 3 months and 60.0% at 6 months in group IV) ($p > 0.05$). Therefore, vaccination of women with subunit adjuvanted influenza vaccines during pregnancy has no further impact on lactation and duration of breastfeeding.

3.4.3. *Body weight and length*

Parameters of physical development of infants of the first 6 months of life from different groups were generally comparable. Body weight and body length at different time points were within the percentile rank (25-50-75). The Ketle 1 index in group I newborns was 65.1 ± 0.67, in group II—63.8 ± 1.22, in group III—65.5 ± 1.72, and in group IV—67.1 ± 1.03 ($p > 0.05$).

In the majority of cases, the proportionality of physical development among infants in their first few months of life had the average values of harmonious development, namely 65–74% in group I, 70–76% in group II, 69–81% in group III, and 69–76% in placebo group ($p > 0.05$). The infants with the average values below harmonious development were found equally often (14–22% in group I, 12–16% in group II, 12–19% in group III, and 18–21% in group IV). The infants with the average values above harmonious development (6–22% in group I, 10–17% in group II, 7–12% in group III, and 6–15% in group IV) were considered as a variant of body constitutional norm ($p > 0.05$). Infants with a disproportional physical development have not been found.

Therefore, our results attest to the sufficiency of basic criteria for infant development and reflect the population maturity in terms of their physical development regardless of vaccination of their mothers during pregnancy with different influenza subunit vaccines.

3.4.4. Neuropsychological development

Parameters of neuropsychological development (NPD) of children born to vaccinated mothers did not differ significantly from those of the placebo group. Overall, no changes of NPD have been observed in 81.6% of group I infants in their first 6 months of life who had been born to mothers vaccinated during pregnancy with a monovalent influenza vaccine. In other clinical groups, this parameter was 83.3% (group II), 78.6% (group III), and 77.1% (group IV) ($p > 0.05$). Within the structure of occasional NPD disorders, there were conditions which number did not exceed the average statistical rate of neurological pathology in a given pediatric age group.

It was noted that infants born to women vaccinated during pregnancy with trivalent influenza vaccines were 1.8-times less likely to develop non-influenza respiratory infections within the first 6 months of life as compared to infants from placebo control group (**Figure 2**).

3.5. Immunogenicity of adjuvanted influenza vaccine "Grippol® Plus" in pregnant women vaccinated during different trimesters of pregnancy

In this study, the level of post-vaccination antibodies to influenza virus was evaluated only in a group of pregnant women and non-pregnant women vaccinated with a trivalent adjuvanted influenza vaccine with the aim of revealing the features of the effect of pregnancy on the synthesis of antibodies. Since it has been already proven that the introduction of subunit unadjuvanted vaccines in pregnant women is accompanied by the formation of antibodies to the influenza virus in values not differing from those in non-pregnant ones, it seemed to us interesting to investigate the interaction of the immunoadjuvant preparation with the transiently altered immune status of the pregnant woman [36].

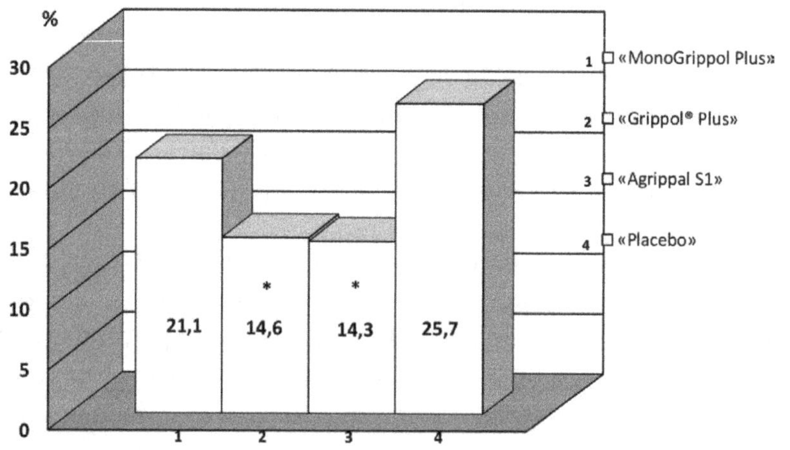

Figure 2. Incidence of morbidity due to non-influenza respiratory infections in infants during their first 6 months of life. *Note:* *- $p < 0.05$ for differences between groups I, II, III and group IV.

It was found that a part of women before immunization had a seroprotective (≥1:40) baseline antibody level to vaccine strains of influenza virus (**Table 6**). In all examined women, the antibody titer was higher to influenza virus B (22.2% of women in the second trimester, 26.1% in the third trimester and 25.7% in non-pregnant women). This is probably due to the duration of its circulation in the population and the formation of natural immunity. It should be noted that none of the participants in the study was vaccinated before and did not confirm an acute illness caused by the influenza virus. One month after vaccination, women of all groups demonstrated a significant rise in antibody titer that fully met one of the CPMP criteria. In the post-vaccination period, the antiviral antibody titer gradually declined reaching a significant difference against baseline by 3 months postpartum in women vaccinated in the second and third trimesters. The observed difference referred only to viral strain A/H1N1/v ($p < 0.05$). It is possible that the loss of antibodies to a pandemic strain is associated with the peculiarities of the formation of immunity after its first administration. Other authors have shown that specific antibodies to this strain in the post-vaccination period can be synthesized at lower values and therefore be accompanied by their faster loss. At 6 and 12 months post-vaccination, there was a marked regression of seroprotection level with regard to antibody titer against strains A/H1N1/v, A/H3N2/and B in women vaccinated during pregnancy in the second and third trimesters ($p < 0.01$). Such trend was also traced in a group of non-pregnant women; however, the changes were less remarkable, with a fairly significant fraction of subjects having a high level of protective antibodies. Similar dynamics of post-vaccination antibodies were noted in pregnant women vaccinated with subunit non-adjuvanted influenza vaccine [37].

The rate of development and intensity of protective immunity include the level and factor of seroconversion across all influenza virus strains. Those were compared between the groups, and it was found that their values met the CPMP criteria (**Table 7**). The majority of data obtained did not differ between the groups. One exception was the seroconversion factor for strain B in pregnant women vaccinated in the third trimester of pregnancy (5.1) when it was compared with the matching parameter in the non-pregnant women group (6.9) ($p < 0.05$).

The dynamics of influenza antibody (AB) titers based on the geometric mean titer (GMT) reflect the decline of antibody level with time in the post-vaccination period (**Table 8**). It was noted that at one month post-vaccination, the value of GMT AB to A/H1N1/v strain in women vaccinated in the second trimester of pregnancy was significantly lower (49.12 ± 0.29) compared to subjects vaccinated in the third trimester of pregnancy (60.99 ± 0.25) ($p < 0.05$). During all subsequent periods, this parameter showed no differences with regard to the trimester of pregnancy.

Pregnant women vaccinated in the third trimester of pregnancy showed at 3 months post-vaccination and throughout the follow-up period lower GMT AB titers to strain B compared to the non-pregnant women ($p < 0.05$ to $p < 0.01$). Similar trend was traced in women of the same group with regard to all influenza virus strains at 6 months postpartum compared to the non-pregnant women ($p < 0.05$ to $p < 0.01$).

Therefore, the post-vaccination immune response in women vaccinated with a trivalent adjuvanted influenza vaccine at different times of pregnancy, during the first month, did not differ

	Periods of observation	Second trimester (n = 27)			Third trimester (n = 23)			Non-pregnant women (n = 19)		
		A/H1N1/v	A/H3N2/	B	A/H1N1/v	A/H3N2/	B	A/H1N1/v	A/H3N2/	B
Seroprotection level (AB titer ≥ 1:40) (%)	Before vaccination (V)	3.7	11.1	22.2	8.7	13.0	26.1	2.6	14.1	25.7
	1 month post-V	77.0*	88.9*	85.2*	87.0*	87.0*	91.3*	83.1*	90.2*	94.4*
	3 months post-V	74.8	88.4	84.2	—	—	—	80.6	88.7	92.0
	6 (3) months post-V 2–3 days postpartum	74.1	81.5	77.8	62.0	76.2	71.4	78.5	83.1	88.2
	9 (6) months post-V 3 months postpartum	57.7 ×	69.2	65.4	57.1 ×	71.4	62.0	71.4	78.6	72.8
	12 (9) months post-V 6 months postpartum	48.2 ∇∇/×	65.4 ∇∇	57.7 ∇∇/×	50.0 ∇∇/×	61.1 ∇∇	55.6 ∇∇/×	67.6 ∇	72.5 ∇	69.1 ∇∇

Note: Time period elapsed since the moment of vaccination of women in the third trimester of pregnancy (group II) is given in brackets.

*: $p < 0.01$—the intra-group difference for the second/third trimesters of pregnancy; non-pregnant in-between pre-vaccination and 1 month post-vaccination.

∇: $p < 0.05$; ∇∇: $p < 0.01$—the intra-group difference for the second/third trimesters of pregnancy; non-pregnant in-between 1 month and 12 (9) months post-vaccination.

×: $p < 0.05$; ××: $p < 0.01$—difference between the second/third trimesters of pregnancy group and non-pregnant group.

Table 6. Seroprotection level in pregnant women vaccinated with "Grippol® Plus," allowing for trimester of pregnancy.

Parameter	Second trimester (n = 27)			Third trimester (n = 23)			Non-pregnant women (n = 19)		
	A/H1N1/	A/H3N2/	B	A/H1N1/	A/H3N2/	B	A/H1N1/	A/H3N2/	B
Seroconversion level (%)	70.4	77.8	74.1	69.6	78.3	65.2	71.5	81.1	70.3
Seroconversion factor	6.5	7.2	6.5	7.1	6.5	5.1*	6.8	7.6	6.9

Note: *$p < 0.05$ for difference between the third trimester group and non-pregnant group.

Table 7. Seroconversion level and seroconversion factor in pregnant women vaccinated with "Grippol® Plus," allowing for the trimester.

	Periods of observation	Second trimester (n = 27)			Third trimester (n = 23)			Non-pregnant (n = 19)		
		A/H1N1/v	A/H3N2/	B	A/H1N1/v	A/H3N2/	B	A/H1N1/v	A/H3N2/	B
Geometric mean antibody titer (log_2GMT AB)	Before vaccination (V)	7.54 ± 0.17	8.79 ± 0.23	13.96 ± 0.26	8.60 ± 0.23	10.62 ± 0.24	14.36 ± 0.25	8.02 ± 0.15	9.12 ± 0.21	14.19 ± 0.21
	1 month post-V	49.12 ± 0.29	63.49 ± 0.28	90.96 ± 0.36	60.99 ± 0.25 *	68.81 ± 0.26	73.08 ± 0.24	52.12 ± 0.22	59.47 ± 0.24	81.11 ± 0.37
	3 months post-V	47.87 ± 0.27	55.85 ± 0.26	65.15 ± 0.35	—	—	—	51.31 ± 0.24	57.73 ± 0.31	73.88 ± 0.26
	6 (3) months post-V 2–3 days postpartum	41.04 ± 0.23	44.33 ± 0.22	47.87 ± 0.32	41.34 ± 0.30	45.64 ± 0.25	42.72 ± 0.30 ×	48.56 ± 0.22	55.53 ± 0.24	63.13 ± 0.36
	9 (6) months post-V 3 months postpartum	30.64 ± 0.23	29.83 ± 0.22 ××	32.32 ± 0.29	30.72 ± 0.31	31.75 ± 0.32 ×	26.92 ± 0.35 ××	44.82 ± 0.25	51.79 ± 0.23	57.71 ± 0.31
	12 (9) months post-V 6 months postpartum	21.67 ± 0.24 ∇∇/×	24.10 ± 0.26 ∇∇/××	25.42 ± 0.25 ∇∇/××	20.79 ± 0.34 ∇∇/×	25.19 ± 0.33 ∇∇/××	19.24 ± 0.35 ∇∇/××	38.17 ± 0.26 ∇	44.47 ± 0.21 ∇	50.03 ± 0.28 ∇∇

Note: Time period elapsed since the moment of vaccination of women in the third trimester of pregnancy is given in brackets.

*: $p < 0.05$—for difference between the second trimester/third trimester groups.

∇: $p < 0.05$; ∇∇: $p < 0.01$—the intra-group difference for the second/third trimesters of pregnancy; non-pregnant between 1 month and 12 (9) months post-vaccination.

×: $p < 0.05$; ××: $p < 0.01$—for difference between the second trimester group, third trimester group and non-pregnant group.

Table 8. Geometric mean antibody titer in pregnant women vaccinated with "Grippol® Plus," allowing for the trimester.

from that in vaccinated non-pregnant women and fully met the CPMP criteria. The level of antibodies to strain A/H1N1/v following administration of a trivalent vaccine was nearly the same as with vaccination of pregnant women with the monovalent, subunit, adjuvanted vaccine [38, 39]

With time the postpartum women demonstrated a more pronounced reduction of seroprotection level, especially against the A/H1N1/v strain. After 6 months postpartum, the rate of regression of seroprotection level in subgroups of vaccinated pregnant women (taking into account the gestational age) has increased 1.6–1.7-fold (A/H1N1/v), 1.4-fold (A/H3N2) and 1.5- to 1.6-fold (B), whereas in the non-pregnant women group same parameter was 1.2-fold (A/H1N1/v), 1.2-fold (A/H3N2) and 1.4-fold (B), respectively. This trend was in line with dynamic reduction of the MGT AB values during the last months of the follow-up [38]. Consequently, the existing physiological immunological changes in the immune system during pregnancy may affect the formation and preservation of post-vaccination antibodies to strains of influenza virus when using subunit immunoadjuvant vaccines. However, this assumption should be confirmed by new data research.

3.6. Immunologic effectiveness of vaccination of pregnant women using "Grippol® Plus" influenza vaccine in mother-infant pairs

Analysis of transplacental immunity in the first months of life of infants born to women vaccinated during pregnancy with "Grippol® Plus" vaccine has shown that the level of seroprotection against influenza virus strains significantly differed only in the mother-infant pairs from the group of subjects vaccinated in the second trimester of pregnancy ($p < 0.05$), while no differences in the number of seroprotected infants have been found ($p > 0.05$) (**Table 9**). At 3 months after birth all infants, regardless of the time of their mothers' vaccination, demonstrated a significant reduction of protective titers of transplacental antibodies to vaccine strains of influenza virus as compared to their antibody titers obtained at birth and antibody titers in their mothers ($p < 0.01$). Further onwards, protective antibodies to vaccine strains of influenza virus completely vanished, and among the 6-month infants, the titer dropped to zero in both groups [40]. It should be noted that by 3 months of life, the rate of regression of antibody titer was higher in the subgroup of infants born to mothers vaccinated in late pregnancy, namely 2.8-fold higher for A/H1N1/v, 2.6-fold higher for A/H3N2/, and 4.0-fold higher for B strain.

Therefore, 52.3–61.9% of babies born to women vaccinated during pregnancy with "Grippol® Plus" vaccine had protective antibody levels against vaccine influenza strains at the time of their birth. This level of protection significantly declined with time and by 3 months of life remained at a protective level in only 14.2–24.0% of infants. At the age of 6 months, protective titers of maternal antibodies completely vanished in all infants. Infants born to women vaccinated in the second trimester of pregnancy had higher activity of protective antibodies and lower rate of reduction of seroprotection level which attests to a better preservation of the post-vaccination transplacental immunity. Thus, the advantage of vaccination of pregnant women with the use of immunoadjuvant subunit vaccine in the II trimester of gestation was revealed.

	Observation periods	Second trimester						Third trimester					
		A/H1N1/v		A/H3N2/		B		A/H1N1/v		A/H3N2/		B	
		M	**I**	**M**	**I**	**M**	**I**	**M**	**I**	**M**	**I**	**M**	**I**
Seroprotection level (%) (AB titer > 1:40)	Day 2–3 postpartum/ newborns	74.1	55.5 ×	81.5	59.3 ×	77.8	60.2 ×	62.0	52.3	76.2	61.9	71.4	57.1 ×
	At 3 months postpartum/3 months old	57.7	20.0 ××/⊗⊗	69.2	24.0 ××/⊗⊗	65.4	20.0 ▲××/⊗⊗	57.1	19.0 ××/⊗⊗	71.4	23.8 ××/⊗⊗	62.0	14.2 ××/⊗⊗
	At 6 months postpartum/6 months old	46.2	0 ⊗⊗	65.4	0 ⊗⊗	57.7	0 ⊗⊗	50.0	0 ⊗⊗	61.1	0 ⊗⊗	55.6	0 ⊗⊗
Geometric mean antibody titer (log_2GMT AB)	Day 2–3 postpartum/ newborns	41.04 ± 0.23	25.85 ± 0.29 ×	44.33 ± 0.22	27.22 ±0.26 ×	47.87 ±0.32	30.94 ±0.31	41.34 ±0.30	23.59 ±0.28 ×	45.64 ±0.25	26.91 ±0.25 ×	42.72 ±0.30	25.19 ±0.28 ×
	At 3 months postpartum/3 months old	30.64 ± 0.23	11.30 ± 0.26 ××/⊗⊗	29.83 ± 0.22	13.86 ±0.24 ××/⊗⊗	32.32 ±0.29	13.19 ±0.32 ××/⊗⊗	30.72 ±0.31	13.46 ±0.25 ××/⊗⊗	31.75 ±0.32	15.87 ±0.24 ××/⊗⊗	26.92 ±0.35	12.59 ±0.24 ××/⊗⊗
	At 6 months postpartum/6 months old	21.67 ± 0.24	7.52 ± 0.26 ××/⊗⊗	24.10 ± 0.26	8.49 ±0.20 ××/⊗⊗	25.42 ±0.25	7.23 ±0.22 ××/⊗⊗	20.79 ±0.34	8.91 ±0.20 ××/⊗⊗	25.19 ±0.33	11.22 ±0.19 ××/⊗⊗	19.24 ±0.35	7.94 ±0.18 ××/⊗⊗

Note: **M**—mother; **I**—infant.

▲: $p < 0.05$—for differences between infants from different observation groups.

×: $p < 0.05$; ××: $p < 0.01$—for differences between "mother-infant" groups.

⊗: $p < 0.05$; ⊗⊗: $p < 0.01$—for infants' intra-group differences versus at birth data.

Table 9. State of transplacental post-vaccination immunity in "mother-infant" pairs following vaccination against influenza using "Grippol® Plus" vaccine.

4. Conclusions

1. Different underlying diseases diagnosed in women of reproductive age are not an impediment to influenza vaccination during pregnancy.
2. Influenza vaccination during pregnancy using Russian-made polymer-subunit monovalent and trivalent vaccines ("MonoGrippol Plus" and "Grippol® Plus") in 58.1–60.0% of cases is accompanied by asymptomatic post-vaccination period. The frequency of systemic (generalized) post-vaccination reactions in immunized women (6.9–14.0%) does not differ significantly from that in placebo control group (10.2–12.2%).
3. Administration of adjuvanted vaccines to pregnant women does not cause disturbances of their metabolic homeostasis, hormonal profile, and cytokine profile.
4. Vaccination of pregnant women against influenza does not affect trophoblast function and fetal growth. Vaccination neither bears the risk of miscarriage nor influences the pattern and duration of breastfeeding.
5. Considering that safety of adjuvanted influenza vaccines has been proven by clinical and laboratory investigations, additional safety studies in pregnant women before and post-vaccination are redundant.
6. Babies born to mothers vaccinated against influenza with adjuvanted vaccines ("MonoGrippol Plus" and "Grippol® Plus") have a high level of physiological maturity. The basic parameters of physical and neuropsychological development in the early postnatal period in such infants do not differ from those of infants from control group.
7. Infants born to women vaccinated during pregnancy with influenza vaccines are 1.8 times less likely to develop non-influenza respiratory infections within the first 6 months of life as compared to infants born to unvaccinated mothers.
8. Administration of adjuvanted trivalent vaccine to pregnant women elicits a pronounced immune response to influenza vaccine strains A and B that fully meets the CPMP criteria for seroprotection levels: A/H1N1/v—82.0%, A/H3N2/—88.0% and B—88.3%.
9. Women vaccinated with the polymer-subunit vaccine in the second trimester of pregnancy benefit from higher seroprotection level and longer retention time of influenza-specific antibodies.
10. Protective titers of transplacental antibodies to different influenza virus strains are found in 52.3–68.9% of infants that is comparable to control figures. Higher levels of protective antibodies to different influenza virus strains are found in infants whose mothers have been vaccinated with adjuvanted vaccine "Grippol® Plus" in the second trimester of pregnancy.
11. Analysis of mother-infant pairs showed a direct correlation in levels of post-vaccination IgG influenza-specific antibodies between mother and infant. However, after 3 months, protective antibodies to influenza virus strains were detectable in 14.2–36.1% of infants followed by their complete disappearance at 6 months of life versus 57.1–71.4% (3 months)

and 48.1–65.4% (6 months) in their mothers. This observation provides substantiation that vaccination against influenza in high-risk infants shall start at the age of 6 months.

12. The results obtained allow us to recommend the "Grippol® Plus" vaccine for use in healthcare practice for specific prevention of seasonal influenza in pregnant women and their offspring up to age 6 months inclusive, using a single-dose vaccination schedule.

Author details

Kostinov Mikhail Petrovich[1,2], Cherdantsev Alexander Petrovich[3], Shmitko Anna Dmitrievna[1], Akhmatova Nelly Kimovna[1], Kostinova Aristitsa Mikhailovna[4], Praulova Darya Alexandrovna[5], Polyschuk Valentina Borisovna[1], Protasov Andrey Dmitrievich[6*], Zhestkov Alexander Victorovich[6] and Tezikov Yuriy Vladimirovich[7]

*Address all correspondence to: crosss82@mail.ru

1 Federal State-Funded Research Institution "Scientific Research Institute of Vaccines and Sera named after I.I. Mechnikov", Moscow, Russia

2 Federal State-Funded Educational Institution of Higher Education "First Moscow State Medical University named after I.M. Sechenov" of Ministry of Healthcare of Russia, Moscow, Russia

3 Federal State-Funded Educational Institution of Higher Education "Ulyanovsk State University", Ulyanovsk, Russia

4 National Research Center–Institute of Immunology Federal Medical-Biological Agency of Russia, Moscow, Russia

5 Dmitriy Rogachev Federal Research Center of Pediatric Hematology, Oncology and Immunology of the Ministry of Health of Russian Federation, Moscow, Russia

6 Federal State-Funded Educational Institution of Higher Education "Samara State Medical University" of Ministry of Healthcare of Russia, Samara, Russia

7 Department of Obstetrics and Gynecology №1, Samara State Medical University, Samara, Russia

References

[1] ECDC scientific advice on seasonal influenza vaccination of children and pregnant women: ECDC Technical report/European Centre for Disease Prevention and Control. Stockholm: ECDC. 2012. 68

[2] Jamieson DJ, et al. H1N1 2009 influenza virus infection during pregnancy in the USA. Lancet. 2009;**374**. P. 451-458

[3] Tarbaeva DA, Kostinov MP, Zagorodnya E D, Josefson SA, Cherdantsev AP. Obstetrical and perinatal outcomes of pregnancy complicated with acute respiratory infection in the second trimester of pregnancy. Obstetrics and Gynecology (Russian). 2012. (2). pp. 67-71

[4] Tarbaeva DA, Kostinov MP, Josefson SA, Zagorodnya E D. Clinical course and outcomes of influenza A (HINI) 2009 infection in pregnant women. Journal of Microbiology, Epidemiology and Immunobiology (Russian). 2011;(4):pp. 71-76

[5] Mullooly JP. Risk of acute respiratory disease among pregnant women during influenza A epidemics [Text]. Mullooly JP, Barker WH, Nolan TF. Public Health Reports. 1986. Vol. 101:pp. 205-211

[6] Fiore AE. Prevention and control of influenza with vaccines: Recommendations of the advisory committee on immunization practices (ACIP). 2010. Fiore AE. et al. MMWR Recommendations and Reports. 2010;Vol. 59: pp. 1-62

[7] Zaman K, et al. Effectiveness of maternal influenza immunisation in mothers and infants. The New England Journal of Medicine. 2008;**359**(15):pp. 1555-1564

[8] Englund JA. Maternal immunization with inactivated influenza vaccine: Rationale and experience. Vaccine. 2003;**21**:pp. 3460-3464

[9] Fiore AE, et al. Prevention and control of influenza with vaccines: Recommendations of the advisory committee on immunization practices (ACIP). MMWR Recommendations and Reports. 2010;(59):pp. 1-62

[10] CDC. Guidelines for Vaccinating Pregnant Women: From Recommendations of the Advisory Committee on Immunization Practices (ACIP) [Electronic resource]. Centers for Disease Control and Prevention. 2007. Mode of access: http://www.cdc.gOv/vaccines/pubs/preg-guide.htm#5/

[11] Zverev VV, Kostinov MP, Cherdantsev AP, Kuselman AI, Kiselev OI, Erofeeva MK, Krasnopolskiy VI, Novikova S V, Serova OF, Briko NI, Chuchalin AG. Vaccination of Pregnant Women Against Influenza: Federal Clinical Guidelines. Moscow (Russian). 2015. p. 42

[12] Cherdantsev AP, Kostinov MP, Kuselman AI. Vaccine Prophylaxis of Influenza in Pregnant Women. Manual for Physicians. M. 4Mpress (Russian). 2013. p. 96

[13] Cherdantsev AP, Kostinov MP, Kuselman AI. Vaccine prophylaxis of influenza in pregnant women/Manual for physicians. 2nd edition with supplement. M. MDV Art Studio «Constellation» (Russian). 2014. p. 112

[14] Tsai T, et al. Exposure to MF59-adjuvanted influenza vaccines during pregnancy–retrospective analysis. Vaccine. 2010;**7**(28):pp. 1877-1880

[15] Kostinov MP, Kostinova TA, Zolotareva TA. Potentials of vaccination against influenza in high-risk patient groups. «Hospital physician» Journal (Russian). 2001;(10). pp.52-54

[16] Clinico-immunologic effectiveness of immunobiological preparations/Reference book. Kostinov MP, Ozeretskovsky NA. Eds. Moscow. 2004–«Miklosh» (Russian). p. 256

[17] Kostinov MP, Lavrov VF. New generation vaccines for the prevention of infectious diseases. 2nd edition, with supplement, M.: MDV (Russian). 2010. p. 192

[18] Chebykina AV, Kostinov MP, Magarshak OO. Evaluation of safety and effectiveness of vaccination against influenza in patients with syndrome of bronchial obstruction. Epidemiology and Vaccinoprophylaxis (Russian). 2010;**6**(55): pp. 50-53

[19] Protasov AD, Zhestkov AV, Lavrentyeva NE, Kostinov MP, Ryzhov AA. Effect of complex vaccination against pneumococcal, haemophilus type B and influenza infections in patients with chronic obstructive pulmonary disease. Journal of Microbiology. Epidemiology and Immunobiology (Russian). 2011;(4):pp. 80-84

[20] Kostinov MP, Yerofeeva MK, Kharit SM. Effectiveness and safety of influenza vaccinoprophylaxis in different populations. All-Russia Interdisciplinary Journal TERRA MEDICA® (Russian). 2011;(2):pp. 7-11

[21] Kostinov MP, Chuchalin AG, Chebykina AV. Particulars of formation of post-vaccination immunity to influenza in patients with chronic broncho-pulmonary pathology. Infectious Diseases (Russian). 2011;**9**(3):pp. 35-40

[22] Vaccination of adults with broncho-pulmonary pathology. Manual for physicians (Kostinov MP., Ed.), M: 2013. Art studio «Constellation» (Russian). p. 109

[23] Vaccination of Children with Impaired Health State. Manual for Physicians (Kostinov MP, Ed.), 4th edition, M.: 4Mpress (Russian). 2013. p. 432

[24] Vaccines and Vaccination. National Manual (brief version, Zverev VV, Khaitov RM, Eds.) M.: Publishing group «GEOTAR-Media» (Russian). 2014: p. 640

[25] Cherdantsev AP. Effectiveness of immunoadjuvanted vaccines against influenza in pregnant women and evaluation of their safety for fetus and newborn/D. Med. Sci. Thesis (Russian), Moscow. 2013: p. 39

[26] Cherdantsev AP, Kuselman AI, Sinitsyna MN, Shalyagina ME, Kostinov MP, Tarbaeva DA. Study of clinical safety of vaccination against influenza in pregnant women. Medical Almanac (Russian). 2011;**4**(17):pp. 120-122

[27] Kostinov MP, Cherdantsev AP, Savisco AA, Tarbaeva DA, Solovieva IL. True and false reactions to influenza vaccine in pregnant women. Problems of Gynecology, Obstetrics and Perinatology (Russian). 2011;**10**(6):pp. 44-48

[28] Serova OF, Semenova SS, Cherdantsev AP, Tsaregorodseva MV. Evaluation of clinic-laboratory parameters in pregnant women vaccinated against influenza. Russian herald of obstetrics and gynecology (Russian). 2015;(2):pp. 75-79

[29] Cherdantsev AP, Kostinov MP, Kuselman AI, Voznesenskaya NV. Vaccination of pregnant women against influenza A(HINI). Journal of microbiology, epidemiology and immunobiology (Russian). 2011;(4):pp. 46-50

[30] Kostinov MP, Cherdantsev AP, Semenova SS, Tarbaeva DA, Savisco AA, Serova OF, Josefson S A, Akhmatova NK, Kostinova TA, Praulova DA. Obstetrical and perinatal

outcomes after vaccination against influenza or past respiratory infection. Gynecology (Russian), 2015;**14**(3):pp. 43-46

[31] Kostinov MP, Cherdantsev AP. Clinical and immunological safety of inactivated, immunoadjuvanted, subunit vaccine against influenza in pregnant women. Obstetrics and Gynecology (Russian). 2016;(2):pp. 64-69

[32] Cherdantsev AP, Kostinov MP, Kuselman AI, Liutaya ZA, Kutbutdinova MH. Analysis of the ante- and postnatal development of infants against a background of vaccination of pregnant women against influenza. Russian Herald of Perinatology and Pediatrics (Russian). 2013;**58**(2):pp. 30-34

[33] Cherdantsev AP, Kuselman AI, Kostinov MP, Liutaya ZA, Deryabina EV, Azizova R Sh, Melnik RH. Postnatal development of infants born to mothers vaccinated against influenza. Ulyanovsk Medico-Biological Journal (Russian). 2012;(3):pp.80-84

[34] Kostinov MP, Cherdantsev AP, Praulova DA, Kostinova AM. Vaccination against influenza—A safe way to protect pregnant women and newborns from consequences of infection. Russian herald of perinatology and pediatrics (Russian). 2015;(5):pp. 69-74

[35] Kostinov MP, Cherdantsev AP. State of health of infants born to mothers vaccinated against influenza during pregnancy. Pediatrics. Journal named after G.N. Speransky (Russian). 2016;(195):pp. 67-71

[36] Kostinov MP, Khromova EA, Savisko AA, Kostinova AM. Features of the immune system functioning during physiological pregnancy and their relationship with vaccination against influenza. CONSILIUM MEDICUM (Russian). 2016;#6.;**18**. pp. 59-62

[37] Mikhail P. Kostinov, Alexander P. Cherdantsev, Anna D Shmitko, Dmitry Pakhomov, Evgenia O Demina. Duration of Preservation of Antibodies to the Flu Virus in the Mother-Child Pairs during the Vaccination of Women Depending on the Trimester of Pregnancy. International Journal of Biomedicine. 2015;**5**(4): 179-183

[38] Kostinov MP, Cherdantsev AP, Briko NI. Mono and trivalent immunoadjuvant influenza vaccines immunologenicity and safety in pregnant women, The Fifth International Conference & Exhibitiom on: Influenza Vaccines for the World, 6-9 October, Albufeira Algarve Portugal, 2015. Posters № 109

[39] Cherdantsev AP, Kostinov MP, Kuselman AI, Dagil Yu A, Savisko AA. Post-vaccination immunity to influenza virus A/California/2009(H1N1)v in immunized pregnant women. Medical Immunology (Russian). 2012;**14**(6): pp. 527-532

[40] Kostinov MP, Cherdantsev AP and Pakhomov DV. Anti-influenza antibody level in mother-infant pairs depending on trimester of vaccination of pregnant women using immunoadjivant vaccine. Vaccines. 2015;**6**:5. http://dx.doi.org/2157-7560.1000297

2

Chronic Obstructive Pulmonary Disease (COPD): Clinical and Immunological Effects of Mono-Vaccination Against Influenza Using an Immunoadjuvant Vaccine of a New Class Versus Combined Administration S. pneumoniae, H. influenzae, and Influenza Vaccines

Andrey Dmitrievich Protasov ,
Mikhail Petrovich Kostinov ,
Alexander Victorovich Zhestkov ,
Mikhail L'vovich Shteiner ,
Svetlana Vyacheslavovna Kazharova ,
Yuriy Vladimirovich Tezikov and
Igor Stanislavovich Lipatov

Abstract

In Russian Federation, 27,300,000–41,200,000 acute upper and lower respiratory infections are reported annually. Patients with chronic obstructive pulmonary disease (COPD) are at higher risk of severe course, complications, and lethal outcomes of influenza. About 30% of COPD exacerbations are due to viral infections, and influenza A and B viruses are among the most common causes. The aim of our study was to assess exacerbation rate, number of courses of antibiotic chemotherapy, pulmonary function, and immunological effects of mono-vaccination with a new immunoadjuvant influenza vaccine vs. combined vaccination against pneumococcal infection, Hemophilus type b infection, and influenza in COPD patients. Both complex vaccination against Streptococcus pneumoniae, Haemophilus influenzae type b, and influenza and mono-vaccination with a new immunoadjuvant influenza vaccine led to statistically significant reduction in the number of COPD exacerbations and of antibiotic chemotherapy courses. Based on the obtained results, widespread implementation of mono-vaccination against influenza with a new immunoadjuvant influenza vaccine, as well as complex vaccination against bacterial respiratory infections and influenza can be recommended for COPD patients, as vaccination is beneficial for their functional status, that is, improves forced expiratory volume in 1 s (FEV1) and 6-minute walk test results. In our study, we evaluated immunogenicity of the new influenza immunoadjuvant vaccine administered as mono-vaccine to COPD patients in accordance with Committee for Proprietary Medicinal Products (CPMP) requirements.

Keywords: chronic obstructive pulmonary disease (COPD), vaccination, influenza, clinical effects, immunological effects

---

1. Introduction

In Russia, 27,300,000–41,200,000 acute upper and lower respiratory infections are reported annually. Patients with chronic obstructive pulmonary disease (COPD) are at higher risk of severe course, complications, and lethal outcomes of influenza. Therefore, influenza prevention in such patients is one of the most urgent tasks.

About 30% of COPD exacerbations are due to viral infections, and influenza A and B viruses are among the most common causes.

The best approach to prophylaxis is provided by vaccination because it combines the advantages of specificity, efficacy, safety, and cost-effectiveness. The GOLD guidelines (Global Initiative for Chronic Obstructive Lung Disease) recommend that influenza vaccination preferentially with split or subunit vaccines must be integrated into treatment strategies for all COPD patients regardless of the disease stage. However, further studies are needed to evaluate the efficacy and immunogenicity of modern adjuvant influenza vaccines [1].

It is not rarely that the risk of COPD exacerbation is associated not directly with the influenza virus as such, but rather with the development of bacterial superinfection, mainly caused by Streptococcus pneumoniae or Haemophilus influenzae type b [2–4].

In the Russian Federation, both inactivated and live vaccines against influenza have been licensed [5]. Antigenic composition of these vaccines is modified annually to adopt current epidemic situation and WHO guidelines. Recently, an innovative new class of immunoadjuvant influenza vaccines has evolved. The use of these vaccines in COPD patients will be outlined below.

According to CPMP criteria (Committee for Proprietary Medicinal Products), a vaccine is considered immunogenic, if at least one of the assessments meets the indicated requirements:

1. Seroconversion rate (at least fourfold increase in anti-hemagglutinin antibody titre): over 40% for individuals aging 18–60 years and over 30% among individuals above 60 years.
2. Seroprotection rate (number of individuals with protective titre of at least 1:40): over 70% for individuals aging 18–60 years and over 60% in individuals above 60 years.

3. Mean titre increase after vaccination: ≥2.5 in individuals aging 18–60 years and ≥2 in individuals above 60 years.

Vaccination against influenza for COPD patients is included into the National Immunization Calendar of the Russian Federation.

S. pneumoniae, H. influenzae, M. catarrhalis, and influenza virus are the most common causes of COPD infective exacerbations [6]. The standard of care for COPD patients includes vaccination against influenza and pneumococcal infection. Several serotypes of H. influenzae are known, and COPD exacerbation may be caused by each of them, including H. influenzae type b. Vaccine against H. influenzae type b is now available; therefore, it is of interest to evaluate a combined vaccination against S. pneumoniae, H. influenzae, and influenza in COPD patients and the effects of these vaccines on exacerbation rate and pulmonary function tests.

In adult COPD patients, the pioneer studies evaluating the therapeutic effect of PPV23 were performed in 2004. Elimination of S. pneumoniae from the sputum was observed in 52.9% cases, that is, at a lower rate compared to children. Other findings include increased levels of IgG against S. pneumoniae serotypes 3, 6B, 9N, 23F; decreased total IgE, and increased Wright's phagocytic index [7].

Immunization of COPD patients with PPV23 contributed to a 2.2-fold decrease in exacerbation rate by 18 months; at 12 months post vaccination, the duration of acute episodes decreased 1.8-fold compared to the control group [8].

Though disputable, the preliminary results regarding therapeutic effects of vaccination against respiratory infections were thus obtained. The common controversy is whether it is possible to improve the respiratory function tests in COPD patients through vaccination.

Study aim—to assess exacerbation rate, number of courses of antibiotic chemotherapy, pulmonary function, and immunological effects of mono-vaccination with a new immunoadjuvant influenza vaccine vs. combined vaccination against pneumococcal infection, Haemophilus type b infection, and influenza in COPD patients.

2. Material and methods

The study enrolled 170 patients with grade 1, 2, 3, 4 COPD (age 30–80 years) who had signed informed consent according to the study protocol approved by the ethics committee of the Samara State Medical University (Russian Federation) and Research Institute of Pulmonology (Moscow, Russian Federation). The diagnosis was determined according to GOLD guidelines (2012) [9].

Patients were divided into four groups. Group I enrolled 50 patients with COPD who continued to receive basic therapy for the main disease and were vaccinated with commercially available vaccines against pneumococcal infection (Pneumo 23, France), H. influenzae type b infection (Hiberix, Belgium), and influenza (new immunoadjuvant vaccine Grippol® plus,

Russian Federation). Vaccines were administered once intramuscularly into various parts of the body. Two patients from Group I did not complete the study per protocol (one patient died after a traffic accident, and one patient died from sudden massive pulmonary embolism). Therefore, the data from these patients were not included into final analysis, and it was based on 48 patients of Group I.

Group II (control for patients who received complex vaccination against pneumococcal infection, Haemophilus type b infection, and influenza) consisted of 80 patients with COPD of similar grade, who were not vaccinated and received only basic therapy.

Group III consisted of 20 COPD patients vaccinated against influenza with a new immunoadjuvant vaccine. Group IV (control for patients who received mono-vaccination against influenza with a new immunoadjuvant vaccine) enrolled 20 unvaccinated COPD patients. Groups II and IV were composed of patients who categorically rejected any vaccination, despite the information provided. Nevertheless, these patients gave their consent to participate in the study. All study patients were followed up for 1 year and subjected to function and immunological tests at baseline and at 12 months.

The use of two control groups was associated with enrollment of patients in two various study centers. Each study center enrolled subjects either to Group I (group of complex vaccination and control group) or to Group III (group of mono-vaccination against influenza and control group). Another reason for the use of two control groups was the probability that baseline characteristics of the patients in Group 1 and Group 3 will not be well balanced, and their comparison with the total control group will be incorrect. Our study is not a direct comparison between the groups of complex vaccination and mono-vaccination. We just compare each of these groups with its own control.

All study patients underwent a history taking (identification of risk factors for COPD, complaints for cough, sputum discharge, dyspnea of any grade worsened by physical exercise). To verify the diagnosis of COPD, all patients were subjected to pulmonary function tests and broncholytic test with 400 μg of salbutamol according to the standard techniques [8]. The study enrolled patients with Tiffeneau index forced expiratory volume in 1 s/forced vital capacity (FEV1/FVC) below 70%.

Inclusion criteria:

- Men and women above 30 years of age.
- Patients with mild/moderate/severe/extremely severe COPD.
- Patient's informed consent.

Exclusion criteria:

- Age below 30 years.
- Vaccination against pneumococcal infection within the previous 3 years.
- Previous vaccination against H. influenzae type b infection.

- Acute infectious diseases and tuberculosis.
- Active phase of chronic virus hepatitis.
- Mental disorders.
- Renal or hepatic failure.
- Malignancies.
- Exacerbation of chronic diseases.
- Hypersensitivity to vaccine components.
- Severe complications of previous vaccination.
- Pregnancy.
- Autoimmune disorders.

Patients were followed up by general practice physicians, pulmonologists, or allergologists-immunologists in the outpatient context or in hospitals, if hospitalization was required. In cases of COPD exacerbation, if necessary, patients were hospitalized to departments of pulmonology.

Patients meeting inclusion/exclusion criteria were divided into four groups. Groups II and IV enrolled patients who categorically rejected any vaccination. Other patients were first recruited to Group I to undergo complex vaccination and then to Group III to be vaccinated against influenza using a new immunoadjuvant vaccine. Sample size was determined by the number of vaccines.

All patients received basic bronchodilatory and anti-inflammatory therapies in accordance with the disease severity and GOLD guidelines (2012). At baseline, groups were well balanced for age, gender, disease severity, and scope of basic therapy, which remained unchanged throughout the study period. Vaccination was performed at remission in the outpatient context, follow-up period lasted for 12 months after vaccination.

PPV23 vaccine is a polyvalent pneumococcal vaccine manufactured by Sanofi aventis (France). It contains purified capsule S. pneumoniae polysaccharides of 23 serotypes. One dose of vaccine is 0.5 ml.

Hiberix is a conjugated vaccine to prevent infections caused by H. influenzae type b (GlaxoSmithKline Biologicals s.a., Belgium). One dose contains 10 μg of purified capsule polysaccharide isolated from str. H. influenzae type b conjugated with 30 μg of tetanus toxoid.

Grippol plus vaccine (NPO Petrovax Pharm, Russia) is a trivalent polymeric subunit immunoadjuvant vaccine (Petrovax, Russia) containing protective antigens isolated from purified influenza type A and B viruses grown in chicken embryos. One immunization dose (0.5 ml) contains at least 5 μg of hemagglutinin of epidemiologically relevant influenza subtype A (H1N1 and H3N2) and type B viruses, and polyoxidonium immunoadjuvant 500 μg in sodium phosphate buffer. Vaccine is free of preservatives.

Clinical efficacy of vaccination was assessed by the number of COPD exacerbations during the year before vaccination and after vaccination. COPD exacerbation was defined as increased dyspnea, cough, and sputum volume requiring medical advice and modification of current therapy documented by primary medical records.

Ventilation function was investigated using a Spiro S-100 spirometer (Russian Federation). The following parameters were measured: forced vital capacity (FVC), forced expiratory volume in 1 s (FEV1), and a calculated ratio of these two parameters (FEV1%/FVC), that is, modified Tiffeneau test. Exercise tolerance was assessed using the 6-minute walk test (6MWT) according to the standard protocol.

The levels of IgG antibodies against influenza virus strains were measured using standard HAI assay (hemagglutination inhibition assay) in accordance with the manufacturer's instructions to the kit.

The results were studied statistically using StatPlus 2009 Professional 5.8.4. Measures of central tendency and dispersion were chosen depending on the data distribution type. Continuous variables corresponding to normal distribution are presented as means (SD); variables differing from normal distribution as medians (interquartile distance). Categorical variables are presented as proportions (%) and absolute values.

The choice of statistical test depends on the data distribution type and evaluation of dispersion equality. The hypothesis of data distribution normality was tested (Shapiro-Wilks test). In cases of normal distribution of data in each sample, dispersion is to be compared between two distributions (Levene's test). If both criteria are met, Student's t test is selected, if no, its non-parametric alternative is used (Mann-Whitney test). The same is applicable to paired tests for comparisons of changing variables (pairwise Student's t test or Wilcoxon test for paired comparisons). Comparative analysis of categorical variables was performed using exact two-sided Fisher's test. Differences were statistically significant at $p < 0.05$ [10].

Prospective study design allows calculating the following statistics:

- Number of patients with exacerbations per year before and after vaccination.
- Absolute risk (AR) of exacerbation per year before and after vaccination.
- Relative risk (RR) of exacerbation per year before and after vaccination.
- Reduction of absolute risk (RAR) of exacerbation after vaccination.
- Reduction of relative risk (RRR) of exacerbation after vaccination.
- Chance of exacerbation.
- Odds ratio (OR) for exacerbation after vaccination compared to no vaccination.
- Number of patients needed to treat to prevent one additional bad outcome (NNTp).

About 95% CI of the difference of absolute risks (AR): the results are statistically significant, if 95% CI will not contain 0.

About 95% CI of the relative risk (RR): the results are statistically significant, if 95% CI will not contain 1.

About 95% CI for the odds ratio (OR): the results are statistically significant, if 95% CI will not contain 1.

3. Results and discussion

3.1. Clinical effects of vaccination in COPD patients

The clinical effects of vaccination (exacerbation rate) in COPD patients are characterized by groups in **Table 1**.

Parameter (formula)	Before vaccination				After vaccination			
	Group I Complex (n=48)	Group II Control I (n=80)	Group III Mono (n=20)	Group IV Control II (n=20)	Group I Complex (n=48)	Group II Control I (n=80)	Group III Mono (n=20)	Group IV Control II (n=20)
Number of COPD exacerbations over 12 months	2 [1,75; 3]	2 [1; 3]	2 [2; 3]	2 [1; 3]	0 [0; 1]***	2 [1; 3]	1 [0; 2]*	2 [1; 3]
Number of patients with exacerbations	44	67	16	17	18	71	10	18
Chance of exacerbation (no. patients with exacerbations /no. patients without exacerbations)	44/4 = 11	67/13 = 5.2	16/4 = 4	17/3 = 5.7	18/30 = 0.6	71/9 = 7.9	10/10 = 1	18/2 = 9
AP (no. patients with exacerbations /no. patients at risk of exacerbation)	44/48 = 0.92 = 92%	67/80 = 0.84 = 84%	16/20 = 0.8 = 80%	17/20 = 0.85 = 85%	18/48 = 0,38 = 38%	71/80 = 0.89 = 89%	10/20 = 0.5 = 50%	18/20 = 0.9 = 90%
	Flu+PPV23+ HIB (n=48)		**Control I (n=80)**		**Flu (n=20)**		**Control II (n=20)**	
OR (AR after vaccination/ AR without vaccination), 95% CI	0.38/0.92 = 0.41 = 41% (0.16; 1.08)		0.89/0.84 = 1.06 = 106% (0.49; 2.29)		0.5/0.8 = 0.63 = 63% (0.23; 1.69)		0.9/0.85 = 1.06 = 106% (0.19; 5.7)	
RAR (AR after vaccinations – AR without vaccination), 95% CI	0.38 – 0.92 = - 0.54 = - 54% (-1.53; 0.45)		0.89 – 0.84 = 0.05 = 5% (-0.76; 0.86)		0.5 – 0.8 = - 0.3 = - 30% (-1.29; 0.69)		0.9 – 0.85 = 0.05 = 5% (-1.63; 1.73)	
RRR (AR difference /AR without vaccination)	(92% - 38%)/92% = 0.59 = 59%		(84% - 89%)/84% = - 0.06 = -6%		(80% - 50%)/80% = 0.38 = 38%		(85% - 90%)/85% = - 0.06 = - 6%	
OR (chance with vaccination / chance without vaccination), 95% CI	0.6/11 = 0.05 = 5% (0.02; 0.17)#		7.9/5.2 = 1.52 = 152% (0.61; 3.78)		1/4 = 0.25 = 25% (0.06; 1.02)		9/5.7 = 1.58 = 158% (0.23; 10.8)	
NNTp (1/RAR)	1/0.54 = **1.9**		-		1/0.3 = **3.3**		-	

Notes: continuous variables are presented as medians and interquartile distances.

* p<0.05 vs. before vaccination in a given group (exact Fisher's test).

*** p<0.001 vs. before vaccination in a given group (exact Fisher's test).

# p<0.05.

Abbreviations: AR – absolute risk, RR – relative risk, RAR – reduction of absolute risk, RRR – reduction of relative risk, OR – odds ratio, NNTp – number of patients needed to treat to prevent unfavorable outcome.

Table 1. Number of exacerbations (calculated statistics) in COPD patients per year before and after vaccination.

Both complex and mono-vaccination resulted in a statistically significant reduction of the number of COPD exacerbations. The risk of COPD exacerbation was reduced by 54% after complex vaccination vs. 30% after mono-vaccination ($p > 0.05$ for all comparisons).

Parameter (formula)	Before vaccination				After vaccination			
	Group I Complex (n=48)	Group II Control I (n=80)	Group III Mono (n=20)	Group IV. Control II (n=20)	Group I Complex (n=48)	Group II Control I (n=80)	Group III Mono (n=20)	Group IV Control II (n=20)
Number of courses of antibiotic chemotherapy (ABC) over 12 months	2 [1; 3]	2 [1; 3]	2 [2; 3]	2 [1; 3]	0 [0; 1]***	2 [1; 3]	0 [0; 1]*	2 [1; 3]
Number of patients treated with ABC	41	62	17	15	15	63	11	18
Chance of ABC (no. patients treated with ABC/no. patients not treated with ABC)	41/7 = 5.9	62/18 = 3.4	17/3 = 5.7	15/5 = 3	15/33 = 0.5	63/17 = 3.7	11/9 = 1.2	18/2 = 9
AR (no. patients treated with ABC/no. patients not treated with ABC)	41/48 = 0.85 = 85%	62/80 = 0.78 = 78%	17/20 = 0.85 = 85%	15/20 = 0.75 = 75%	15/48 = 0.31 = 31%	63/80 = 0.79 = 79%	11/20 = 0.55 = 55%	18/20 = 0.9 = 90%
RR (AR with vaccination – AR without vaccination), 95% CI	**Combined (n=48)**		**Control I (n=80)**		**Mono (n=20)**		**Control II (n=20)**	
	0.31/0.85 = 0.36 = 36% (0.18; 0.73)#		0.79/0.78 = 1.01 = 101% (0.56; 1.82)		0.55/0.85 = 0.65 = 65% (0.21; 2.06)		0.9/0.75 = 1.2 = 120% (0.26; 5.48)	
RAR (AR with vaccination – AR without vaccination), 95% CI	0.31 – 0.85 = - 0.54 = - 54% (-1.25; 0.17)		0.79 – 0.78 = 0.01 = 1% (-0.58; 0.6)		0.55 – 0.85 = - 0.3 = - 30% (-1.45; 0.85)		0.9 – 0.75 = 0.15 = 15% (-1.37; 1.67)	
RRR (difference AR/AR without vaccination)	(85% - 31%)/85% = 0.64 = 64%		(78% - 79%)/78% = - 0.01 = -1%		(85% - 55%)/85% = 0.35 = 35%		(75% - 90%)/75% = - 0.2 = - 20%	
OR (chance with vaccination/chance without vaccination), 95% CI	0.5/5.9 = 0.08 = 8% (0.03; 0.22)#		3.7/3.4 = 1.09 = 109% (0.49; 2.41)		1.2/5.7 = 0.21 = 21% (0.05; 0.96)#		9/3 = 3 = 300% (0.49; 18.03)	
NNTp (1/RAR)	1/0.54 = **1.9**		-		1/0.3 = **3.3**		-	

Notes: continuous variables are presented as medians and interquartile distances.
* - $p<0.05$ vs. baseline value in a given group (exact Fisher's test).
*** - $p<0.001$ vs. baseline value in a given group (exact Fisher's test).
# - $p<0.05$.
Abbreviations: AR – absolute risk, RR – relative risk, RAR – reduction of absolute risk, RRR – reduction of relative risk, OR – odds ratio, NNTp – number of patients needed to treat to prevent unfavorable outcome.

Table 2. Number of courses of antibiotic chemotherapy (calculated statistics) in COPD patients per year before and after vaccination in the groups considered.

As compared to unvaccinated patients, complex vaccination reduced the risk of COPD exacerbation by 59 vs. 38% reduction after mono-vaccination vs. increase by 6% in unvaccinated patients.

In the group of complex vaccination against pneumococcal, Haemophilus type b infection, and influenza, the chance of COPD exacerbation was 5% of that in unvaccinated patients ($p < 0.05$). In the group of mono-vaccination, the chance of COPD exacerbation was 25% of that without vaccination ($p > 0.05$).

Table 2 presents characteristics of the clinical effect of vaccination (i.e., number of courses of antibiotic chemotherapy) in different groups of COPD patients.

Both complex and mono-vaccination led to statistically significant reduction in the number of antibacterial chemotherapy courses.

The risk of antibiotic chemotherapy was reduced by 54% in the group of complex vaccination against pneumococcal, Hemophilus type b infection, and influenza vs. 30% in the group of mono-vaccination ($p > 0.05$ for all comparisons).

As compared to no vaccination, complex vaccination reduced the risk of antibiotic chemotherapy in patients with COPD by 64%, whereas mono-vaccination reduced it by 35%.

In the group of complex vaccination against pneumococcal, Hemophilus type b infection, and influenza, the chance of antibiotic chemotherapy was 8% of that in unvaccinated patients ($p < 0.05$). In the group of mono-vaccination, the chance of antibiotic chemotherapy was 21% of that in unvaccinated ($p < 0.05$).

3.2. The effect of vaccination on the pulmonary function tests in COPD patients

In COPD patients from Groups I and II, FVC changes did not undergo any statistically significant changes over 12 months (**Table 3**). In Group I (patients vaccinated against pneumococcal, Hemophilus type b infection, and influenza), forced expiratory volume in 1 s (FEV1) increased to 57.4% (2.0%) at 12 months vs. 53.9% (2.7%) at baseline ($p < 0.05$). In unvaccinated patients (Group II), these parameters remained unchanged: 54.1% (1.9%) at baseline vs. 50.4% (2.8%) at 12 months ($p > 0.05$), indicating that the rate of FEV1 decrease was lower in vaccinated COPD patients (Group I). Detailed characteristics of FEV1 changes in Groups I and II depending on the disease severity are given in **Table 4**, and **Table 5** outlines the same for Tiffeneau index.

COPD grade	At baseline		At 12 months	
	Abs., ml	%	Abs., ml	%
1 (n = 3/n = 24)	3611 (466)	100.7 (3)	3724 (489)	104 (0.4)
	3608 (206)	97.8 (3.2)	3572 (176)	95.6 (2.9)
2 (n = 23/n = 25)	2943 (180)	78.9 (3.3)	2867 (169)	79.3 (3.3)
	2936 (173)	77.9 (4.1)	2918 (167)	76.9 (3.5)
3 (n = 18/n = 25)	2301 (129)	55.2 (2.8)	2173 (208)	53.3 (3.5)
	2311 (128)	55.2 (2.7)	2086 (96.2)	51.2 (2.6)
4 (n = 4/n = 6)	1854 (116)	46.6 (5.6)	2158 (119)&	55.8 (3.8)&
	1845 (129)	45.2 (5.1)	1778 (106)	43.3 (2.2)
Total (n = 48/n = 80)	2653 (119)	68.7 (2.9)	2602 (131)	68.3 (2.9)
	2648 (122)	67.9 (2.5)	2562 (131)	64.8 (2.2)

Data are presented as means (standard deviation).
Group I patients in the numerator, Group II patients in the denominator.
& $p < 0.05$—differences between Groups I and II (Student's test).

Table 3. FVC changes in COPD patients from Groups I and II over 12 months.

COPD grade	At baseline		At 12 months	
	Abs., ml	%	Abs., ml	%
1 (n = 3/n = 24)	2412 (236)	86.7 (1.6)	2597 (337)	90.5 (1.1)&&
	2399 (205)	85.8 (2.0)	2384 (136)	85.4 (1.2)
2 (n = 23/n = 25)	1954 (112)	66.1 (2.1)	1985 (109)	69.9 (2.6)&
	1959 (110)	66.4 (2.7)	1916 (102)	62.9 (1.4)
3 (n = 18/n = 25)	1274 (65.1)	39.1 (1.4)	1314 (101)	42.0 (2.2)
	1280 (69.3)	40.0 (1.3)	1204 (76.3)	37.2 (1.6)
4 (n = 4/n = 6)	876 (106.5)	26.9 (1.4)	951 (106.5)	28.6 (2.7)
	883 (115.5)	27.9 (1.2)	826 (97.2)	25.9 (1.0)
Total (n = 48/n = 80)	1638 (86.6)	53.9 (2.7)	1685 (95.4)	57.4 (2.0)&
	1642 (92.5)	54.1 (1.9)	1574 (94.4)	50.4 (2.8)

Data are presented as means (standard deviation).
Group I patients in the numerator, Group II patients in the denominator.
& $p < 0.05$; && $p < 0.01$—differences between Groups I and II (Student's test).

Table 4. FEV1 changes in COPD patients from Groups I and II over 12 months.

COPD grade	At baseline	At 12 months
	%	%
1 (n = 3/n = 24)	67.27 (1.95)	69.8 (0.1)
	66.34 (2.18)	68.4 (0.89)
2 (n = 23/n = 25)	67.14 (2.04)	69.9 (2.29)&
	66.85 (1.95)	64.24 (1.58)
3 (n = 18/n = 25)	56.68 (2.59)	62.39 (2.61)
	55.43 (2.12)	58.4 (2.53)
4 (n = 4/n = 6)	47.85 (6.69)	44.2 (4.95)
	47.38 (5.12)	45.84 (2.53)
Total (n = 48/n = 80)	61.62 (1.73)	64.93 (1.94)&
	60.98 (1.85)	59.13 (2.15)

Data are presented as means (standard deviation).
Group I patients in the numerator, Group II patients in the denominator.
& $p < 0.05$—differences between Groups I and II (Student's test).

Table 5. Tiffeneau index changes in COPD patients from Groups I and II over 12 months.

One year post vaccination, vaccinated COPD patients (Group I) showed 6MWT results that were 75.2% (2.8%) of the desired values vs. 60.4% (2.3%) in Group II patients ($p < 0.001$). Detail characteristics of the dynamics of the 6-minute walk test depending on the disease severity are given in **Table 6**.

COPD grade	At baseline		At 12 months	
	Abs., m	%	Abs., m	%
1 (n = 3/n = 24)	440 (49.0)	86.1 (8.6)	450 (54.5)	92.8 (4.3)
	434 (52.8)	84.7 (9.1)	429 (41.2)	83.5 (4.2)
2 (n = 23/n = 25)	355 (13.1)	71.8 (2.4)	401 (15.8)$^{*,\&\&\&}$	81.2 (3.1)$^{*,\&\&\&}$
	351 (10.2)	70.9 (2.6)	324 (8.7)$^{\#}$	64.1 (1.2)$^{\#}$
3 (n = 18/n = 25)	314 (21.1)	64.0 (3.8)	338 (26.4)	69.7 (4.3)$^{\&}$
	319 (20.3)	64.1 (3.6)	296 (17.1)	59.4 (1.7)
4 (n = 4/n = 6)	230 (45.2)	47.4 (13)	266 (37.3)	54 (12.3)
	235 (40.3)	48.6 (10.3)	213 (10.5)	44.2 (2.3)
Total (n = 48/n = 80)	335 (12.6)	67.8 (2.4)	369 (14.5)$^{\&\&\&}$	75.2 (2.8)$^{*,\&\&\&}$
	332 (18.4)	66.3 (2.6)	305 (10.5)	60.4 (2.3)

Data are presented as means (standard deviation).
Group I patients in the numerator, Group II patients in the denominator.
* $p < 0.05$ vs. baseline values in Group I (Student's test).
# $p < 0.05$ vs. baseline values in Group II (Student's test).
& $p < 0.05$; &&& $p < 0.001$—differences between Groups I and II (Student's test).

Table 6. Dynamics of 6MWT in COPD patients from Groups I and II over 12 months.

Detailed characteristics of spirometry data in COPD patients from Groups III and IV are presented in **Table 7**.

Parameter		Vaccinated against influenza (Group III, n = 20)		Unvaccinated (Group IV, n = 20)	
		At baseline	At 12 months	At baseline	At 12 months
FVC	Abs.	1.62 (0.18)	1.71 (0.13)	2.05 (0.12)	1.88 (0.16)
	%	37.69 (3.61)	42 (2.74)	47.06 (2.9)	41.94 (3.05)
FEV1	Abs.	1.13 (0.13)	1.17 (0.08)	1.48 (0.1)	1.38 (0.11)
	%	33.65 (3.43)	35.76 (2.16)	42.25 (2.76)	40.83 (3.46)
FEV1/FVC	%	52.7 (3.42)	46.46 (3.2)$^{\&}$	55.8 (2.18)	57.9 (2.66)

Data are presented as means (standard deviation).
& $p < 0.05$—differences between Groups III and IV at 12 months (Student's test).

Table 7. Spirometry values in COPD patients vaccinated against influenza (Group III) and in unvaccinated control patients (Group IV).

The analysis of the 6-minute walk test results showed a trend to distance increase by 13 m (+3.7%) 1 year after mono-vaccination ($p > 0.05$, Student's test).

Thus, the study demonstrated statistically significant increase in FEV1 [57.4% (2.0%)] at 12 months after complex vaccination when compared to unvaccinated COPD patients [50.4% (2.8%)]. This FEV1 increase was 3.5%, that is, not statistically significant vs. baseline value, although the positive trend was observed.

The group of mono-vaccination against influenza also demonstrated the positive trend of FEV1 increase, but the increase was only 2.11%, which is less than 3.5% in the group of complex vaccination.

In the group of complex vaccination, patients demonstrated significantly improved 6MWT results at 12 months vs. baseline distance. In Group I, the increase was 7.4% (+34 m), that is, statistically significant ($p < 0.05$). In patients vaccinated against influenza, 6MWT increase approached trend levels of significance.

3.3. Immunological effect of vaccination in patients with COPD

Previously, we have reported the dynamics of specific antibodies against influenza virus in COPD patients after complex vaccination against S. pneumoniae, H. influenzae type b, and influenza [11].

Combined vaccination against pneumococcal, H. influenzae type b and influenza is accompanied by production of antibodies to these infections, which persist during 1 year (observation period), regardless of disease severity. In patients with stage 4 COPD, the level of antibodies to influenza virus (strains A/H1N1, A/H3N2 and B) in post-vaccination period was lower than in patients with stages 1, 2, and 3. Probably, these patients should be vaccinated against influenza twice. Despite the fact that patients with COPD had lower levels of post-vaccination antibodies than control, they demonstrated apparent clinical effect throughout 12 months, which was recorded as reduction of both exacerbation number and the need in antibacterial medications. Combined vaccination against bacterial and viral infections contributes to the achievement of antibody levels leading to the development of significant clinical effect in patients with COPD.

Table 8 demonstrates lists immunogenicity parameter of the new immunoadjuvant vaccine against influenza after mono vaccination of COPD patients.

No statistically significant differences in immunogenicity were found between COPD patients and healthy participants vaccinated only against influenza, the latter, however, demonstrated a trend toward higher immune response to vaccination.

In the comparative analysis of COPD patients, in whom antibodies to all three influenza virus strains were detected at arbitrarily protective titres (≥1:40) at 6 months after vaccination, and patients, in whom, despite vaccination, antibody titres were <1:40, COPD patients at risk of low response to vaccination were identified. These patients had a long history of COPD with frequent respiratory infections and COPD exacerbations requiring hospitalization and systemic glucocorticosteroids or antibiotic chemotherapy.

Vaccine strains	Seroconversion, % (N ≥ 40%)		Seroprotection, % (N ≥ 70%)		Mean geometric antibody titre (N ≥ 40)		
	6 months	12 months	6 months	12 months	At baseline	6 months	12 months
A/H1N1/ Brisbane/ 59/07	60 ± 16	40 ± 16	58 ± 14	67 ± 14	20 (log_2 4.32 ± 0.36)	30.64 (log_2 4.94 ± 0.38)	33.64^p(log_2 5.07 ± 0.28)
A/H3N2/ Uruguay/ 716/2007	70 ± 15	50 ± 16	75 ± 13	83.3 ± 11	24.75 (log_2 4.63 ± 0.63)	71.91 (log_2 6.17 ± 0.62)	59.93 (log_2 5.91 ± 0.38)
B/Florida/ 4/2006	30 [15; 45]	10 [1; 20]	100 ± 0	100 ± 0	46.94 (log_2 5.55 ± 0.30)	84.38 (log_2 6.4 ± 0.33)	59.9 (log_2 5.91 ± 0.38)

Marked values meet CPMP requirements.

Table 8. Immunogenicity parameters of the new immunoadjuvant vaccine against influenza after mono-vaccination of COPD patients (n = 15).

4. Conclusions

During post-vaccination period, treating physicians and patients as well focus their attention on the main disease course. The clinical course of the disease may be characterized by number of COPD exacerbations and the need for antibiotic chemotherapy. Both complex vaccination against S. pneumoniae, H. influenzae type b, and influenza and mono-vaccination with a new immunoadjuvant influenza vaccine led to statistically significant reduction in the number of COPD exacerbations and of antibiotic chemotherapy courses.

Our study had some limitations, that is, its pilot character, absence of randomization and blinding, and small sample size. As follows from the study results, complex vaccination of COPD patients against bacterial and viral respiratory infections have more expressed beneficial effects on their functional status when compared to mono-vaccination against influenza. Further well-designed multicenter clinical studies devoid of these limitations are needed to refine the hypothesis. Nevertheless, based on the obtained results, widespread implementation of mono-vaccination against influenza with a new immunoadjuvant influenza vaccine, as well as complex vaccination against bacterial respiratory infections and influenza can be recommended for COPD patients, as vaccination is beneficial for their functional status, that is, improves FEV1 and 6-minute walk test results.

Mono-vaccination of COPD patients using immunoadjuvant vaccines of a new class as well as combined vaccination against S. pneumoniae, H. influenzae, and influenza is associated with protective antibody titres. In our study, we evaluated immunogenicity of the new influenza immunoadjuvant vaccine administered as mono-vaccine to COPD patients in accordance with CPMP requirements. Immune response to vaccine strains of influenza virus was more intense and durable in initially seropositive patients compared to seronegative.

Combined vaccination against pneumococcal, H. influenzae type b and influenza is accompanied by production of antibodies to these infections. In patients with stage 4, COPD the level of antibodies to influenza virus (strains A/H1N1, A/H3N2 and B) in post-vaccination period was lower than in patients with stages 1, 2, and 3. Probably, these patients should be vaccinated against influenza twice. Combined vaccination against bacterial and viral infections contributes to the achievement of antibody levels leading to the development of significant clinical effect in patients with COPD.

Influenza prophylaxis in COPD patients implies annual influenza vaccination of all individuals having no contraindications regardless of the disease severity. Influenza vaccine prophylaxis must be included into patient's care plan and into the list of recommendations given by a pulmonologist at an outpatient visit or at discharge from hospital. If possible, simultaneous vaccination against S. pneumoniae, H. influenzae type b, and influenza is recommended as early as possible before the season of respiratory infections starts. Combined vaccination against respiratory infections has more significant effects on clinical characteristics and functional status of COPD patients and promotes production of specific antibodies not only against vaccine strains of influenza virus but also against S. pneumoniae and H. influenzae antigens contained in the corresponding vaccines.

Author details

Andrey Dmitrievich Protasov[1,2*], Mikhail Petrovich Kostinov[1,2],
Alexander Victorovich Zhestkov[1,2], Mikhail L'vovich Shteiner[1,2],
Svetlana Vyacheslavovna Kazharova[1,2], Yuriy Vladimirovich Tezikov[1,2] and
Igor Stanislavovich Lipatov[1,2]

*Address all correspondence to: crosss82@mail.ru

1 Samara State Medical University, Samara, Russian Federation

2 Mechnikov Research Institute of Vaccines and Sera, Moscow, Russian Federation

References

[1] Chebykina A.V. Clinico-functional status and anti-influenza immune response in vaccinated patients with bronchial asthma and chronic obstructive pulmonary disease (COPD). [thesis]. Moscow:2012. 26 p. (In Russ.)

[2] Protasov A.D., Zhestkov A.V., Lavrenteva N.E., Kostinov M.P., Ryzhov A.A. Effect of complex vaccination against pneumococcal, Haemophilus type b infections and influenza in patients with chronic obstructive pulmonary disease. Journal of Microbiology, Epidemiology and Immunobiology. 2011;4:80–84. (In Russ.)

[3] Protasov A.D. Immunologic and clinical effects of combined use of pneumococcal vaccine, haemophilus influenzae type B vaccine and influenza vaccine in patients with COPD. [thesis]. Moscow: Right; 2012. 26 p. (In Russ.)

[4] Protasov A.D. The grounds for the development and introduction of the vaccine against M. catarrhalis for patients with chronic obstructive pulmonary disease. Medical Almanac. 2013;2(26):66–68. (In Russ.)

[5] Kostinov M.P., editor. Vaccination of adult subjects with bronchopulmonary pathology. A guide for physicians. Moscow: Art-studio "Constellation"; 2013. 112 p. (In Russ.)

[6] Protasov A.D., Zhestkov A.V., Kostinov M.P., Ryzhov A.A.. Changes in sputum bacterial landscape after vaccination against Streptococcus pneumoniae, Haemophilus influenzae type b and influenza in patients with chronic obstructive pulmonary disease. Pulmonology. 2012;5:23–27. (In Russ.)

[7] Dubinina V.V., Markelova E.V., Kostinov M.P. Immune response after "Pneumo-23" vaccination in persons of different age groups. Medical Immunology. 2005;7(2–3):259. (In Russ.)

[8] Chuchalin A.G, editor. Chronic obstructive pulmonary disease. Moscow: Atmosphere; 2008. 568 p. (In Russ.)

[9] Belevskii A.S., editor. Global strategy for the diagnosis, management, and prevention of chronic obstructive pulmonary disease. Moscow: Russian Respiratory Society; 2012. 80 p. (In Russ.)

[10] Lang T.A., Sesik M. How to describe statistical analysis in medicine. A manual for authors, editors and reviewers. Moscow: Applied medicine; 2011. 480 p. (In Russ.)

[11] Kostinov M.P., Protasov A.D., Zhestkov A.V., Pakhomov D.V., Chebykina A.V., Kostinova T.A. Post-vaccination immunity to pneumococcal, Haemophilus influenzae type B infection and influenza in patients with chronic obstructive pulmonary disease (COPD). J Vaccines Vaccin. 2014;5(2):1-5. doi:10.4172/2157-7560.1000221.

3

Influenza Diagnosis with a Specific Emphasis on the M2e Antigen as a Diagnostic Tool

Yasemin Budama-Kilinc and Rabia Cakir-Koc

Abstract

The therapy, observation, inclusiveness, and preclusion of related diseases all influence the diagnosis of influenza. Particularly, the pandemic duration and diagnosis time for influenza are extremely important. After the appearance of symptoms, antiviral medication must be initiated within 48 h. Cell culture, real-time polymerase chain reaction (PCR), flow cytometry, direct and indirect immunofluorescence methods, and the quick diagnosis test are all valuable approaches for the diagnosis of influenza. Different instruments, different time durations for the results, and different specialists characterize all these approaches. Antigen selection is of critical importance with regard to the specificity and sensitivity of these methods, especially the serological and rapid diagnosis tests. M2e, the highly conserved external domain of the influenza A M2 protein, is a potential differential diagnostic marker for influenza virus infection. This chapter reviews the studies that use M2e as a diagnosis agent, and it illuminates the role and importance of M2e in the diagnosis of influenza.

Keywords: M2e, diagnosis, peptide, antigen, virus culture, rapid immunochromotographic test, serological test, ELISA, PCR

1. Introduction

Influenza viruses can cause respiratory infections, and it is a major cause of morbidity and mortality worldwide [1]. Influenza is typically a mild disease that lasts for 1–2 weeks in most people [2], although in some cases it can be fatal [3]. The likelihood of developing complications is higher in certain risk groups, such as people with chronic health problems, children under 2 years old, and the elderly [4]. While 45–77% of those hospitalized due to influenza are under 65 years old, the patients who are older than 65 years are the most likely (60–90%) to die as a result of influenza [5–8].

The variable nature of the influenza has already caused several pandemics. The accurate and rapid diagnosis of influenza is therefore of great importance to the effective management of epidemic and pandemic periods [4]. As there are several respiratory pathogens that may cause clinical symptoms similar to those caused by influenza, a final diagnosis is difficult for doctors to establish [9]. As a result, sensitive and rapid diagnosis methods are needed to confirm the clinical diagnosis of influenza, as well as to improve the quality of monitoring systems. A variety of laboratory methods for the diagnosis of influenza are available (**Table 1**). Each of these methods has both advantages and disadvantages, and some or all of these factors may affect the selection of an appropriate diagnosis method [2].

Diagnosis method	Average acquisition time	Mechanism	Application opportunity	Sample required
Viral culture	3–7 days	Virus isolation	Limited	Bronchoalveolar lavage Nose and throat swab Nasopharyngeal aspirate
Molecular tests	1–2 days	RNA detection	Limited	Post-mortem tissue Bronchoalveolar lavage Nose and throat swab Nasopharyngeal aspirate
Rapid immunochromatographic tests	15–30 min	Antigen detection	Widespread	Bronchoalveolar lavage Nose and throat swab Nasopharyngeal aspirate
Serological tests	2 days	Antigen/antibody detection	Widespread	Serum

Table 1. Comparison of the diagnostic methods available for the influenza A virus.

In this chapter, the methods that have developed and used in the diagnosis of influenza will be evaluated in terms of their principles, sensitivity, specificity, time, advantages and disadvantages, and the antigens used for the diagnosis of influenza A.

2. Diagnosis methods for influenza A

There are four basic methods available for the diagnosis of influenza [10], each of which is detailed in **Table 1**.

2.1. Virus cultures

2.1.1. Classic virus cultures

Symptoms such as the deformation of cell morphology, cell necrosis, pouring from the cell location to the cell culture, and fusion in cells that are infected with the virus are, depending on the virus proliferation, referred to as the cytopathic effects (CPE) [11].

Virus cultures that use primary rhesus monkey kidney cells (PMK) or Madin-Darby canine kidney cells (MDCK) are commonly accepted to be one of the "gold standards" for laboratory diagnosis. Whether or not the cells are infected with the virus is determined by the cytopathic effects in the cell cultures and hemadsorption using immunofluorescence monoclonal antibodies against influenza [10].

2.1.2. Rapid shell vial virus cultures

Coverglasses are used in the rapid shell vial cell culture method to passage the cell lines onto them. The specimens are inoculated after the monolayer cell lines occur. The coverglasses are then stained with cause-specific FITC-marked monoclonal antibodies for about 24–48 h. Cytopathic effects are not expected with this method, unlike in standard tube cultures [12].

Influenza isolation with the rapid shell vial culture method provides an advantage with regard to its simplicity and speed when compared to traditional culture method [13]. Influenza shell vial cultures show results within 1–3 days after virus inoculation [12] (**Figure 1**).

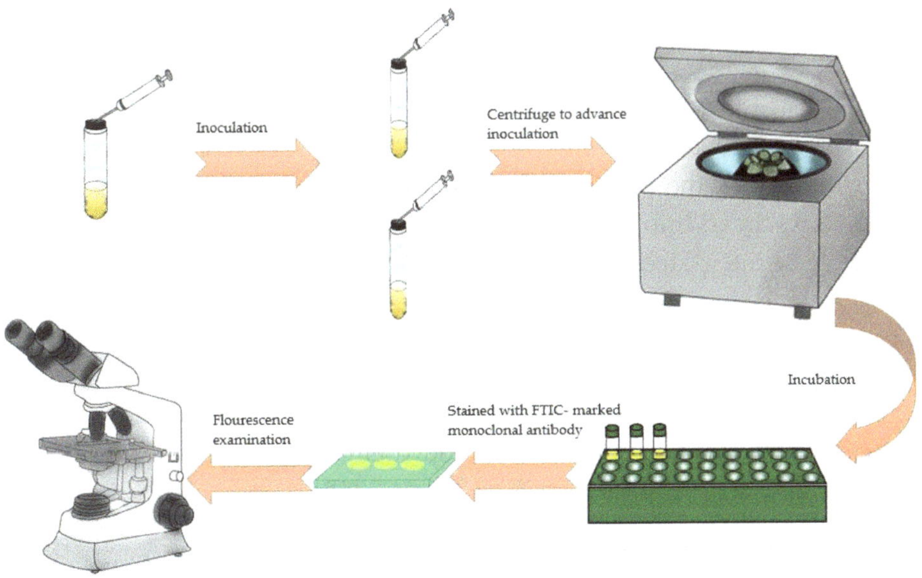

Figure 1. Schematic presentation of shell vial method.

The specificity of the rapid shell vial test is 100%. Although the time necessary to obtain the results is much shorter in this method than in traditional cell cultures, in many cases, the time is actually insufficient to begin optimal antiviral treatment [10].

2.2. Molecular methods

The genome of the influenza viruses consists of eight different parts of single-stranded negative sense RNA. This structure changes continuously and it contributes to the evaluation of the virus [14]. Major changes occur in the genes encoding the two major surface glycoproteins, namely the hemagglutinin (HA) and neuraminidase (NA) antigens. The HA antigens play a role in the connection of the virus to the cell, NA plays an essential role in release and spread of progeny virions, following the intracellular viral replication cycle [15]. There are 18 different hemagglutinin subtypes and 11 different neuraminidase subtypes, H1–H18 and N1–N11, respectively [16]. The high mutation rate causes the development of subtypes [17].

The extreme genetic variability of the influenza viruses leads to challenges in the design of molecular-based diagnosis tests. Most conserved sequences in the genome used to determine the RT-PCR primers can be used to identify individual strains of influenza virus [12]. A PCR that has been modified by the addition of the reverse transcription step is known as a reverse transcription-PCR (RT-PCR). In addition, the use of specific primers for significant types of HA and NA antigens can aid in the identification of subtypes of influenza viruses [17].

A RT-PCR can be performed in two different ways: (1) the one-step approach (reverse transcription and PCR), which is performed in a single tube; and (2) the two-step approach, which involves the transformation of RNA to cDNA and the amplification of the tested sequences. The two-step reaction process is more sensitive when compared with the one-step reaction. On the other hand, the one-step RT-PCR reaction is fast, and the minimal number of steps reduces the risk of contamination and so improves the reproducibility of the obtained results [12].

Many RT-PCR tests of the subtypes of influenza have shown greater sensitivity than other rapid diagnosis tests and conventional cell cultures. The RT-PCR activity does not change depending on the age of the patients. The rotation period of the RT-PCR for influenza is between 1 and 2 days. In addition, molecular tests require considerable skill and expertise, and they should hence be integrated into the laboratory processes [10].

2.3. Rapid immunochromatographic tests

Rapid diagnosis kits are immunochromatographic methods that include the use of monoclonal antibodies against preserved antigens or nucleoproteins that are localized with a membrane or impregnated onto a strip of influenza A or A and B [18].

Briefly put, according to these methods, the respiratory specimen is primarily treated with an extraction buffer and it is then applied to a filter paper or test strip depending on the test format. If influenza viral antigens are available, a visible color change is generated by the reaction of the antigens and influenza-specific monoclonal antibodies [19].

The sensitivity of the rapid diagnostic kits is approximately 70%, depending on the particular test kit used, the patient's age, and the sample collection time [20]. The specificity of the rapid diagnostic kits ranges from 76 to 100% [21]. In addition, many kits can distinguish between the influenza A and B strains, although they cannot subtype further [20].

Influenza A has a higher sensitivity in the rapid diagnosis test kits when compared with influenza B. Such rapid diagnosis kits are very convenient, and they have a high positive predictive value because of the spread of influenza in the community [21]. The most important advantage of these tests is the fact that they can provide results in approximately 10–30 min [10].

However, during periods of low influenza activity, the predictive value of the rapid diagnostic kits is also low, and false positive results are more likely. Therefore, the use of these tests during periods of high influenza activity is suggested [21]. In addition, more specific testing methods must be performed on patients who present with negative results according to the rapid influenza diagnostic kits during high influenza periods. The major disadvantage of these tests is their limited shelf life of approximately 1–2 years. The inadequate collection of samples and the misinterpretation of test strips by inexperienced personnel may also lead to errors [10].

2.4. Serological tests

Serological methods are all based on determining the antibody response in the sera or specific antigens or gene sequences of influenza virus. Specific, sensitive, and validated serological assays can be used for diagnosis of influenza, the identification of the source of infection, the epidemiology studies, and the identification of asymptomatic cases. Serological methods have also been utilized at prescreening of influenza disease [22].

The immunology of tested population and sensibility and specificity of the tests have major role on interpret results of serological tests [23]. Each type of serological methods have own advantages, disadvantages, and unique characteristics [24]. The serological diagnosis of influenza infection is based on agar gel immunodiffusion, radioimmunoassay, immunofluorescence antibody tests, hemagglutination inhibition, enzyme-linked immunoassay (EIA), complement fixation, and an increase of specific antibody titer between acute and healing serum samples as measured by neutralization tests [10, 17, 25].

2.4.1. Direct immunofluorescence antibody test (DFA)

In this method, antibodies are labeled with fluorescent compounds called fluorophores. Fluorophores are generally organic molecules with cyclic structure. Fluorescein and rhodamine are examples of the most used molecules.

In this method, the antigen in the suspected material is fixed on slides and specifically labeled antibodies placed onto the antigen. Fluorescence labeled (FITC) "monoclonal antibodies" are considered positive due to the luminescence in the presence of agent in patients' samples [12, 25–27]. DFA test is developed for antigen detection in tissue or body fluids and used successfully for diagnosis of influenza. Among children who have high fever and spread lots of influenza viruses, DFA sensitivity is commonly higher [26] (**Figure 2**).

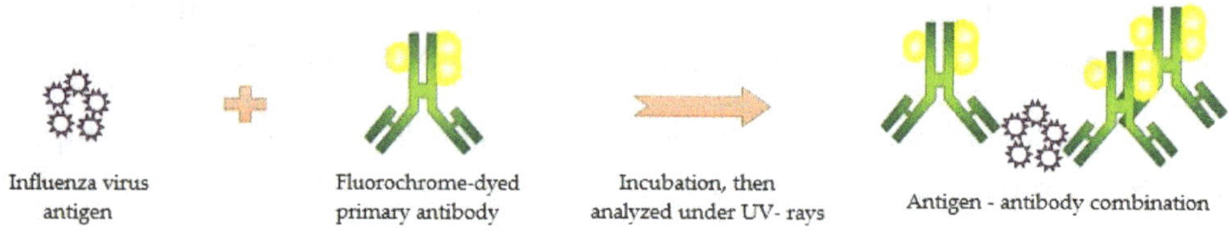

Figure 2. Schematic presentation of direct immunofluorescence antibody test.

2.4.2. *Indirect immunofluorescence antibody test (IFAT)*

In an indirect immunofluorescence assay, antibodies against influenza labeled with fluorescence dyes are used [10, 27, 28]. Influenza A virus particles are fixed on a slide and then the suspected serum is added. FITC conjugated anti-human IgG antibodies are added and examination is made under a microscope [29]. If there is a homologous antibody against the virus on the slide in the influenza suspected serum, a yellow-green glow is seen under a microscope (i.e., a positive reaction) [10, 12].

In principle, the serum antibodies react with immunofluorescence allow for the rapid diagnosis. The sensitivity of the IFA test is 70–90%, while the specificity is above 90% for diagnosis of influenza [20]. There are individual differences in the reporting methods for the different immunofluorescence tests, since this test faces the issue of subjectivity in the reading of slides. To overcome this problem, the IFAT should be reported by experienced clinical laboratorians [30, 31] (**Figure 3**).

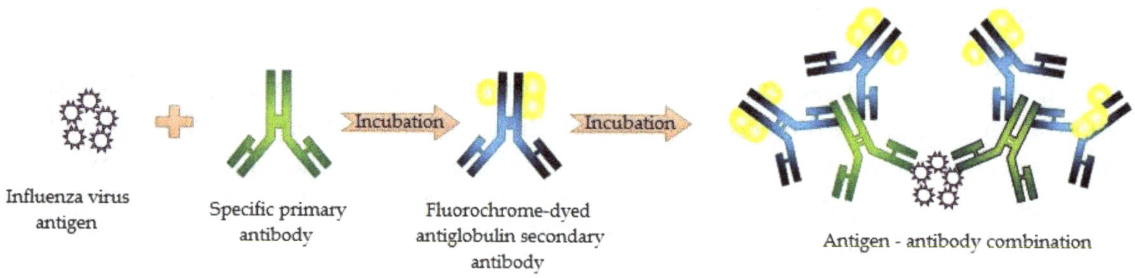

Figure 3. Schematic presentation of indirect immunofluorescence antibody test.

2.4.3. *Radioimmunoassay (RIA)*

Radioimmunoassay test is used to search for both an antibody against influenza and virus or viral antigen, immunoglobulins are conjugated with radioactive material (radioisotopes ^{14}C, ^{125}I, etc.). In positive reactions, the immune complex that occurs when the influenza antigen and specific antibody couple gains radioactivity. This radioactivity is determined by special counters (such as a gamma counter detector). When the results are evaluated according to a curve known as the standard curve, an overall result can be seen. The degree of determined

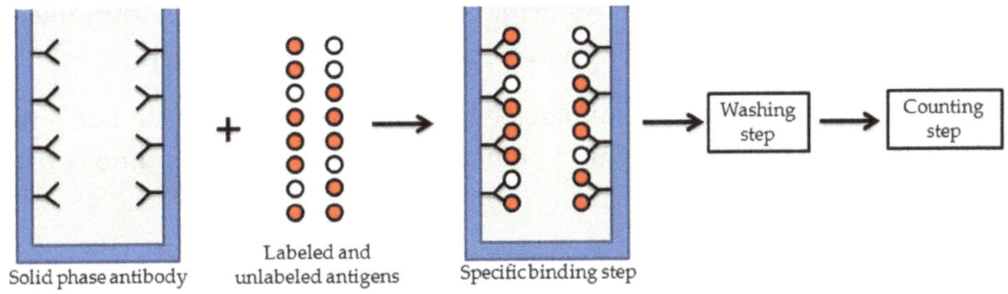

Figure 4. Principle of RIA. Labeled antigen competes with patient antigen for a limited number of binding sites on solid-phase antibody.

radioactivity could be measured in this way. In negative reactions, radioactivity cannot be detected [27, 32].

RIA is a very sensitive and precise technique for detection low amounts of analytes. Otherwise, the health hazard of radioactive substances is most important limitation of all RIA techniques due to disposal problems, short half-life, and the need for expensive equipment [31] (**Figure 4**).

2.4.4. *Agar gel immunodiffusion (AGID)*

The AGID detects antibodies against all influenza A viruses, regardless of subtype. The principle of the AGID test is the simultaneous migration of antigen and antibodies toward each other through an agar gel matrix. Influenza antigens and antibodies form a precipitate in to gel matrix and precipitation line is visualized. Various parameters such as electrolyte concentration, pH, and temperature can affect precipitate formation [33]. Also, concentrations of the antigen or antibodies cause shift the location of the line [34]. The immunodiffusion method can be performed in three different ways, namely simple diffusion (the Oudin method), unidirectional diffusion (the Mancini method), and bidirectional diffusion (Ouchterlony) [35]. The advantages of this method are simplicity, low cost, and inessential specialized laboratory equipment [36].

2.4.5. *Neutralization test*

The neutralization assay determines that patients' antibody can neutralize the infectivity of a given influenza virus strain. Sera that contain specific neutralizing antibodies prevent the cytopathic effects of influenza virus [27]. Influenza viruses cause CPE via proliferation in cells form plaques (i.e., the CPE focus) on nutrient agarose-coated cells [19]. If the virus is cultured on monolayer cells after being stirred with antiviral homologous antibodies formed against itself and then left at room temperature for 30–40 min, plaques either do not form (i.e., plaque neutralization) or else the number of plaques decreases in those cells coated with nutrient agar (i.e., plaque reduction). A reduction in the number of plaques of 50% or more is considered a positive reaction. If the virus encounters a homologous antibody carrying serum, then plaque formation is seen because the neutralization does not occur [12].

The influenza subtypes can be defined by using a type-specific antiviral immune serum. The neutralization reaction is also utilized as a protection test in animals [27].

The neutralization test has several advantages which it can identify functional, strain-specific antibodies in sera [37]. However, it cannot be used routinely since it is time-consuming and laborious.

2.4.6. Complement fixation (CF) test

The complement fixation test (CFT) is one of the classical influenza diagnostic assays, which mainly detects IgG antibodies [38].

In this test, the primarily influenza suspected serum (titrated), then the known viral antigen (titrated), and later the complement (fresh guinea pig serum titer) are added. They are thoroughly mixed and then allowed to stand. At this stage, if a homologous antibody against influenza is present in the serum, the antibody couples with the antigen and the complement binds with this complex. If there is no antibody present, coupling with the antigen does not occur and hence the complement cannot connect and so remains free. A mixture known as the hemolytic system (hemolytic serum + sheep red blood cells) is added to the tubes to determine whether or not the complement is attached. If there is no hemolysis in the erythrocytes, the complement is held in the first stage or, in other words, in the antibody-antigen complex. This indicates the presence of an antibody in the influenza suspected patient's serum (i.e., a positive reaction) [12, 39].

CFT is useful test for diagnosis of acute virus infection, however, it is quite complex, less sensitive, very labor intensive, and is not suitable for automation.

2.4.7. Hemagglutination (HA) vs. hemagglutination inhibition (HI)

The hemagglutination inhibition test is an important diagnostic tool in certain infections especially influenza. The hemagglutinin protein on the surface of the virus may cause agglutination in the presence of erythrocytes [40]. Blocking of this aggregation by specific antibodies in the patient's serum is named as hemagglutination inhibition test [37].

The HA agglutination test is the conventional method for the determination of influenza viruses, while the HI test is commonly used for typing [40]. If the sera from individuals suspected of carrying the disease have virus-specific antibodies against the virus, then these antibodies prevent HA by neutralizing the HA property of the virus when the antibodies and the virus come into contact with each other. In test tubes, erythrocyte aggregate occurs on the bottom in the form of a round point [19].

In the HI test, the numbers of antibodies within the serum are proportional to the amount of HI titers. The HI titers in the serum may remain at the initial dilution if there is less antibody present, although the titers in the serum will reach different dilutions if there is too much antibody present [39, 41].

The hemagglutination inhibition assay is a reliable, relatively simple, and inexpensive technique to antigenically characterize isolates of influenza viruses [37]. Whereas the HI test is very useful in epidemiological surveys, it is not suitable for routine diagnosis of influenza [42]. Nowadays, this assay is widely used and is replaced by more modern immunoassays [38].

2.4.8. Enzyme-linked immunosorbent assay (ELISA)

In enzyme immunoassays, enzyme-conjugated antibodies are generally used for detection of viral antigens. These groups of tests, antigen or antibody are bound to solid phase as microtiter plates, nitrocellulose membranes, and magnetic latex beads [31]. Patient serum is added to antigen bounded solid phase and an enzyme-labeled antiglobulin is added. If anti-influenza antibody is present in patient's serum, enzyme-labeled secondary antibody reacts and chromogenic substrate causes color change [27].

The specific antigens as HA, NA, NP, and M protein of influenza are widely used ELISA. The sensitivity of EIA varies between 64 and 78% [43]. Because of the high specificity, sensitivity, simplicity, and low cost, ELISA is one of the most common used immunoassays in the clinical laboratory [31].

3. Antigens that are used in diagnosis

The methods used in the diagnosis of influenza (except for viral cultures) are based on the determination of the antigen of the virus, the determination of antibodies against the antigen in the patient, or the determination of the gene region of the selected antigen as in molecular methods [40]. In all these methods, the target antigenic structures are used as important selection criteria that affect the specificity and sensitivity of the method. Nucleoproteins and neuraminidase are used in the viral commercial diagnostic kits (rapid tests) popular in commercial studies and academic research. Due to the virus undergoing changes, the use of these antigens in the diagnosis tests affects the obtained results. For this reason, it is also important to use the conserved regions of influenza A in diagnosis [44].

Therefore, in this part of the chapter, the M2 protein, the most conserved structure of influenza A, will be evaluated in terms of its diagnostic importance by considering its biological functions.

3.1. Definition of M2e protein

In influenza A viruses, one of the most important structural proteins is matrix protein 2 (M2) [45]. The M2 protein, the internal membrane protein, is made up of an ectodomain part, which is a single membrane spanning domain located at the N-terminus, and a cytoplasmic tail, which is found in the C-terminal [46].

While the N-terminus domain is 24 amino acids long, part of it is located at the outer side of the membrane surface (M2e), while the 54 amino acids long C-terminus is situated in the cytoplasmic side and the remaining 19 amino acids sequence the lipid bilayer [46] (**Figure 5**).

From the first human influenza A strain that was isolated in 1933 to the present day, no amino acid mutation has been found in the extracellular domain of the M2 protein [47]. In all subtypes of the influenza A viruses, the extracellular domain of the M2 protein, M2e, is significantly conserved with an unchanged SLLTEVET (residues 2e9) sequence at the N-terminal [48]. The M2e protein consists of a homotetramer structure with disulfide linkages that are held together by noncovalent interactions [49]. The M2e protein is conserved in all types of influenza A viruses. Despite appearing in small amounts on the surface of mature virions, this protein is majorly expressed on the surface of infected cells [46].

The peptide epitope of the influenza A virus M2e protein is: Met-Ser-Leu-Leu-Thr-Glu-Val-Glu-Thr-Pro-Ile-Arg-Asn-Glu-Trp-Gly-Cys-Arg-Cys-Asn-Asp-Ser-Ser.

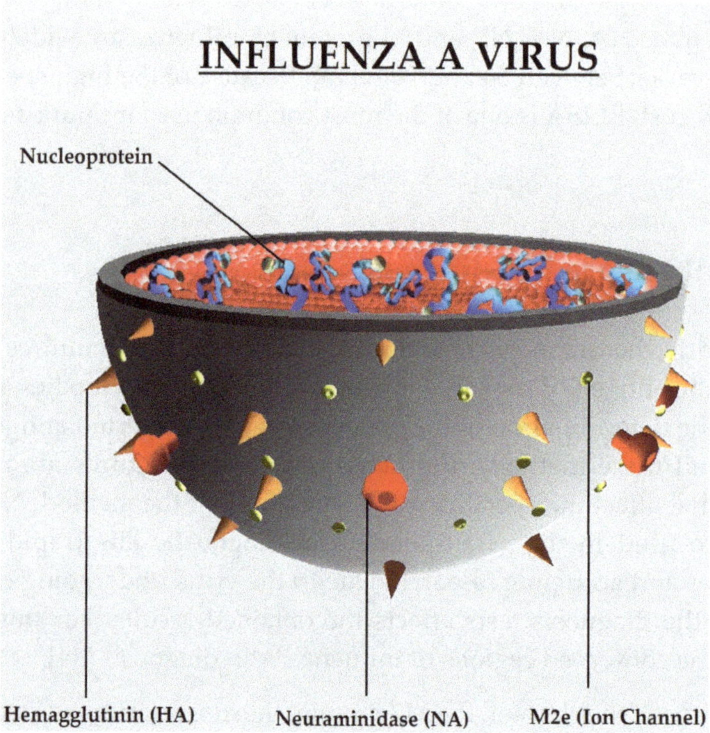

Figure 5. Schematic presentation of influenza A virus structure.

3.2. Biological function of M2e

The main functions of the M2e protein are: (i) functioning as a proton channel; (ii) playing a role in viral replication; and (ii) defending the maturation of HA and structural integrity [48].

The M2e protein is not required for viral replication, but during viral disintegration, it does act as an ion channel that allows the entry of protons into the virions [50]. M2 also plays an effective role in virus morphogenesis and assembly.

M2e stabilizes the newly synthesized HA molecules by adjusting the pH toward the secretion pathway [51]. M2 transport protons reduce the interior pH of the virions via a receptor-mediated endocytosis procedure during the entry of the virus [52].

3.3. Immunological responses against M2e

Mucosal and systemic immunity play a role in the body's resistance to infection. Influenza-specific lymphocytes have been detected in the blood and lower respiratory secretions of influenza patients [53]. A short-term primary cytotoxic T-cell response can be detected after 1–2 weeks (infection with influenza viruses leads to virus-specific B cell as well as T-cell responses) [54]. Antibodies occur against type-specific internal proteins, NA, and M1, as well as against viral surface glycoproteins such as HA and NA. The neutralizing antibodies against HA are the first immune constituents to protect the host from infections caused by the influenza viruses [55, 56].

M2 is a significantly expressed structural protein on the surface of infected cells. M2e is a small portion with a low immunogenicity in its native form [52]. The relatively small size of M2e and its low abundance in virions when compared to other glycoproteins like HA and NA are possible explanations for the low reactivity of M2e [57]. Anti-M2e antibodies can develop in some infected patients [52]. The host's adaptive immune system attracts the virus. At the same time, the infection of humans with influenza A viruses stimulates a weak anti-M2 antibody response for a short duration of time [58]. The anti-M2e antibodies' seroprevalence is increased with age, which is an auxiliary factor in this pre-existing immunity against M2 [59].

M2e-specific antibodies act through the antibody dependent cell cytotoxicity, and the innate or complementary immune system promotes the killing of infected cells. Specific M2e antibodies prevent the release of viral particles toward the extracellular fluid or else stimulate the uptake by phagocytic cells through the Fc receptors via connecting to the viral cell [44, 52].

3.4. Studies that have used M2e in the diagnosis of influenza

Ingrole et al. chose to use M2e in their study based on its preserved region. The use of an elastin-like particle led to the increase in size of the produced antibody. M2e can easily be recognized by the M2e-specific antibodies due to the conjugation of M2e and ELP (elastin-like particles) [60].

Khurana et al. conducted an experiment based on HA2 (488–516), PB1-F2 (2–75), and M2 (2–24) peptides, which have the most conserved regions of the H5N1 strain. In their study, experiments were carried out with ELISA and rapid diagnostic kits, and the effects of these peptides were investigated. In the study that used rapid diagnostic kits, the attachment to the HA2 and M2 peptide bands was observed to be positive in the serum of infected patients. In the ELISA study, there was no reactivity against H5N1 in patients who were vaccinated with a vaccine that did not include the M2e peptide [61].

Denis et al. investigated the use of the papaya mosaic virus as a carrier of the conserved and small amount M2 peptide instead of HA and NA peptides in a vaccine study. Papaya mosaic virus conjugated virus-like particles have been observed to increase the production of the antibody against the M2 peptide. Specific bindings were observed against M2e in both ELISA and MCDK cell culture experiments [62].

Wolf examined the effect of M2e-based multiple antigenic peptides on the production of antibodies via ELISA and ELISPOT techniques. The specificity to the M2e peptide was measured in antibody secreting cells by ELISPOT assay and, as a result, a higher formation of immunoglobulin levels was observed [63].

Hadifar et al. used an ELISA method based on the distracted intravenous access (DIVA) test against H5N1 in their study. The M2e antigenicity of the monomers that form when infected in a natural way to be limited is developed with the DIVA test method. The use of the tetramer structure of M2e instead of the M2e monomer increased the efficiency of the ELISA and other tests mentioned in this study [64].

Tarigan et al. used the single M2e peptide (sp-M2e) ELISA and multiple antigenic forms of the M2e ELISA methods, and the sensitivity of these tests in the diagnosis of M2e was compared. The degrees of M2e were measured by ELISA in order to use the M2e as a target in the DIVA test during pandemics. Although both ELISA techniques have specificity in the diagnosis of the M2e peptide, the MAP-M2e ELISA technique has higher specificity and sensitivity in the diagnosis of M2e [65].

Black et al. determined the influenza A (H2N2) M2 expression of recombinant baculovirus via an indirect immunofluorescent antibody assay (IFA) in a study conducted in 1993. The formation of an antibody against M2e was determined using the EIA test [54].

4. Future aspects

In a study conducted by the US Food and Drug Administration (FDA), the analytical performance of the 11 most widely used influenza diagnostic tests on the market was evaluated in a comprehensive manner. In experiments conducted using 23 different influenza subtypes that have been in circulation recently, although most brands could detect the viral antigen in samples that included a high concentration of influenza virus, it was found that detection based on subtypes of the virus is limited in lower concentrations. It was further suggested that physicians should be careful of negative results when using rapid diagnosis tests for the diagnosis of influenza [66].

Peptide-based enzyme immunoassays are widely used in the sero-diagnosis of bacterial and viral infections. These tests can be easily applied due to their enhanced advantages, namely simplicity, specificity, sensitivity, and relative inexpensiveness.

Despite the genetic differentiation of the influenza A virus, it has been shown that the peptide region formed by the 24 amino acids of the M2e protein located on the surface of the virus is the most conserved region in all strains, and it has therefore been used as a potential diagnosis marker in various studies [56, 57, 67, 68]. Although M2e is normally found in small quantities on virus particles, it is secreted abundantly on the cell surface infected by the virus and, in particular, it will provide a significant advantage in the detection of the disease during pandemic periods [61]. Therefore, diagnosis tests that are developed based on M2e will be able to detect different subtypes of the influenza viruses.

Acknowledgements

The authors would like to thank The Scientific and Technological Research Council of Turkey (TUBİTAK) for their support the named "Development of Rapid Diagnostic Kit with Immunochromatographic Method of Depending on IgY Antibody Specific in (M2e) Peptide for Diagnosis of Influenza A Infection" (Project No. 115S132).

Author details

Yasemin Budama-Kilinc* and Rabia Cakir-Koc

*Address all correspondence to: yaseminbudama@gmail.com

Department of Bioengineering, Chemical and Metallurgical Engineering Faculty, Yildiz Technical University, Esenler, Istanbul, Turkey

References

[1] Kunisaki, K.M. and E.N. Janoff, Influenza in immunosuppressed populations: a review of infection frequency, morbidity, mortality, and vaccine responses. The Lancet Infectious Diseases, 2009. 9(8): p. 493–504.

[2] Ellis, J.S. and M.C. Zambon, Molecular diagnosis of influenza. Reviews in Medical Virology, 2002. 12(6): p. 375–389.

[3] Morens, D.M., J.K. Taubenberger, and A.S. Fauci, Predominant role of bacterial pneumonia as a cause of death in pandemic influenza: implications for pandemic influenza preparedness. Journal of Infectious Diseases, 2008. 198(7): p. 962–970.

[4] Steininger, C., et al., Effectiveness of reverse transcription-PCR, virus isolation, and enzyme-linked immunosorbent assay for diagnosis of influenza A virus infection in different age groups. Journal of Clinical Microbiology, 2002. 40(6): p. 2051–2056.

[5] Irwin, D.E., et al., Impact of patient characteristics on the risk of influenza/ILI-related complications. BMC Health Services Research, 2001. 1(1): p. 1.

[6] Barker, W.H., Excess pneumonia and influenza associated hospitalization during influenza epidemics in the United States, 1970–78. American Journal of Public Health, 1986. 76(7): p. 761–765.

[7] Bridges, C.B., et al., Prevention and control of influenza. Recommendations of the Advisory Committee on Immunization Practices (ACIP). MMWR. Recommendations

and Reports: Morbidity and Mortality Weekly Report. Recommendations and Reports/ Centers for Disease Control, 2002. 51(RR-3): p. 1–31.

[8] Perrotta, D.M., M. Decker, and W.P. Glezen, Acute respiratory disease hospitalizations as a measure of impact of epidemic influenza. American Journal of Epidemiology, 1985. 122(3): p. 468–476.

[9] Montalto, N.J., An office-based approach to influenza: clinical diagnosis and laboratory testing. American Family Physician, 2003. 67(1): p. 111–118.

[10] Gavin, P.J. and R.B. Thomson, Review of rapid diagnostic tests for influenza. Clinical and Applied Immunology Reviews, 2004. 4(3): p. 151–172.

[11] Albrecht, T., et al., Effects on cells. 1996.

[12] Kim, D.-K. and B. Poudel, Tools to detect influenza virus. Yonsei Medical Journal, 2013. 54(3): p. 560–566.

[13] Espy, M., et al., Rapid detection of influenza virus by shell vial assay with monoclonal antibodies. Journal of Clinical Microbiology, 1986. 24(4): p. 677–679.

[14] Webster, R.G., et al., Evolution and ecology of influenza A viruses. Microbiological Reviews, 1992. 56(1): p. 152–179.

[15] Matrosovich, M.N., et al., Neuraminidase is important for the initiation of influenza virus infection in human airway epithelium. Journal of Virology, 2004. 78(22): p. 12665–12667.

[16] Quan, F.-S., et al., Progress in developing virus-like particle influenza vaccines. Expert Review of Vaccines, 2016: p. 1–13.

[17] Wozniak-Kosek, A., B. Kempińska-Mirosławska, and G. Hoser, Detection of the influenza virus yesterday and now. Acta Biochimica Polonica, 2014. 61(3): p. 465–470.

[18] Hurt, A.C., et al., Performance of six influenza rapid tests in detecting human influenza in clinical specimens. Journal of clinical virology, 2007. 39(2): p. 132–135.

[19] Chen, H., et al., Evaluation of a rapid detection influenza virus A antigens kit using paired serum antibody test. Yonsei Medical Journal, 2013. 54(2): p. 476–479.

[20] Foo, H. and D.E. Dwyer, Rapid tests for the diagnosis of influenza. Australian Prescriber, 2009. 32(3).

[21] Boivin, G., I. Hardy, and A. Kress, Evaluation of a rapid optical immunoassay for influenza viruses (FLU OIA test) in comparison with cell culture and reverse transcription-PCR. Journal of Clinical Microbiology, 2001. 39(2): p. 730–732.

[22] Vemula, S.V., et al., Current approaches for diagnosis of influenza virus infections in humans. Viruses, 2016. 8(4): p. 96.

[23] Miller, E., et al., Incidence of 2009 pandemic influenza A H1N1 infection in England: a cross-sectional serological study. The Lancet, 2010. 375(9720): p. 1100–1108.

[24] Desvaux, S., et al., Evaluation of serological tests for H5N1 avian influenza on field samples from domestic poultry populations in Vietnam: consequences for surveillance. Veterinary Microbiology, 2012. 156(3): p. 277–284.

[25] Aksakal, B.B.Z.İ.A., Avian İnfluenza Tip A Virüsleri: Etiyoloji, Teshis ve Korunma.

[26] Nitsch-Osuch, A., A. Wozniak-Kosek, and L.B. Brydak, Accuracy of rapid influenza diagnostic test and immunofluorescence assay compared to real time RT-PCR in children with influenza A (H1N1) pdm09 infection Wiarygodność szybkiego testu diagnostycznego i metody immunofluorescencji bezpośredniej w odniesieniu do real-time RT-PCR u dzieci z grypą wywołaną wirusem typu A (H1N1) pdm09. Journal Cover, 2016. 70.

[27] di BS, K., C. Hoffmann, and W. Preiser, Influenza Report 2006.

[28] Wang, B., et al., Protective efficacy of a broadly cross-reactive swine influenza DNA vaccine encoding M2e, cytotoxic T lymphocyte epitope and consensus H3 hemagglutinin. Virology Journal, 2012. 9(1): p. 1.

[29] Allwinn, R., et al., Determination of serum antibodies against swine-origin influenza A virus H1N1/09 by immunofluorescence, haemagglutination inhibition, and by neutralization tests: how is the prevalence rate of protecting antibodies in humans? Medical Microbiology and Immunology, 2010. 199(2): p. 117–121.

[30] Read, M.C., Influenza Report 2006.

[31] Stevens, C.D., Clinical immunology & serology: a laboratory perspective. 2009: FA Davis.

[32] Sarkkinen, H., P. Halonen, and A. Salmi, Detection of influenza A virus by radioimmunoassay and enzyme-immunoassay from nasopharyngeal specimens. Journal of Medical Virology, 1981. 7(3): p. 213–220.

[33] Beard, C., Demonstration of type-specific influenza antibody in mammalian and avian sera by immunodiffusion. Bulletin of the World Health Organization, 1970. 42(5): p. 779.

[34] Harlow, E. and D. Lane, A laboratory manual. New York: Cold Spring Harbor Laboratory, 1988: p. 579.

[35] Grist, N.R., et al., Diagnostic methods in clinical virology. 1979: Blackwell Scientific Publications, Osney Mead, Oxford OX2 OEL.

[36] Jenson, T.A., Agar Gel immunodiffusion assay to detect antibodies to type A influenza virus. Animal Influenza Virus, 2014: p. 141–150.

[37] Klimov, A., et al., Influenza virus titration, antigenic characterization, and serological methods for antibody detection. Influenza Virus: Methods and Protocols, 2012: p. 25–51.

[38] Vainionpää R., W.M., Leinikki P., Diagnostic techniques: serological and molecular approaches, in Reference module in biomedical sciences. 2015, Elsevier.

[39] Julkunen, I., R. Pyhälä, and T. Hovi, Enzyme immunoassay, complement fixation and hemagglutination inhibition tests in the diagnosis of influenza A and B virus infections. Purified hemagglutinin in subtype-specific diagnosis. Journal of Virological Methods, 1985. 10(1): p. 75–84.

[40] Amano, Y. and Q. Cheng, Detection of influenza virus: traditional approaches and development of biosensors. Analytical and Bioanalytical Chemistry, 2005. 381(1): p. 156–164.

[41] Serter, P.D.N., Genel Mikrobiyoloji Ve Immünoloji: Anadolu Universitesi.

[42] Garin, B., E. Plateau, and S. Gillet-Forin, Serological diagnosis of influenza A infections in the horse by enzyme immunoassay. Comparison with the complement fixation test. Veterinary Immunology and Immunopathology, 1986. 13(4): p. 357–363.

[43] Allwinn, R., et al., Laboratory diagnosis of influenza–virology or serology? Medical Microbiology and Immunology, 2002. 191(3–4): p. 157–160.

[44] Staneková, Z. and E. Varečková, Conserved epitopes of influenza A virus inducing protective immunity and their prospects for universal vaccine development. Virology Journal, 2010. 7(1): p. 1.

[45] Cho, K.J., et al., Structure of the extracellular domain of matrix protein 2 of influenza A virus in complex with a protective monoclonal antibody. Journal of Virology, 2015. 89(7): p. 3700–3711.

[46] Liu, W., H. Li, and Y.-H. Chen, N-terminus of M2 protein could induce antibodies with inhibitory activity against influenza virus replication. FEMS Immunology & Medical Microbiology, 2003. 35(2): p. 141–146.

[47] Stepanova, L.A., et al., Protection against multiple influenza A virus strains induced by candidate recombinant vaccine based on heterologous M2e peptides linked to flagellin. PLoS One, 2015. 10(3): p. e0119520.

[48] Du, L., Y. Zhou, and S. Jiang, Research and development of universal influenza vaccines. Microbes and Infection, 2010. 12(4): p. 280–286.

[49] Holsinger, L.J. and R. Alams, Influenza virus M2 integral membrane protein is a homotetramer stabilized by formation of disulfide bonds. Virology, 1991. 183(1): p. 32–43.

[50] Lamb, R. and R. Krug, Orthomyxoviridae: the viruses and their replication. Fields Virology, 2001. 1: p. 1487–1531.

[51] Webby, R. and R. Webster, Emergence of influenza A viruses. Philosophical Transactions of the Royal Society of London. Series B: Biological Sciences, 2001. 356(1416): p. 1817–28.

[52] Ebrahimi, S.M. and M. Tebianian, Influenza A viruses: why focusing on M2e-based universal vaccines. Virus Genes, 2011. 42(1): p. 1–8.

[53] Huleatt, J.W., et al., Potent immunogenicity and efficacy of a universal influenza vaccine candidate comprising a recombinant fusion protein linking influenza M2e to the TLR5 ligand flagellin. Vaccine, 2008. 26(2): p. 201–214.

[54] Black, R.A., et al., Antibody response to the M2 protein of influenza A virus expressed in insect cells. Journal of General Virology, 1993. 74(1): p. 143–146.

[55] Cox, N.J., et al., Orthomyxoviruses: influenza. Topley and Wilson's microbiology and microbial infections, 1998.

[56] Tompkins, S.M., et al., Matrix protein 2 vaccination and protection against influenza viruses, including subtype H5N1. Matrix, 2007.

[57] Neirynck, S., et al., A universal influenza A vaccine based on the extracellular domain of the M2 protein. Nature Medicine, 1999. 5(10): p. 1157–1163.

[58] De Filette, M., et al., Improved design and intranasal delivery of an M2e-based human influenza A vaccine. Vaccine, 2006. 24(44): p. 6597–6601.

[59] Fiers, W., et al., M2e-based universal influenza A vaccine. Vaccine, 2009. 27(45): p. 6280–6283.

[60] Tao, W. and H.S. Gill, M2e-immobilized gold nanoparticles as influenza A vaccine: Role of soluble M2e and longevity of protection. Vaccine, 2015. 33(20): p. 2307–2315.

[61] Khurana, S., et al., H5N1-SeroDetect EIA and rapid test: a novel differential diagnostic assay for serodiagnosis of H5N1 infections and surveillance. Journal of Virology, 2011. 85(23): p. 12455–12463.

[62] Denis, J., et al., Development of a universal influenza A vaccine based on the M2e peptide fused to the papaya mosaic virus (PapMV) vaccine platform. Vaccine, 2008. 26(27): p. 3395–3403.

[63] Wolf, A.I., et al., Vaccination with M2e-based multiple antigenic peptides: characterization of the B cell response and protection efficacy in inbred and outbred mice. PLoS One, 2011. 6(12): p. e28445.

[64] Hadifar, F., et al., Multimeric recombinant M2e protein-based ELISA: a significant improvement in differentiating avian influenza infected chickens from vaccinated ones. PLoS One, 2014. 9(10): p. e108420.

[65] Tarigan, S., et al., Characterization of the M2e antibody response following highly pathogenic H5N1 avian influenza virus infection and reliability of M2e ELISA for

identifying infected among vaccinated chickens. Avian Pathology, 2015. 44(4): p. 259–268.

[66] Shively, R. Evaluation of 11 commercially available rapid influenza diagnostic tests — United States, 2011–2012. Morbidity and Mortality Weekly Report (MMWR) 2012. Available from: http://www.cdc.gov/mmwr/preview/mmwrhtml/mm6143a3.htm.

[67] Liu, W., et al., Sequence comparison between the extracellular domain of M2 protein human and avian influenza A virus provides new information for bivalent influenza vaccine design. Microbes and Infection, 2005. 7(2): p. 171–177.

[68] Fiers, W., et al., A "universal" human influenza A vaccine. Virus Research, 2004. 103(1): p. 173–176.

4

Influenza Inactive Virus Vaccine with the Fusion Peptide (rTα1-BP5) Enhances Protection Against Influenza through Humoral and Cell-Mediated Immunity

Chen Wang, Chengshui Liao, Wufan Zhang,
Deyuan Li and Puyan Chen

Abstract

Thymosin α1 (Tα1) and Bursopentin (BP5) are both immunopotentiators. To explore whether the thymosin α1-Bursopentin (rTα1-BP5) is an adjuvant or not, we cloned the gene of Tα1-BP5 and provided evidence that the gene of Tα1-BP5 in a recombinant prokaryotic expression plasmid was successfully expressed in *Escherichia coli* BL21. To evaluate the immune adjuvant properties of rTα1-BP5, chickens were immunized with rTα1-BP5 combined with H9N2 avian influenza whole-inactivated virus (WIV). The titers of HI antibody, antigen-specific antibodies, Avian influenza virus (AIV)-neutralizing antibodies, levels of Th1-type cytokines (gamma interferon (IFN-γ)) and Th2-type cytokines (interleukin 4 (IL-4)), and lymphocyte proliferation responses were determined. We found that rTα1-BP5 enhanced HI antibody and antigen-specific immunoglobulin G (IgG) antibodies titers, increased the level of AIV-neutralizing antibodies, induced the secretion of Th1- and Th2-type cytokines, and promoted the proliferation of T and B lymphocyte. Furthermore, virus challenge experiments confirmed that rTα1-BP5 contributed to the inhibition replication of the virus (H9N2 AIV (A/chicken/Jiangsu/NJ07/05) from chicken lungs. Altogether, these findings suggest that rTα1-BP5 is a novel adjuvant suitable for H9N2 avian influenza vaccine.

Keywords: thymosin α1 (Tα1), Bursopentin (BP5), fusion peptide, avian influenza vaccine, adjuvant

1. Introduction

Avian influenza virus (AIV) is an enveloped virus that belongs to the *Orthomyxoviridae* family and has an eight-segmented, single-stranded, negative-sense RNA genome. Among the proteins encoded by the genome, there are two surface glycoproteins, hemagglutinin (HA) and neuraminidase (NA) [1]. AIVs are classified into subtypes according to the combination of 16 HA and nine NA molecules. Among the many subtypes of AIV, H9N2 is thought to have originated from shorebirds and gulls, and has rapidly spread to become one of the most prevalent diseases in domestic poultry worldwide. It also causes serious economic loss in the poultry industry [2] (see **Table 1**).

Abbreviation	Full name
Tα1	Thymosin α1
BP5	Bursopentin
rTα1-BP5	Thymosin α1-Bursopentin
WIV	Whole-inactivated virus
AIV	Avian influenza virus
HA	Hemagglutinin
NA	Neuraminidase
BRM	Biological response modifier
MIF	Macrophage migration inhibitory factor
BF	Bursa of Fabricius
BLP	Bursin-like epitope peptide
HI	Hemagglutination inhibition assay
IFN-γ	Interferon-γ
IL-4	Interleukin-4
TNF-α	Tumor necrosis factor-α
Th	T-helper type
Th1	T-helper type 1
Th2	T-helper type 2
MDCK	Madin-Darby canine kidney
FBS	Fetal bovine serum
MTT	3-(4,5-dimethylthiazol-2-yl)2,5-diphenyltetrazolium bromide
IPTG	Isopropyl-β-D-thiogalactoside
ConA	Concanavalin A
PMA	Phorbol-12-myristate-13-acetate

Abbreviation	Full name
TMB	Tetramethyl benzidine
HRP	Horseradish peroxidase
SPF	Specific pathogen-free
SOE-PCR	Splicing overlap extension PCR method
TRX	Thioredoxin
$TCID_{50}$	50% tissue culture infective dose
PBS	phosphate-buffered saline
pfu	Plaque-forming unit
OD	Optical density
IgG	Immunoglobulin G
ELISA	Enzyme-linked immunosorbent assay
$PRNT_{50}$	50% plaque-reducing neutralizing titer

Table 1. Abbreviations for full name.

In domestic avian species in North America, H9N2 influenza viruses occur primarily in turkeys, occasionally in quail, and rarely if ever in chickens. The H9N2 virus subtype was first isolated from turkeys in 1966 [3], when the virus was associated with mild respiratory disease. In Asia, long-term surveillance in live poultry markets in Hong Kong from 1975 to 1985 detected H9N2 influenza viruses in apparently healthy ducks but not in chickens [4]. Since the early 1990s, H9N2 influenza viruses have become widespread in domestic chickens in Asia [5]. Among the avian influenza A virus subtypes, H9N2 viruses have the potential to cause an influenza pandemic because they are widely prevalent in avian species in Asia and have demonstrated the ability to infect humans [6]. In April 1999, two World Health Organization reference laboratories independently confirmed the isolation of avian influenza A (H9N2) viruses for the first time in humans [7].

The best protection against influenza virus infection remains effective vaccination [8]. Inactivated vaccines have been undergoing clinical trials as pandemic vaccine candidates, and it has been shown that inactivated vaccines elicit strong humoral responses; however, it is commonly accepted that no adequate mucosal or cellular immunity is achieved [9]. Adjuvants are able to improve the quantity and quality of innate immune responses by enhancing their speed and duration, and by inducing adequate adaptive immunity [10]. To improve methods for influenza vaccine production, the current strategy of many investigators is to increase the efficacy of pandemic influenza vaccines by the addition of adjuvants to boost immune responses, such as aluminum salts, MF59, IC31®, and chitosan [11–14].

A defined peptide sequence able to stimulate specific immune cell subsets has the potential to act as an adjuvant for a variety of immunogens. The thymus is an important central immune organ for T-lymphocyte differentiation and maturation [15]. It is capable of secreting many peptides with the functions of regulating the development of different phenotypic markers and lymphocyte [16]. Thymosin alpha 1 (Tα1), an immunomodulatory peptide consisting of 28 amino acid residues, was isolated originally from calf thymus [17]. As a biological response modifier (BRM), Tα1 has multiple biological activities in the immune system. It can promote specific lymphocyte functions, stimulate the production of lymphokines such as gamma interferon (IFN-γ), tumor necrosis factor-α (TNF-α), interleukin 2 (IL-2), macrophage migration inhibitory factor (MIF), and precursor stem cell into the CD4+/CD8+ T cells, increase T-cell proliferation, differentiation and maturation, and so on [18, 19]. Furthermore, it has the activities of antitumor and protection against oxidative damage [20]. Consequently, Tα1 is widely used in clinic treating various diseases including immunodeficiency diseases, severe sepsis, and systemic infectious disorder [21].

The bursa of Fabricius (BF) is a primary humoral immune organ unique to birds and is the site of B-lymphocyte development and differentiation. The tripeptidebursin (LysHisGlyNH2) has been described as an endogenous B-cell stimulant or differentiation factor [22]. BS and bursin-like peptide T-X-N-L-K-H-G significantly enhance the JEV subtype vaccine-induced immune response in immunized mice [23]. Bursin-like epitope peptide (BLP) is one of bursin-like peptides and enhances immune responses in mice immunized with inactivated H9N2 avian influenza vaccine [24]. Our previous study has been reported that Bursopentin (BP5) is a small peptide separated from BF, which amino acid sequence is CKDVY. We found that BP5 not only promotes T-cell and B-cell proliferation, enhances humoral immunity and cellular immunity but also balances Th1 and Th2 immune responses [25, 26].

Although both Tα1 and BP5 have the potent adjuvant effects, this study designed and synthesized Tα1-BP5 fusion gene according to the preferential codons of *Escherichia coli*, fused with prokaryotic expression vector pET-32a, and then transferred into *E. coli* BL21 to induce its expression. Then, we tested whether rTα1-BP5 could enhance immune responses in chicken upon vaccination with H9N2 avian influenza whole-inactivated virus (WIV).

2. Materials and methods

2.1. Plasmid, viruses, and reagents

pET-32a (+), *E. coli* DH5α, *E. coli* BL21 (DE3), pET32a (+)-BP5, and avian influenza virus A/Chicken/Jiangsu/JS-1/2002(H9N2) were maintained in our laboratory. Avian influenza virus A/Chicken/Jiangsu/NJ08/05(H9N2) was kindly provided by Dr. Qi-Sheng Zheng. Virus titers were determined in MDCK cells. H9N2 avian influenza whole-inactivated virus (WIV) was prepared by diluting the virus 1:4000 (v/v) in formalin [27, 28]. All restriction enzymes and *Taq* polymerase were purchased from TakaRa Biotechnology (Dalian, China). RPMI 1640 medium and fetal bovine serum (FBS) were purchased from Gibco (New York, NY, USA). Isopropyl-β-D-thiogalactoside (IPTG), 3-(4,5-dimethylthiazol-2-yl)2,5-diphenyltetrazolium bromide (MTT), TEMED, dNTP, Concanavalin A (ConA), Phorbol-12-myristate-13-acetate (PMA), and tetramethylbenzidine (TMB) were purchased from Jiu Shi Corporation (Zhengzhou, China). Horseradish peroxidase (HRP)-conjugated goat anti-mice IgG was obtained from Boshide Corporation (Wuhan, China). Control Standard Tα1 and BP5 peptides were synthesized by

Shanghai Science Peptide Biological Technology Co., Ltd. (Shanghai, China), and the purity was over 95%.

2.2. Chicken embryos, animals, and vaccines

Specific pathogen-free (SPF) Roman chicken and chicken embryos were obtained from the Henan Experimental Animal Research Center. Avian influenza virus A/Chicken/Jiangsu/NJ08/05(H9N2) (10^7 $TCID_{50}$/0.1 mL) was inoculated into the allantoic cavities of 10-day-old SPF chicken embryos; the embryos that died within 24 h were discarded, and the allantoic fluids were harvested from the infected embryos at 48 h postinfection and inactivated by treatment with 0.2% formalin. The inactivated virus was emulsified with mineral oil to make an oil-formulated inactivated H9N2 AIV vaccine. One dose of the vaccine contained 10^7 $TCID_{50}$/0.1 mL, which was equal to it before inactivation. Procedure and test of inactivated vaccine were described according to OIE Terrestrial Manual 2012 [29].

2.3. Gene cloning and expression of the recombinant fusion peptide Tα1-BP5

Gene of the recombinant fusion peptide thymosin α1-Bursopentin (Tα1-BP5) was designed according to the preferential codons of *E. coli* and amplified by splicing overlap extension polymerase chain reaction (SOE-PCR) method [30]. Sequences of the primers used for the synthetic Tα1-BP5 are as follows: F1: 5′-CCG GAA TTC AGC GAC GCT GCT GTT GAC ACT AGC AGC GAA ATC ACT ACTA AAG ACT TG-3′; F2: 5′-GTT CGG GGT GCTG CCG CCG CCG CCG TTT TCA GCT TCT TCA ACA ACT TCT TTT TTT TCT TTC AAG TCT TTA GTA GT-3′; and F3: 5′-GGC GGC GGC GGC AGC TGC AAA AAT GTG TAT TAA GTC GAC TCG-3′, with *Eco*R I and *Sal* I site (underlined). The genes of Tα1 and BP5 were connected with the gene of the GGGGS linker to form the Tα1-BP5 fusion gene. And then, the amplified DNA fragment was digested by *Eco*R I and *Sal* I, and then ligated into the expression vector pET32a. The ligation mix was transformed into competent DH5α cells and the single bacterial colony was selected by overnight growth on Luria broth (LB) agar plates containing 100-μg/mL ampicillin. The obtained recombinant plasmid pET32a-Tα1-BP5 was confirmed by restriction endonuclease digestion and DNA sequencing. The pET32a-Tα1-BP5 plasmid was transformed into *E. coli* BL21 (DE3) for inducing expression. The expression products were examined by sodium dodecyl sulfate-polyacrylamide gel electrophoresis (SDS-PAGE). And the recombinant proteins were purified on a Ni-affinity chromatography column (Amersham Bioscience HiTrap chelating HP 5 mL × one column) following the manufacturer's instructions.

2.4. Activity testing of fusion peptide Tα1-BP5 (rTα1-BP5) in vitro

Thymus and spleens from 4 to 6-week-BALB/c mice with (20 ± 2) g were collected aseptically, put them at 200-mesh stainless screen mesh cells, and gently minced into single cell suspension with a syringe followed by adding Hank's solution. The red blood cells were removed by centrifugation at 500 rpm for 5 min. The supernatant was centrifuged at 500 rpm for 5 min. The obtained pellet was washed with Hank's solution twice. The density of lymphocytes was adjusted to around 5 × 10^6 cells/mL using RPMI-1640 medium containing 10% FBS. ConA and PMA were added into thymic lymphocytes and splenic lymphocytes to make the concentrations reach 5 μg/mL and 300 ng/mL, respectively. The two kinds of solutions were subpackaged into a 96-well plate with 100 μL/well, respectively, and three parallel samples were set for each well. The plates were incubated in CO_2 incubator at 37°C for 6 h, followed by adding 100-μL/well rTα1-BP5 (affinity chromatography purified through Ni column) with different concentrations (1.25, 2.5, 5.0, 10.0, and 20.0 μg/mL) and continued culturing for 72 h. Control groups (phosphate-buffered saline (PBS), 10.0 μg/mL thioredoxin, 10.0 μg/mL Tα1, and 10.0 μg/mL BP5) were used following the same procedures. MTT method was used to test the effect of rTα1-BP5 effect on thymic and splenic lymphocytes proliferation. Relative ratio of cell proliferation (%) = (experimental group OD_{570}/control group OD_{570}) × 100% [31, 32].

2.5. Immunization of chickens

All animal experiments were approved by the Henan University of Science and Technology Animal Care and Use Committee. Twenty-one-day-old SPF Roman chickens were randomly divided into six experimental groups of 25 chickens each and intramuscularly immunized two times on days 0 and 14 with (i) 100 μL PBS as a negative control, (ii) 100 μL H9N2 WIV (A/Chicken/Jiangsu/NJ08/05, 10^7 $TCID_{50}$/0.1 mL), (iii) a mixture of 100 μL H9N2 WIV and Tα1 (50 μg), (iv) a mixture of 100 μL H9N2 WIV and BP5 (50 μg), (v) a mixture of 100 μL H9N2 WIV and rTα1-BP5 (50 μg), and (vi) 100 μL oil-formulated inactivated H9N2 AIV vaccine (A/Chicken/Jiangsu/NJ08/05, 10^7 $TCID_{50}$/0.1 mL) as a positive control (**Table 2**).

Group	Vaccination on days 0 and 14[a]
1	100 μL PBS
2	10^7 $TCID_{50}$ H9N2 WIV
3	10^7 $TCID_{50}$ H9N2 WIV + 50 μg Tα1
4	10^7 $TCID_{50}$ H9N2 WIV + 50 μg BP5
5	10^7 $TCID_{50}$ H9N2 WIV + 50 μg rTα1-BP5
6	10^7 $TCID_{50}$ H9N2 AIV vaccine

[a] H9N2 WIV, inactivated H9N2 avian influenza whole-inactivated virus; H9N2 AIV vaccine, H9N2 avian influenza virus vaccine prepared with oil/water as an adjuvant.

Table 2. Animal groups and the experimental design.

The details of the animal experiment time points are shown in **Figure 1**.

2.6. Detection of antibodies in serum

Chicken (n = 5 per group) sera were collected on 7 and 21 days after the first immunization. Serum antibody (HI and antigen-specific antibodies) titers were determined using standard HI microliter and enzyme-linked immunosorbent assay (ELISA) as described [25, 33]. Briefly, to detect the HI titers in chicken serum, sera were inactivated by incubation for 30 min at 56°C and serially diluted twofold in PBS, then transferred in duplicate to 96-well round-bottomed

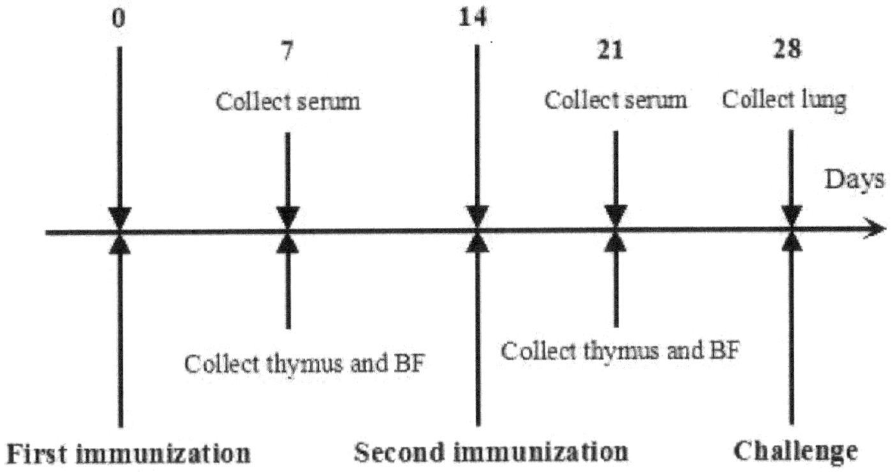

Figure 1. Experimental scheme of immunization, sample collection, and challenge.

plates. Standard avian influenza virus (A/Chicken/Shandong/6/96(H9N2)) antigen with four units was then added to each diluted serum samples in a volume of 50 μL, and followed by an equal volume of 0.5% chicken erythrocyte suspensions. The mixture was incubated for 1 h at room temperature before the results were read. The HI titers were defined as the highest serum dilution capable of preventing hemagglutination.

To evaluate the antigen-specific antibodies titers, ELISA plates were coated with 10-μg/mL recombinant influenza HA protein (expressed in *E. coli* BL21) and blocked with 1% bovine serum albumin (BSA) for 2 h at 37°C. Aliquots of diluted chicken sera were added to the plates, which were then incubated overnight, washed, and incubated with HRP-conjugated goat anti-chicken IgG. Finally, TMB was added and the reaction was stopped by the addition of 2N H_2SO_4 and the absorbance was read at OD_{450}. Each serum sample was repeated in quintuplicate. The results were plotted as OD versus dilution (log scale). Titers at half maximal OD were determined by linear interpolation [34].

2.7. Determination of AIV-neutralizing antibodies

Inactivated sera were incubated with 100 plaque-forming unit (pfu) of avian influenza virus (A/Chicken/Jiangsu/JS-1/2002(H9N2), and the titers of AIV-neutralizing antibodies determined as described [35].

2.8. Cytokine assays

On 7 and 21 days after the first immunization, the serum levels of Th1-type cytokine (IFN-γ) in chickens were determined using commercial Chicken cytokines gamma interferon ELISA kits (Cusabio Biotech, MD, USA), whereas Th2-type cytokine (IL-4) was determined with another commercial Chicken cytokines interleukin 4 ELISA kits (Cusabio Biotech, USA). The procedure followed the manufacturer's instructions.

2.9. Lymphocyte proliferation response

To detect changes in cellular immunity, lymphocyte proliferation response was performed. Thymus and bursa of Fabricius were collected from immunized chickens at 7 and 21 days after the first immunization. The thymus and BF lymphocytes were isolated and maintained in 1640 medium supplemented with 10% FBS at 37°C with 5% CO_2. The thymus lymphocytes (5×10^6 cells/mL) were seeded in a 96-well plate and incubated with 50 μL of ConA (40 μg/mL) at 40°C/5% CO_2 for 48 h, whereas the BF lymphocytes (5×10^6 cells/mL) were treated with 50 μL of PMA (1 μg/mL) in a 96-well plate at 40°C/5% CO_2 for 24 h. Then, the lymphocyte proliferation assay was performed using a standard MTT method as described previously [36, 37]. Then, the plate was incubated with 10 μL of 5 mg/mL MTT for 3 h. Finally, 100 μL of 10% (w/v) SDS in 0.01 M HCl was added into the plate and allowed to incubate for 2 h. A spectrophotometric measurement was taken at A_{570}.

2.10. Virus challenge experiment

Two weeks after the second vaccination, chickens (n = 15 per group) were intranasally challenged with 2.5×10^6 $TCID_{50}$ avian influenza virus A/chicken/Jiangsu/JS-1/2002(H9N2) in 100 μL PBS. Five chickens per group were humanely sacrificed at 3, 5, and 7 days after virus challenge and the viral titers in their lungs assessed by plaque formation assays using MDCK cells as described [35].

2.11. Statistical analysis

Statistical analyses were performed using unpaired t-tests or one-way analysis of variance (ANOVA) F-statistics followed by GraphPad Prism 6 software. Data are presented as the mean ± standard deviation (SD). Turkey multiple comparison tests were used to assess differences among the five experimental groups, with differences being considered significant at $P < 0.05$ or $P < 0.01$.

3. Results

3.1. Expression of the recombinant fusion peptide Tα1-BP5

The gene of Tα1-BP5 was amplified by SOE-PCR with the primers F1, F2, and F3. The PCR products were identified by electrophoresis, and then about 114bp strip was observed. The recombinant plasmid was extracted and identified with *Hind* III enzyme. The results showed that the recombinant plasmid was not digested by *Hind* III, indicating that the recombinant plasmid had deleted the *Hind* III restriction site (**Figure 2A**). Sequencing result showed that the gene of the recombinant fusion peptide Tα1-BP5 was inserted into pET32a vector, and it was consistent to the expected size (**Table 3**), which was suggested that the recombinant expression vector was constructed successfully, and it was named pET32a-Tα1-BP5. Then, pET32a-Tα1-BP5 was transferred into *E. coli* BL21 (DE3) for its expression, and the expressed products were detected by using SDS-PAGE. The result showed that Tα1-BP5 was expressed and purified with the molecular weight of 31.4 kDa (**Figure 2B**), which is consistent with its predicted molecular weight.

Name	Amino acid sequence
Tα1-BP5	Ser Asp Ala Ala Val Asp Thr Ser Ser Glu Ile Thr Thr Lys Asp Leu Lys Glu Lys Lys Glu Val Val Glu Glu Ala Glu Asn Gly Gly Gly Gly Ser Cys Lys Asp Val Tyr

Table 3. Amino acid sequence of recombinant fusion peptide Tα1-BP5.

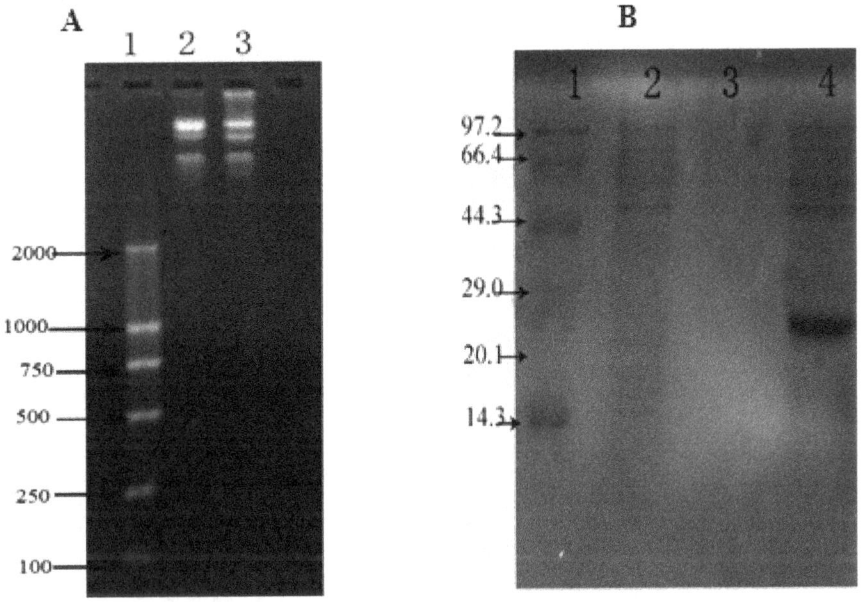

Figure 2. Identification of the recombinant plasmid pET32a-Tα1-BP5 and the expression of fusion peptide Tα1-BP5 in *E. coli*. (A) 1: DL2000 marker; 2: the recombinant plasmid pET32a-Tα1-BP5 after *Hind* III enzyme digestion; and 3: the recombinant plasmid pET32a-Tα1-BP5. (B) 1: low molecular weight protein marker; 2: not induced *E. coli* BL21 (DE3); 3: Not induced recombinant *E. coli* BL21 (DE3)/pET32a-Tα1-BP5; 4: induced recombinant *E. coli* BL21 (DE3)/pET32a-Tα1-BP5.

3.2. Activity of rTα1-BP5 in vitro

The expressed product of TBP5 recombinant bacteria was affinity chromatography purified through protein Ni column and quantified through spectrophotometer. MTT method was used to test the effect of rTα1-BP5 on the proliferation of mouse thymic and splenic lymphocytes. The results showed that all rTα1-BP5 with different concentrations (1.25, 2.5, 5.0, 10.0, and 20.0 μg/mL) could promote the proliferation of thymic and splenic lymphocytes compared to PBS group. rTα1-BP5 could stimulate thymic and splenic lymphocytes proliferation stronger than TP5 and BP5. The differences were significant ($P < 0.05$) on the concentrations of 5.0 and 20.0 μg/mL, and the differences were more significant ($P < 0.01$) on the concentrations of 10.0 μg/mL (**Figure 3A** and **B**). All these data demonstrated that rTα1-BP5 could promote the proliferation of mouse thymic T lymphocytes and splenic B lymphocytes.

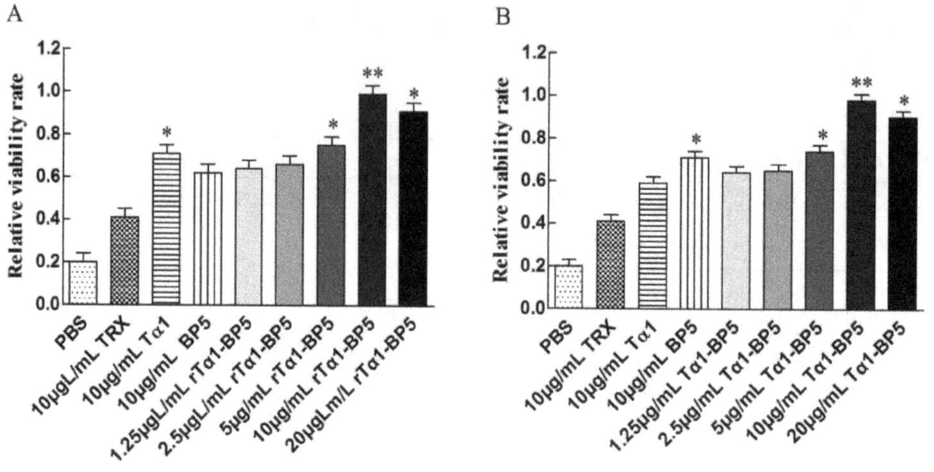

Figure 3. The effects of rTα1-BP5 on the proliferation of thymic lymphocytes (A) or splenic lymphocytes (B) from immunized mice. The data presented are of five replicates. *, $P < 0.05$, compared with mice immunized with PBS, and **, $P < 0.01$, compared with mice immunized with BP5 or Tα1.

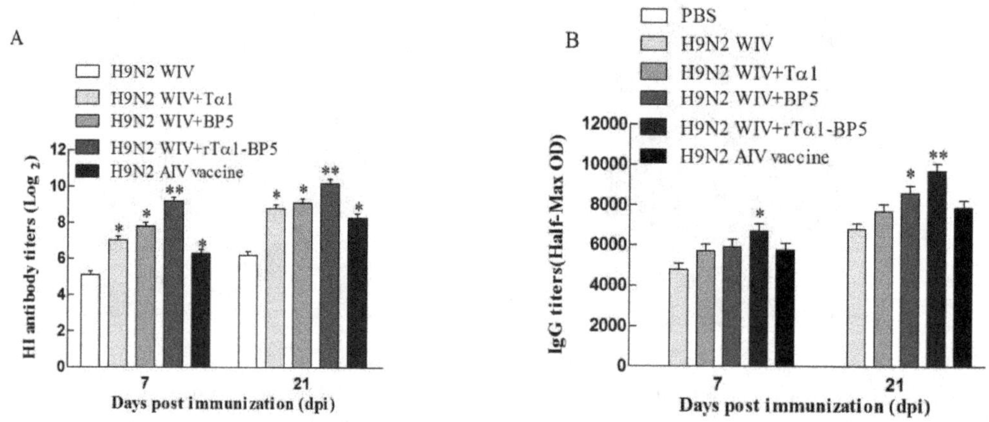

Figure 4. Effect of rTα1-BP5 to H9N2 AIV vaccination on antigen-specific HI titers and anti-HA IgG antibodies. Chickens were immunized two times, and chicken sera were collected on days 7 and 21 after the first immunization, and the serum HI titers (A) and IgG titers (B) were analyzed by HI assay and ELISA, respectively. The data presented are means ± SD of results from five replicates. *, $P < 0.05$, and **, $P < 0.01$, compared with chickens immunized with H9N2 WIV alone.

3.3. rTα1-BP5 stimulates significant antigen-specific immune responses

To determine antigen-specific immune responses to immunization, chickens were immunized two times, then sera were taken on days 7 and 21 after the first immunization and detected for HI and anti-HA antibody titers. HI antibody titers of chickens immunized with inactivated vaccine, Tα1 combined with H9N2 WIV and BP5 combined with H9N2 WIV increased significantly compared with chickens immunized with the H9N2 WIV alone at days 7 and 21 ($P < 0.05$). However, HI antibody titers in chickens immunized with rTα1-BP5 combined with H9N2 WIV were significantly higher than in chicken immunized with BP5 combined with

H9N2 WIV at days 7 and 21 ($P < 0.05$) (**Figure 4A**). Anti-HA IgG antibody was observed in immunized chickens on days 7 and 21 after the first immunization. rTα1-BP5 enhanced the secretion of IgG antibody on day 7 after the first immunization, and the effect was greater than that induced by H9N2 AIV vaccine, Tα1 combined with H9N2 WIV and BP5 combined with H9N2 WIV. On day 21 after the first immunization, BP5 significantly enhanced IgG antibody secretion levels compared with that induced by H9N2 vaccine, Tα1 combined with H9N2 WIV ($P < 0.05$), while the effect of rTα1-BP5 was the greatest than the other groups ($P < 0.01$) (**Figure 4B**). These results suggested that rTα1-BP5 stimulates significant antigen-specific immune responses.

3.4. rTα1-BP5 promoted the production of AIV-neutralizing antibody

To assess whether rTα1-BP5 can effectively enhance virus-neutralizing antibodies, chicken sera were collected on days 7 and 21 after the first immunization and the titers of AIV-neutralizing antibody were assessed. The result showed that the titers of neutralizing antibody of chickens immunized with Tα1 plus H9N2 WIV, BP5 plus H9N2 WIV, and H9N2 AIV vaccine were higher than that in chickens immunized with H9N2 WIV alone on day 7, while it was higher in chickens immunized with Tα1-BP5 plus H9N2 WIV than that of other groups. Consistent with this, AIV-neutralizing antibody titers of chicken injected with rTα1-BP5 plus H9N2 WIV were the highest on day 21 (**Table 4**). These results indicated that rTα1-BP5 significantly stimulates the production of AIV-neutralizing antibodies.

Treatment	PRNT50[a]	
	First boost	Second boost
PBS	–	–
H9N2 WIV	10 ± 0.38	19 ± 0.21
H9N2 WIV + Tα1	15 ± 0.30*	22 ± 0.25*
H9N2 WIV + BP5	18 ± 0.32*	28 ± 0.43*
H9N2 WIV + rTα1-BP5	22 ± 0.24**	32 ± 0.19**
Inactivated H9N2 AIV vaccine	16 ± 0.15*	25 ± 0.54**

a Chickens were vaccinated on days 0 (first boost) and 14 (second boost). Chicken sera ($n = 5$) were collected on days 7 and 21, and plaque-reducing neutralizing antibody titers were determined. The 50% plaque-reducing neutralizing titer ($PRNT_{50}$) was reported as the geometrical reciprocal of the serum dilution resulting in a 50% reduction in plaques. The data presented are means ± SD of results from five replicates.
*, $P < 0.05$, and
**, $P < 0.01$, compared with chickens immunized with H9N2 WIV alone.

Table 4. Titers of plaque-reducing neutralizing antibody in groups of chicken.

3.5. rTα1-BP5 increases the production of both Th1- and Th2-type cytokines

We then examined the levels of Th1 (IFN-γ) and Th2 (IL-4) cytokines from immunized chickens. Compared with stimulation with H9N2 WIV alone, both IFN-γ and IL-4 secretion were remarkably increased after immunization with inactivated H9N2 AIV vaccine, Tα1 plus

H9N2 WIV and BP5 plus H9N2 WIV at days 7 and 21, and the highest level of IFN-γ secretion was observed in the vaccination group with rTα1-BP5 plus H9N2 WIV ($P < 0.01$) (**Figure 5A** and **B**). Taken together, the results suggested that rTα1-BP5 promoted the secretion of both Th1 and Th2 cytokines.

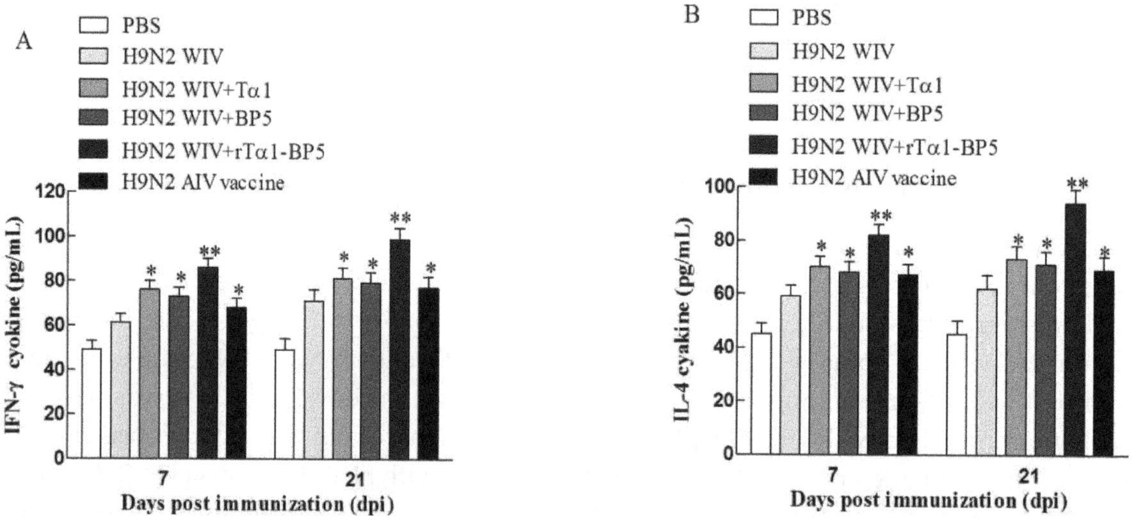

Figure 5. Effect of rTα1-BP5 to H9N2 AIV vaccination on cytokine production in chicken sera. Chickens were immunized two times, and chicken sera were collected on days 7 and 21 after the first immunization. Cytokine release was measured by using commercial chicken cytokines gamma interferon (IFN-γ) and interleukin 4 (IL-4) ELISA kits. The data presented are means ± SD of results from five replicates. *, $P < 0.05$, and **, $P < 0.01$, compared with chickens immunized with H9N2 WIV alone.

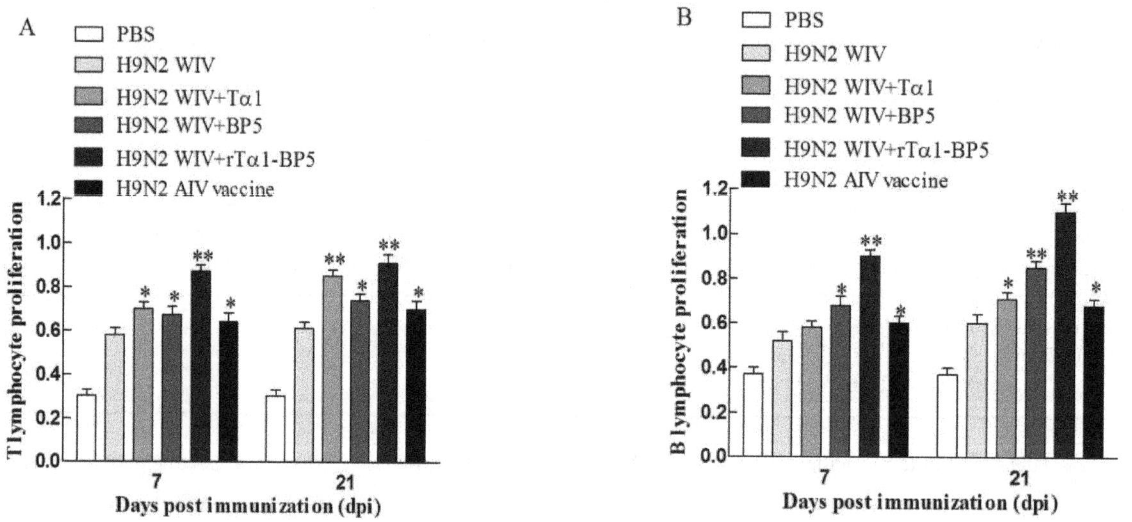

Figure 6. rTα1-BP5 significantly stimulates chicken T- and B-lymphocyte proliferation. Chickens were immunized two times, and chicken thymus and bursa of Fabricius were collected on days 7 and 21 after the first immunization. T- (A) and B (B)-lymphocyte proliferation assays were evaluated by MTT method. The data presented are means ± SD of results from five replicates. *, $P < 0.05$, and **, $P < 0.01$, compared with chickens immunized with H9N2 WIV alone.

3.6. rTα1-BP5 significantly enhances T- and B-lymphocyte proliferation

To investigate the effects of rTα1-BP5 on T- and B-lymphocyte proliferation, thymus and BF were collected from chickens immunized with rTα1-BP5 plus H9N2 WIV. T-lymphocyte proliferation responses of chickens immunized with Tα1 plus H9N2 WIV, BP5 plus H9N2 WIV, and H9N2 AIV vaccine were enhanced at 7 days compared with chickens immunized with H9N2 WIV alone ($P < 0.05$), whereas it was higher for that immunized with rTα1-BP5 plus H9N2 WIV ($P < 0.01$). On day 21, T-lymphocyte proliferation responses of chickens immunized with Tα1 plus H9N2 WIV and H9N2 AIV vaccine were higher than chickens immunized with H9N2 WIV alone ($P < 0.05$), while it was highest for that immunized with rTα1-BP5 plus H9N2 WIV ($P < 0.01$) (**Figure 6A**). Similarly, B-lymphocyte proliferation responses of chickens immunized with BP5 plus H9N2 WIV and H9N2 AIV vaccine were enhanced at 7 and 21 days compared with chickens immunized with H9N2 WIV alone ($P < 0.05$), whereas, it was highest for that immunized with rTα1-BP5 plus H9N2 WIV ($P < 0.01$) (**Figure 6B**). The data indicated that rTα1-BP5 promoted T- and B-lymphocyte proliferative responses.

3.7. rTα1-BP5 significantly promotes immune protection against H9N2 AIV challenge

To evaluate whether rTα1-BP5 promotes immune protection against H9N2 AIV infection, viral titers in chicken lungs were evaluated at 3, 5, and 7 days after viral challenge by plaque formation assays. Chickens immunized with Tα1 plus H9N2 WIV, BP5 plus H9N2 WIV, and H9N2 AIV vaccine showed significant virus removal from the lungs at 3, 5, and 7 days after challenge compared with H9N2 WIV groups ($P < 0.05$), while the viral titers of lungs from chicken immunized with rTα1-BP5 plus H9N2 WIV were significantly lower than that in the H9N2 AIV vaccine group ($P < 0.01$). Moreover, chickens immunized with rTα1-BP5 plus H9N2 WIV had almost no detectable virus particles in the lungs 7 days after challenge (**Figure 7A–C**). The data indicated that rTα1-BP5 significantly promoted immune protection against H9N2 AIV challenge.

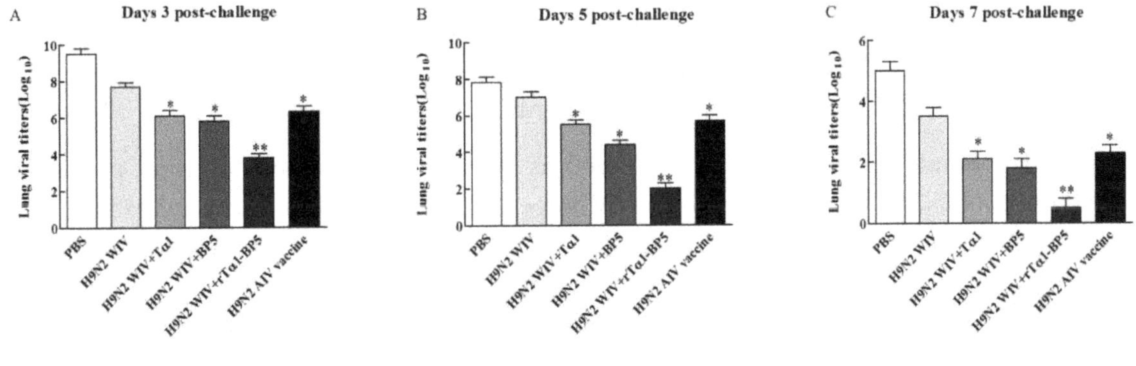

Figure 7. AIV-viral titers of lung in chickens. Lung samples from individual chicken in each group ($n = 5$) were collected on days 3, 5, and 7 post challenge with 2.5 × 106 $TCID_{50}$ avian influenza virus (A/chicken/Jiangsu/JS-1/2002(H9N2)). Each lung sample was diluted to 1 mL with 1640 media. The titers are presented as pfu per mL. The data presented are means ± SD of results from five replicates. *, $P < 0.05$, and **, $P < 0.01$, compared with chickens immunized with H9N2 WIV alone.

4. Discussion

In the event of an influenza pandemic, vaccination is one of the most effective ways of intervention in terms of reducing cost, disease, and even death. Appropriate adjuvant can enhance the immunogenicity of the vaccine and improve the immune responses [38, 39]. However, most of the adjuvants used in conjugation with antigen have unacceptable levels of side effects, only a few of them are used clinically [40]. Thus, we need to find new and optimal adjuvant candidates for vaccine. In recent years, some small peptide immunostimulants were reported in use for vaccine adjuvants [41–43]. Both Tα1 and BP5 are associated with immune regulation. Previous studies showed that both Tα1 and BP5 had high potential as an adjuvant for vaccines [26, 44].

In this study, the fusion peptide of rTα1-BP5 was designed and synthesized, and to investigate it as an adjuvant for inducing immune responses in chickens upon vaccination with inactivated H9N2 avian influenza virus (WIV). An effective adjuvant should be able to enhance the levels of both humoral and cell-mediated immunity. To investigate the effect of rTα1-BP5 on humoral responses, chickens were immunized with H9N2 WIV combined with Tα1-BP5, and then titers of HI antibody, antigen-specific antibodies, and AIV-neutralizing antibodies were assessed. Then, we found that rTα1-BP5 significantly enhanced HI antibody and antigen-specific IgG antibodies titers, promoted the secretion of AIV-neutralizing antibodies, which suggested that rTα1-BP5 enhanced the levels of humoral immune responses in chickens when it was co-immunized with H9N2 WIV.

In addition to humoral immune responses, cellular immunity also plays an important role in fighting influenza virus infections [45]. The levels of Th1- and Th2-type cytokines are important references to measure cellular immunity. And lymphocyte homeostasis is required for the maintenance of normal immune function [46]. Th1-type cytokines mainly include IL-2, TNF-α, and IFN-γ, whereas Th2-type cytokines include IL-4, IL-5, and IL-10 [47]. Our study though analyzed the production of Th1 (IFN-γ)- and Th2 (IL-4)-type cytokines, and T- and B-lymphocytes proliferation in vaccinated chickens post immunization to evaluate the cell-mediated immunity. The results suggested that rTα1-BP5 promoted the secretion of both Th1 and Th2 cytokines and T- and B-lymphocyte proliferative responses. Overall, this study found that rTα1-BP5 not only enhanced the humoral immune responses but also promoted the cell-mediated immune responses, and it had the potential to use as an adjuvant.

To further evaluate the influence of rTα1-BP5 as an adjuvant on the immunity protection provided by H9N2 AIV vaccine against AIV infection, chickens were intramuscularly challenged with H9N2 AIV (A/chicken/Jiangsu/JS-1/2002) on day 28 post immunization. After 3 days post challenge, the PBS group chickens that received the challenge virus were mildly depressed. No other clinical signs were observed in that group or any of the other groups, which is typical of low-pathogenicity AIV in chickens [48, 49]. At 7 days post challenge, only the PBS-challenged group had mild, grossly detectable lesions in both the respiratory and gastrointestinal tract. And we found that the viral titers of lungs from chicken immunized with rTα1-BP5 plus H9N2 WIV were significantly lower than all the other groups at 3 days. Chickens immunized with rTα1-BP5 plus H9N2 WIV had almost no detectable virus particles in the lungs at 7 days after challenge. Our data indicated that rTα1-BP5 could effectively inhibit the replication of H9N2 AIV in chickens and promote virus clearance in the lungs of chickens. Thus, rTα1-BP5 had the potential to be used in vaccine formulations to provide improved protection against H9N2 AIV infection in poultry.

In summary, this study demonstrated that inactivated H9N2 AIV vaccine with Tα1-BP5 as an adjuvant enhanced strong immune responses at both humoral and cellular levels against AIV infection in chickens. These data may provide a novel insight to find new adjuvant in vaccines.

Acknowledgements

This work was supported by Grant no. 31101792 from the National Natural Science Foundation of China and no. 2012GGJS-077 from the Foundation for University Key Teacher by Higher Education of Henan Province.

Author details

Chen Wang[1*], Chengshui Liao[1], Wufan Zhang[1], Deyuan Li[2] and Puyan Chen[2]

*Address all correspondence to: wangchen2001@126.com

1 Key Laboratory of Veterinary Oncological Immunology, Henan University of Science and Technology, Luoyang, China

2 Key Laboratory of Animal Bacteriology of China's Department of Agriculture, Nanjing Agricultural University, Nanjing, China

#C.WANG and C.S.LIAO equally contributed to this work.

References

[1] Fouchier RA, Munster V, Wallensten A, Bestebroer TM, Herfst S, Smith D, Rimmelzwaan GF, Olsen B, Osterhaus AD. Characterization of a novel influenza A virus hemagglutinin subtype (H16) obtained from black-headed gulls. Journal of Virology. 2005; 79: 2814–2822. DOI: 10.1128/JVI.79.5.2814-2822.2005

[2] Banet-Noach C, Perk S, Simanov L, Grebenyuk N, Rozenblut E, Pokamunski S, Pirak M, Tendler Y, Panshin A. H9N2 influenza viruses from Israeli poultry: a five-year outbreak. Avian Diseases. 2007; 51: 290–296. DOI: 10.1637/7590-040206R1.1

[3] Homme PJ, Easterday BC. Avian influenza virus infections. IV. Response of pheasants, ducks, and geese to influenza A-turkey-Wisconsin-1966 virus. Avian Diseases. 1970; 14: 285–290. DOI: 10.2307/1588473

[4] Shortridge KF. Pandemic influenza: a zoonosis? Seminars in Respiratory Infections. 1992; 7: 11–25.

[5] Sun Y. Proceedings of the Fourth International Symposium on Avian Influenza: avian influenza, a global problem: Georgia Center for Continuing Education, the University of Georgia, Athens, Georgia, USA, May 28–31, 1997. pp. 47–49.

[6] Alexander DJ. Proceedings of the Fourth International Symposium on Avian Influenza: Avian Influenza, A Global Problem: Georgia Center for Continuing Education, the University of Georgia, Athens, Georgia, USA, May 28–31, 1997. pp. 9–13

[7] Li C, Yu K, Tian G, Yu D, Liu L, Jing B, Ping J, Chen H. Evolution of H9N2 influenza viruses from domestic poultry in Mainland China. Virology. 2005; 340: 70–83. DOI: 10.1016/j.virol.2005.06.025

[8] Nicholson KG, Wood JM, Zambon M. Influenza. Lancet. 2003; 362: 1733–1745. DOI: 10.1016/S0140-6736(03)14854-4

[9] Nichol KL, Treanor JJ. Vaccines for seasonal and pandemic influenza. The Journal of Infectious Diseases. 2006; 194:S111–S118. DOI: 10.1086/507544

[10] Wareing MD, Tannock GA. Live attenuated vaccines against influenza; an historical review. Vaccine. 2001; 19: 3320–3330. DOI: 10.1016/S0264-410X(01)00045-7

[11] Singh M, O'Hagan D. Advances in vaccine adjuvants. Nature Biotechnology. 1999; 17(11): 1075–1781. DOI: 10.1038/15058

[12] Bungener L, Geeraedts F, Ter Veer W, Medema J, Wilschut J, Huckriede A. Alum boosts TH2-type antibody responses to whole-inactivated virus influenza vaccine in mice but does not confer superior protection. Vaccine. 2008; 26: 2350–2359. DOI: 10.1016/j.vaccine.2008.02.063

[13] Riedl K, Riedl R, von Gabain A, Nagy E, Lingnau K. The novel adjuvant IC31 strongly improves influenza vaccine-specific cellular and humoral immune responses in young adult and aged mice. Vaccine. 2008; 26: 3461–3468. DOI: 10.1016/j.vaccine.2008.04.029

[14] O'Hagan DT. MF59 is a safe and potent vaccine adjuvant that enhances protection against influenza virus infection. Expert Review of Vaccines. 2007; 6: 699–710. DOI: 10.1586/14760584.6.5.699

[15] Li J, Zheng L, Li P, Wang F. Intein-mediated expression, purification, and characterization of thymosin alpha 1-thymopentin fusion peptide in *Escherichia coli*. Protein Expression and Purification. 2012; 84: 1–8. DOI: 10.1016/j.pep.2012.04.013

[16] Lunin SM, Glushkova OV, Khrenov MO, Novoselova TV, Parfenyuk SB, Fesenko EE, Novoselova EG. Thymic peptides restrain the inflammatory response in mice with

experimental autoimmune encephalomyelitis. Immunobiology. 2013; 218: 402–407. DOI: 10.1016/j.imbio.2012.05.023

[17] Goldstein AL, Low TL, McAdoo M, McClure J, Thurman GB, Rossio J, Lai CY, Chang D, Wang SS, Harvey C, Ramel AH, Meienhofer J. Thymosin alpha1: isolation and sequence analysis of an immunologically active thymic polypeptide. Proceedings of the National Academy of Sciences of the United States of America.1977; 74: 725–729. DOI: 10.1073/pnas.74.2.725

[18] Ahmed A, Wong DM, Thurman GB, Low TL, Goldstein AL, Sharkis SJ, Goldschneider I. T-lymphocyte maturation: cell surface markers and immune function induced by T-lymphocyte cell-free products and thymosin polypeptides. Annals of the New York Academy of Sciences. 1979; 332: 81–94. DOI: 10.1111/j.1749-6632.1979.tb47100.x

[19] Hadden JW, Verastegui E, Hadden E. IRX-2 and thymosin alpha 1 (zadaxin) increase T lymphocytes in T lymphocytopenic mice and humans. Thymosins in Health and Disease: First International Symposium. Annals of the New York Academy of Sciences. 2007; 1112: 245–255. DOI: 10.1196/annals.1415.032

[20] Lao X, Liu M, Chen J, Zheng H. A tumor-penetrating peptide modification enhances the antitumor activity of thymosin alpha 1. PLoS One. 2013; 8: e72242. DOI: 10.1371/journal.pone.0072242

[21] Li YM, Chen H, Li X, Zhou WC, He MY, Chiriva-Internati M, Wachtel MS, Frezza EE. A new immunomodulatory therapy for severe sepsis: Ulinastatin Plus Thymosin {alpha} 1. Journal of Intensive Care Medicine. 2009; 24: 47–53. DOI: 10.1177/0885066608326970

[22] Audhya T, Kroon D, Heavner G, Viamontes G, Goldstein G. Tripeptide structure of bursin, a selective B-cell-differentiating hormone of the bursa of fabricius. Science. 1986; 231: 997–999. DOI: 10.1126/science.3484838

[23] Wang C, Wen WY, Su CX, Ge FF, Dang ZG, Duan XG, Cao RB, Zhou B, Chen PY. Bursin as an adjuvant is a potent enhancer of immune response in mice immunized with the JEV subunit vaccine. Veterinary Immunology and Immunopathology. 2008; 122: 265–274. DOI: 10.1016/j.vetimm.2007.11.010

[24] Wang C, Li XK, Wu TC, Li DY, Niu MF, Wang Y, Zhang CJ, Cheng XC, Chen PY. Bursin-like peptide (BLP) enhances H9N2 influenza vaccine induced humoral and cell mediated immune responses. Cellular Immunology. 2014; 292: 57–64. DOI: 10.1016/j.cellimm.2014.09.003

[25] Li DY, Xue MY, Wang C, Wang JB, Chen PY. Bursopentine as a novel immunoadjuvant enhances both humoral and cell-mediated immune responses to inactivated H9N2 avian influenza virus in chickens. Clinical and Vaccine Immunology. 2011; 18(9): 1497–1502. DOI: 10.1128/CVI.05133-11

[26] Li DY, Geng ZR, Zhu HF, Wang C, Miao DN, Chen PY. Immunomodulatory activities of a new pentapeptide (Bursopentin) from the chicken bursa of Fabricius. Amino Acids. 2011; 40(2): 505–515. DOI: 10.1007/s00726-010-0663-7

[27] Novak M, Moldoveanu Z, Schafer DP, Mestecky J, Compans RW. Murine model for evaluation of protective immunity to influenza virus. Vaccine. 1993; 11: 55–60. DOI: 10.1016/0264-410X(93)90339-Y

[28] Sha Z, Compans RW. Induction of CD4 (+) T-cell-independent immunoglobulin responses by inactivated influenza virus. Journal of Virology. 2000; 74: 4999–5005. DOI: 10.1128/JVI.74.11.4999-5005.2000

[29] OIE 2012. Manual of diagnostic tests and vaccines for terrestrial animals. Paris: Office International des Epizooties. [Internet]. Available from: http://www.oie.int/manual-of-diagnostic-tests-and-vaccines-for-terrestrial-animals/

[30] Horton RM, Hunt HD, Ho SN, Pullen JK, Pease LR. Engineering hybrid genes without the use of restriction enzymes: gene splicing by overlap extension. Gene. 1989; 77: 61–68. DOI: 10.1016/0378-1119(89)90359-4

[31] Mosmann T. Rapid colorimetric assay for cellular growth and survival: application to proliferation and cytotoxicity assays. Journal of Immunological Methods.1983; 65: 55–63. DOI: 10.1016/0022-1759(83)90303-4

[32] Yu L, Li JR, Huang YW, Liang XY, Meng SS. Enhanced immunogenicity of plasmid encoding polyprotein gene of infectious bursal disease virus by co-administration of chicken interleukin 2 (IL-2). Sheng Wu Gong Cheng Xue Bao. 2001; 17: 652–657. DOI: 10.3321/j.issn:1000-3061.2001.06.013

[33] Haan L, Verweij WR, Holtrop M, Brands R, van Scharrenburg GJ, Palache AM, Agsteribbe E, Wilschut J. Nasal or intramuscular immunization of mice with influenza subunit antigen and the B subunit of Escherichia coli heat-labile toxin induces IgA- or IgG-mediated protective mucosal immunity. Vaccine. 2001; 19: 2898–2907. DOI: 10.1016/S0264-410X(00)00556-9

[34] Fritz JH, Brunner S, Birnstiel ML, Buschle M, Gabain AV, Mattner F, Zauner W. The artificial antimicrobial peptide KLKLLLLLKLK induces predominantly a TH2-type immune response to co-injected antigens. Vaccine. 2004; 22: 3274–3284.DOI: 10.1016/j.vaccine.2004.03.007

[35] Rimmelzwaan GF, Baars M, van Beek R, van Amerongen G, Lovgren-Bengtsson K, Claas EC, Osterhaus AD. Induction of protective immunity against influenza virus in a macaque model: comparison of conventional and iscom vaccines. The Journal of General Virology. 1997; 78: 757–765. DOI: 10.1099/0022-1317-78-4-757

[36] Du L, Lyle CS, Obey TB, Gaarde WA, Muir JA, Bennett BL, Chambers TC. Inhibition of cell proliferation and cell cycle progression by specific inhibition of basal JNK activity:

evidence that mitotic Bcl-2 phosphorylation is JNK-independent. The Journal of Biological Chemistry. 2004; 279: 11957-11966. DOI: 10.1074/jbc.M304935200

[37] Wang C, Li XK, Zhang CJ, Wu TC, Li YJ, Cheng XC. A eukaryotic expression plasmid carrying chicken interleukin-18 enhances the response to Newcastle disease virus vaccine. Clinical and Vaccine Immunology. 2015; 22: 56–64. DOI: 10.1128/CVI.00636-14

[38] Bhardwaj N. Processing and presentation of antigens by dendritic cells: implications for vaccines. Trends in Molecular Medicine. 2001; 7: 388–394. DOI: 10.1016/S1471-4914(01)02101-3

[39] Schijns VE. Immunological concepts of vaccine adjuvant activity. Current Opinion in Immunology. 2000; 12: 456–463. DOI: 10.1016/S0952-7915(00)00120-5

[40] Petrovsky N, Aguilar JC. Vaccine adjuvants: current state and future trends. Immunology and Cell Biology. 2004; 82: 488–496. DOI: 10.1111/j.0818-9641.2004.01272.x

[41] Cai MH, Zhu F, Wu HC, Shen PP. A new recombinant hybrid polypeptide and its immunologic adjuvant activity for inactivated infectious bursal disease vaccine. Biotechnology Letters. 2014; 36: 1431–1437. DOI: 10.1007/s10529-014-1499-0

[42] Charoenvit Y, Goel N, Whelan M, Rosenthal KS, Zimmerman DH. CEL-1000—a peptide with adjuvant activity for Th1 immune responses. Vaccine. 2004; 22: 2368–2373. DOI: 10.1016/j.vaccine.2003.11.062

[43] Gagnon L, DiMarco M, Kirby R, Zacharie B, Penney CL. D-LysAsnProTyr tetrapeptide: a novel B-cell stimulant and stabilized bursin mimetic. Vaccine. 2000; 18: 1886–1892. DOI: 10.1016/S0264-410X(99)00374-6

[44] Li WY, Lu HM, Guo Q, Hu WM, Zhang ZD. Effects of thymosin alpha1 on immune effector molecules of mouse. Sichuan da xue xue bao Yi xue ban = Journal of Sichuan University Medical science edition. 2014; 45: 400–404.

[45] Kreijtz JH, Bodewes R, van Amerongen G, Kuiken T, Fouchier RA, Osterhaus AD, Rimmelzwaan GF. Primary influenza A virus infection induces cross-protective immunity against a lethal infection with a heterosubtypic virus strain in mice. Vaccine. 2007; 25: 612–620. DOI: 10.1016/j.vaccine.2006.08.036

[46] Wen L, Chen SJ, Zhang W, Ma HW, Zhang SQ, Chen L. hsBAFF regulates proliferation and response in cultured CD4(+) T lymphocytes by upregulation of intracellular free Ca(2+) homeostasis. Cytokine. 2011; 53: 215–222. DOI: 10.1016/j.cyto.2010.11.006

[47] Kumar DA, Manikandan P, Sumitra M, Raju KV, Gayathri C, Arutselvan N, Puvanakrishnan R. A novel peptide derivative exhibits anti inflammatory and antioxidant activity in adjuvant induced arthritis in rats. Molecular and Cellular Biochemistry. 2002; 229: 9–17. DOI: 10.1023/A:1017980024029

[48] Lee CW, Song CS, Lee YJ, Mo IP, Garcia M, Suarez DL, Kim SJ. Sequence analysis of the hemagglutinin gene of H9N2 Korean avian influenza viruses and assessment of the

pathogenic potential of isolate MS96. Avian diseases. 2000; 44: 527–535. DOI: 10.2307/1593091

[49] Soda K, Asakura S, Okamatsu M, Sakoda Y, Kida H. H9N2 influenza virus acquires intravenous pathogenicity on the introduction of a pair of di-basic amino acid residues at the cleavage site of the hemagglutinin and consecutive passages in chickens. Virology Journal. 2011; 8: 64. DOI: 10.1186/1743-422X-8-64

5

Application of the New Generation of Sequencing Technologies for Evaluation of Genetic Consistency of Influenza A Vaccine Viruses

Ewan Peter Plant, Tatiana Zagorodnyaya,
Elvira Rodionova, Alin Voskanian-Kordi,
Vahan Simonyan, Zhiping Ye and Majid Laassri

Abstract

For almost half a century, Sanger sequencing has been the conventional method for sequencing DNA. However, its utility for sequencing heterogeneous viral populations is limited because it can only detect mutations that are present in a significant portion of the DNA molecules. Several molecular methods that quantify mutations present at low levels in viral populations were proposed for evaluation of genetic consistency of viral vaccines; however, these methods are only suitable for single site polymorphisms, and cannot be used to screen for unknown mutations.

Next-generation (deep) sequencing methods have enabled the determination of sequences of the entire viral population, including minority components. They enable not only sequencing, but also accurate quantification of mutations. This technique has great value for monitoring the genetic consistency of viral vaccines. Recently, a number of new deep sequencing platforms were introduced (MiSeq, Iron Torrent, etc.) that made such an analysis quite affordable for individual research labs. Here, we review the use of current deep sequencing approaches for influenza virus studies, focusing on the evaluation of the genetic consistency of influenza A vaccine viruses. We also describe a new bioinformatic tool to analyze deep sequencing data and identify artifacts from the true mutants.

Keywords: deep sequencing, DNA and RNA libraries, influenza viruses, mutational profiles, sequence heterogeneity

1. Introductory comments on influenza viruses and vaccines

1.1. Influenza viruses

Influenza A viruses are the causative agents of seasonal epidemics and periodic pandemics. There are many serotypes that infect birds, especially waterfowl, and a few serotypes that infect mammals, including humans. Although some influenza A strains from birds and pigs have jumped the species barrier to infect humans, the majority of human infections are caused by the spread of endemic strains. The endemic strains are continually evolving being one of the reasons that influenza A infections remain a persistent problem. Strains of influenza virus that are used in vaccine production are prone to mutations during the manufacturing process, which can cause breaches in the consistency of vaccine quality. Such mutations can lead to changes in the antigenic structure of the virus and thus affect vaccine effectiveness.

Influenza A viruses belong to the Orthomyxoviridae family of viruses [1]. There are several common features shared among the viruses in this family: they are all negative sense, single-stranded RNA viruses that replicate in the nucleus of the host cell. The influenza A virus genome is comprised of eight RNA segments that encode more than 11 proteins. Two of the segments each encode a major antigenic protein. The fourth largest segment encodes a hemagglutinin (HA) protein and the sixth largest segment encodes a neuraminidase (NA) protein. The different subtypes and strains of influenza A viruses are distinguished by the HA and NA proteins that coat the surface of the virus. There are at least 18 different HA types and 11 NA types [2]. The segmented nature of the viral genome enables two viruses co-infecting the same cell to exchange their segments to produce reassortant progeny. Replication of influenza A viruses also results in mutated viral genomes because of the high error frequency of the RNA polymerase and actions by host defensive elements [3, 4]. Mutations contribute to the emergence of new endemic strains and reassortment may lead to the emergence of epidemic or pandemic strains.

The presence of mutations in influenza A populations has been examined in a variety of contexts. Several groups have isolated clones and used Sanger sequencing to identify mutations. Isolation of a sufficient number of clones has resulted in estimates of the mutation frequencies ranging from 6×10^{-4} to 2×10^{-6} [3, 5, 6]. Although the information about heterogeneity is of great interest, caution must be exercised to ensure that it is accurately reflected in sequence databases. The presence of errors in influenza databases has been noted [7, 8]. To limit discrepancies, some groups have used next-generation sequencing (NGS) to identify sequence heterogeneities [9–12]. Additional technologies such as multisegment reverse-transcription PCR have also been employed [13]. These studies revealed several interesting things. For example, it has been found that differences in viral sequences may occur after a single passage [14], that the same antigenic variants can be detected in different individuals [15], and that oseltamivir resistant and sensitive viruses can be found together as part of heterogeneous viral populations [16].

Most human infections are caused by influenza B viruses and the influenza A serotypes H1N1 and H3N2. In addition to the endemic human influenza transmission, there are cases reported each year of influenza A infections originating from an animal. Influenza A (H3N2) variant viruses from swine are sometimes transmitted to humans, especially those in close contact with pigs in agricultural settings [17]. Poultry workers are also frequently seropositive for a variety of different avian influenza strains [18–20] suggesting infrequent but detectable transmission. In most cases, there is no person-to-person transmission of the animal viruses. Nevertheless candidate vaccine viruses (CVVs) are prepared each year against some of these viruses to provide a prophylactic option in the event of an outbreak (http://www.who.int/influenza/en/). The CVVs for vaccines against endemic strains and potentially pandemic strains are provided to vaccine manufacturers for use as seed viruses in the manufacturing process.

1.2. Influenza vaccine production

There are several different methods that are used to produce influenza vaccines. Errors may be introduced into the antigenic protein during the replication of the seed virus, no matter which production method is used. The different licensed vaccines are produced from influenza virus grown in eggs or cell culture, or from recombinant viruses expressing the influenza HA from an alternative viral backbone grown in cell culture. Contemporary strains isolated from patients during the current epidemic season normally do not always grow well in cell substrates used for vaccine production. To increase virus yields they are recombined with reference high-growth strains, such that the CVVs have HA and NA-coding RNA segments from the contemporary strain, and RNA segments coding for replicative proteins from the high-growth reference virus. HA is the primary protective antigen and is responsible for binding the cellular receptor. Receptor properties in human and chicken cells differ, forcing the virus HA to adapt to the new receptor, leading to changes in the antigenic specificity potentially affecting vaccine potency.

The most common manufacturing process used in FDA-licensed vaccines is to grow influenza virus in eggs and then inactivate the virus. The inactivated virus is purified and then diluted to the desired potency for filling vials or syringes. Live attenuated influenza vaccines (LAIV) are also grown in eggs but are administered as a nasal spray. Codon deoptimization has also been proposed as a method for creating attenuated viruses [21, 22]. Unlike the current licensed products these may be grown in cell culture.

Some inactivated influenza vaccines are grown in cells. Production of cell-grown vaccines currently uses the same egg isolated seed virus that is used for egg inactivated vaccine production. The cell-grown viruses are harvested, inactivated, and filled into vials or syringes for distribution in a similar manner to the egg grown viruses. The production of recombinant viruses to prepare HA does not require a live seed virus. The HA sequence is cloned into the virus used for production. Although the frequency of errors during replication may differ from that of an influenza virus, the concern still remains. Even if vaccine strains are produced using cloned DNA sequences or synthetic sequences, there is still the possibility of errors arising during amplification of the seed virus. Errors may emerge because of inaccuracies inherent in the replication system or as a response to the host cell defenses.

1.3. Influenza vaccine seed viruses

The seed viruses used to produce influenza vaccines are derived from different sources. Because the influenza virus spreads throughout the world and strains are continually evolving, a network of academic, governmental, and commercial organizations work together to produce new seed viruses. New virus isolates are collected by National Influenza Centers and sent to the World Health Organization Collaborating Centers (WHO CCs). The viruses are typed according to strain and subtype using antigenic and genetic analyses. Viruses are usually isolated in Madin-Darby Canine Kidney Epithelial Cells (MDCK cells) and then amplified in eggs. It is important that the seed virus is as close in sequence and antigenicity to the original isolate as possible. To this end, the egg-amplified virus is used to immunize ferrets for the production of antiserum. The antiserum is then used for antigenic typing of viruses. Such analyses are used to determine how well the strains used in the influenza vaccine are matched to the currently circulating strains.

To produce sufficient quantities of vaccine, the CVVs must have good growth characteristics. Ideally, the viruses should replicate efficiently, have a high antigen (primarily hemagglutinin) to total protein ratio and not have increased pathogenicity. Many viruses do not produce high yields in eggs without adaptation. Some viruses have been propagated for many years and have well-known growth characteristics. They include the influenza A strains Puerto Rico/8/1934, cold-adapted A/Ann Arbor/6/1960, A/Leningrad/134/17/1957 and variants of these viruses. Where appropriate these strains have been used as a backbone for influenza A CVVs. Combining the high yield characteristics with the antigenic characteristics of contemporary strains facilitates vaccine production. Reassortant viruses with the desired antigenicity and growth characteristics are produced by two different methods; classical reassortment and genetic reassortment. Dr. Kilbourne of the New York Medical College (NYMC) developed the classical method to create reassortant viruses that expressed the HA and NA from a seasonal strain in the background of a high-growth virus [23]. This method involves co-culture of a contemporary virus and a high yield strain with antibodies to select against the HA and NA of the high yielded strain. Although the resulting viruses have the desired HA and NA genomic segments, the remaining segments may come from either the high-growth strain or the contemporary strain. Another approach based on genetic engineering allows the production of viruses from plasmids expressing the eight influenza virus segments. Genetic engineering also allows the expression of HA and NA proteins in a vector-based system such as a baculovirus. The desired genetic sequence of HA engineered in this system may be incompatible with baculovirus components, which can result in changes as more efficient mutants displace the parental virus (the so-called gene constellation effect) [24].

All CVVs go through several rounds of replication at manufacturers' facilities as they produce their own virus stocks, working seed, and the final product. Some changes to the virus may occur during manufacture so tests to verify the identity, purity, potency and stability of vaccine lots are required. The potency of inactivated influenza vaccines and influenza vaccine produced from recombinant viruses is determined using standardized reagents supplied by national regulatory authorities. The potency of a live-attenuated virus is calculated from the amount of viable attenuated virus. Genetic characterization of the vaccine viruses is currently achieved by partial genome sequencing or restriction analysis.

It has been suggested that most of the differences between natural isolates and vaccine seed viruses occur during the selection and clonal isolation of the candidate virus prior to manufacture [25]. The fidelity of replication will vary among viruses and es and will depend on other factors such as the host cell line and multiplicity of infection used. There are some limits on the number of times that seed viruses may be passaged so that mutations are less likely to occur. The European Pharmacopoeia monograph 0158 for inactivated influenza vaccines states that the seed virus should not be passaged more than 15 times. However, because regulations tend to lag behind scientific development, there is no universally accepted guideline for influenza vaccine manufacture that covers egg-derived, cell-derived, and synthetic reassortant viruses.

2. Importance of the evaluation of genetic consistency of influenza A vaccine viruses

Virus populations are comprised of genetically variable viruses and this can affect their replication, evolution, attenuation, and pathogenesis [26, 27]. Having an understanding of the mutations present, even at low levels, in a virus population is important for our understanding of how the viruses grow and cause infections. It has recently been shown that an influenza population containing two variants involved in cell exit grows better than populations containing either variant alone [28]. Although good growth properties are a desirable feature in vaccine seed viruses, it is critical that other parts of the genome, such as those causing attenuation or encoding the major antigenic regions, remain stable. Consistency of manufacture is important and having suitable means to assess genetic consistency is valuable. New assays capable of assessing entire viral genomes, and detecting mutations present at a low level, are needed.

The emergence of mutations in the course of vaccine manufacture was shown to contribute to partial reversion to virulence in the oral polio vaccine (OPV). Mutant analysis by PCR and restriction enzyme cleavage (MAPREC) is used to control batches of oral polio vaccine for the presence of neurovirulent mutations [29, 30] and has been expanded to be used for other viruses [31, 32]. Mutations emerging during virus growth may also change antigenic properties and therefore affect protective potency of live and inactivated vaccines. New approaches that can be used not only for monitoring genetic stability of live vaccines, but also for controlling consistency of inactivated vaccines are needed. Influenza vaccines are manufactured in embryonated chicken eggs or cell culture. There is evidence that vaccine seed viruses adapt to grow efficiently in the different substrates and this can lead to changes in the receptor-recognition site of viral hemagglutinin, which is the major protective antigen [33–36]. For this reason, it is important to monitor the changes that may take place in major protective epitopes of the virus. It is also important to know that mutations responsible for attenuated phenotypes are maintained. Knowing which mutations are emerging during virus growth in production substrates could also be used to optimize genetic structure of vaccine strains. Consistently accumulating mutations have higher fitness, and if they have no deleterious properties, their incorporation into the genome of vaccine virus could increase its yield and improve vaccine potency. Given these concerns it is imperative to screen genomes of viral vaccines for emerging mutations.

3. Methods used for evaluation of genetic consistency of vaccine viruses

As mentioned above viral populations are highly heterogeneous, and even small quantities of mutants in virus stocks may affect their biological properties. Although PCR and restriction analysis of reassortant influenza viruses can demonstrate which parental strain each genomic segment was derived from, it cannot detect new mutations. Even traditional sequencing methods are not sensitive enough to detect small amounts of mutants, and highly sensitive PCR-based methods can only analyze one or few known mutations at a time.

Conventional sequencing approaches are suitable for discovery of mutations that are present in substantial amounts, usually around 20–25% [37]. Determining the actual frequency using conventional sequencing requires the labor- and time-intensive analysis of a large number of virus clones (plaques).

There are indirect approaches based on analysis of electrophoretic mobility in gels [38], which are insufficiently sensitive and do not allow mutations to be located accurately. Mass spectrometry (MALDI-TOF) [39] and hybridization with microarrays of short oligonucleotides [40–42] are sensitive, but are laborious and may require follow-up by direct sequencing. A highly sensitive mutant analysis by PCR and MAPREC [29–31] can detect and quantify mutants at levels as low as 0.1% of the viral population. Recently we developed a quantitative allele-specific PCR (asqPCR) [43] for detection of a low level of mutants in viral vaccines. RT-PCR has been proposed as a method for checking the homogeneity of influenza vaccine seed candidates [44]. However, these methods are only suitable for analysis of one known mutation at a time.

Several versions of high-throughput sequencing technology, known also as deep or massively parallel sequencing (MPS) have been used to assess influenza vaccine viruses. These technologies enable rapid generation of large amounts of sequence information [45]. Three different platforms for deep sequencing are used widely at present time: the Roche/454 FLX [46] (http://www.454.com/) (http://454.com/products/technology.asp), the Illumina/Solexa Genome Analyzer [47]) (http://www.illumina.com/technology/next-generation-sequencing/sequencing-technology.html), and the Applied Biosystems SOLiD TM System (http://www.thermofisher.com/us/en/home/brands/applied-biosystems.html). Two new sequencing platforms that are improved to sequence long reads have been developed recently: the Pacific Biosciences SMRT Sequencing (http://www.pacb.com/smrt-science/smrt-sequencing/) [48] and Oxford Nanopore Technologies MinION (https://www.nanoporetech.com/technology/the-minion-device-a-miniaturised-sensing-system/the-minion-device-a-miniaturised-sensing-system).

These systems are also called "single molecule" sequencers and do not require any amplification of DNA fragments prior to sequencing.

The deep sequencing technologies were shown to be suitable for analysis of heterogeneities in viral populations [49]. It can produce huge sequencing information in one run. They are used for *de novo* sequencing of large genomes, metagenomics studies (virome, microbiome, etc.), screening for genomic markers, and many other applications [50–58]. Previously, it was demonstrated that deep sequencing can be used to monitor the genetic stability of oral polio vaccines, and could replace the WHO-recommended MAPREC assay for lot release of OPV [59]. Recently we showed that deep sequencing is suitable for evaluation of genetic consistency of influenza vaccine viruses [36, 60].

4. Description of the most used deep sequencing platforms

Deep or massively parallel sequencing refers to several high-throughput methods for DNA sequencing that are often referred to as NGS. They have dramatically improved the ability of biotechnology, scientific, and healthcare researchers to analyze viruses by allowing users to have massive sequencing information for the entire genomes. The high-throughput sequencing field has witnessed the rise of many technologies capable of massive genomic analysis. In the virology field, deep sequencing has made it simple to sequence full viral genomes. Likewise, identification and classification of novel and known viruses, unbiased characterization of viral populations without the need for virus culturing (viromes), molecular epidemiology, viral diversity and evolution, transmission and pathogenesis, and medical virology have greatly benefited from the use of deep sequencing. The cost of deep sequencing has decreased to an affordable price due to the competition between vendors and the ability to analyze multiple samples run in one lane of the sequencing flow cell. This has allowed virologists to study a huge number of viral samples, including mixture of viral populations, and study low-level mutants in a wide range of viruses [36, 59–61].

There are several platforms for deep sequencing. The most widely used sequencing platforms are the Roche/454 FLX [46] (http://www.454.com/), the Illumina/Solexa Genome Analyzer [47] (http://www.illumina.com/technology/next-generation-sequencing/solexa-technology.html), and the Applied Biosystems SOLiD System (http://www.appliedbiosystems.com/absite/us/en/home/applications-technologies/solid-next-generation-sequencing/next-generation-systems/solid-4-system.html?CID=FL-091411_solid4).

The differences between these platforms include DNA library preparation procedures and chemistry, the sequencing reactions on the amplified strands, the length of reads, the amount of data generated per run, the hardware, the software engineering and the technology used to amplify single strands of a fragment from the library.

In general the DNA libraries of fragment targets are generated, and adaptors containing universal priming sites are ligated to the fragmented target ends, allowing complex genomes to be amplified with PCR primers. After ligation, the DNA is separated into single strands and attached or immobilized to a solid surface or support. The immobilization of spatially separated template sites allows thousands to billions of sequencing reactions to be performed simultaneously.

Immobilization and separation of the millions of molecules to different surfaces can be achieved by a variety of methods including the Polonator and PicoTiter Plate [47, 62–64]. Attachment of forward and reverse primers to a slide and use of solid-phase amplification also result in the enrichment and amplification of separate template strands [47] (Illumina/Solexa).

Two newer sequencing platforms with longer reads differ from those described above. They are sometimes referred to as "single molecule" sequencers because they sequence molecule by molecule and do not require any amplification of DNA fragments prior to sequencing. The Pacific Biosciences system involves the attachment of a DNA polymerase to the DNA molecule. During the sequencing phase the polymerase adds bases labeled with a fluorophore. The fluorescence unique to each base is recorded and, as each new base is added, the fluorescent label is removed [48]. It generates long sequencing reads (10–15 kb long) from single molecules of DNA, very quickly.

The Oxford Nanopore system runs the sample through very small (1 nm wide) pores. As the DNA passes through these nanopores, the Oxford machine records the electrical charge that is associated with each individual base pair of DNA, like a signature. It produces longer reads (>100 kb long).

A detailed description of the most used two deep sequencing platforms for analysis of influenza viruses and their vaccines is given below.

4.1. Roche/454 FLX pyrosequencer

The Roche/454 FLX sequencing [46] is based on the use of the pyrosequencing technology (http://my454.com/products/technology.asp), in which the incorporation of each nucleotide by DNA polymerase results in the release of pyrophosphate that initiates a cascade of enzymatic reactions that converts the pyrophosphate to a light signal. This light is recorded by CCD camera. This approach, as with most NGS procedures, starts with DNA library preparation; the library DNAs with 454-specific adaptors are denatured into single strands and mixed with agarose beads whose surfaces carry oligonucleotides complementary to the 454-specific adapter sequences on the fragment library, so each bead is associated with a single fragment. The DNA fragments captured by beads are amplified by emulsion PCR (ePCR) [65] to produce approximately one million copies of each DNA fragment on the surface of each bead. These amplified single molecules are then sequenced on a picotiter plate (a fused silica capillary structure) that holds a single bead in each of several hundred thousand single wells, which provides a fixed location at which each sequencing reaction can be monitored.

Individual dNTPs are added to the template in the presence of a DNA polymerase. The sequencing reaction releases pyrophosphate (PPi) after the incorporation of a complementary nucleotide. The released PPi is used by an ATP sulfurylase to release ATP from adenosine 5'-phosphosulfate. The ATP is then used to generate light by converting luciferin into oxyluciferin [66]. Unincorporated dNTPs are degraded by an apyrase, and dATPαS (which is not a substrate for luciferase) is used instead of dATP. This pyrosequencing reaction is repeated during the sequence of the entire target DNA. This sequencing technology can now produce sequencing reads with up to 1000 bp in length (http://454.com/products/gs-flx-system/).

These raw reads are processed by the 454 analysis software and then filtered to remove poor-quality sequences, mixed sequences, and sequences without the initiating TCGA sequence. Recently, the 454-FLX system was upgraded to reach 99.9% of accuracy after filter and an output of 14 Gb of data per run within 24 h.

4.2. Illumina genome sequencer

The Illumina sequencing [47] method begins with Illumina library preparation flanked with Illumina-specific adapters. Sequencing templates are immobilized on a proprietary flow cell surface that contains immobilized oligos with sequence complementary to those of the adapters, and designed to present the DNA in a manner that facilitates access to enzymes while ensuring high stability of surface-bound template and low non-specific binding of fluorescently labeled nucleotides. Solid-phase amplification of each single strand DNA from library is performed by bridge amplification, which results in the generation of several million dense clusters of single-stranded DNA in each channel of the flow cell.

The Illumina system sequences DNA in the presence of four reversible terminator-bound dNTPs [47]. At each sequencing step, a fluorescently labeled dNTP is added to the molecule. The fluorescent signal is recorded and then the fluorophore is removed to allow sequencing to continue. The base calls correlate with the signal intensity. Illumina sequencing technology can now produce sequencing reads with up to 600 bp in length (http://www.illumina.com/systems/sequencing.html). The sequencing results are generated in files in which each raw read base has an assigned quality score so that the software can apply a weighting factor in calling differences and generating confidence scores. Illumina data collection software enables users to align sequences to a reference in resequencing applications. This software suite includes the full range of data collection, processing, and analysis modules to streamline collection and analysis of data.

4.3. Deep sequencing data analysis

The massively parallel scale of sequencing implies a similarly massive scale of computational analysis. The conventional pipeline for analysis of next-generation sequencing data includes the following stages: quality control and source data filtering; alignment (mapping); reference profiling (variant-calling, pileup); followed by single-nucleotide polymorphism (SNP) calling (genotyping); and some form of clusterization or classification analysis of samples to discover up or down expression of genes, detect overabundance of SNP positions and correlate those with function and phenotype. Because of the sheer size of the data and amount of calculations needed, such analyses place significant demands on the information technology (IT) infrastructure. Lack of computational power, insufficiency of actively accessible storage facilities in laboratory information management systems (LIMS) and deficiency in network capacity to move data add significantly to the overhead required for high-throughput data production.

The hardware aspect of next-generation sequencing is complicated by the imperfections of current sequence analysis tools, which are suited to shorter sequence read data. There are multiple implementations for all of the stages of the analysis, and some of those are considered to be industry standard tools, running formidable amount of bio-medical analytics. Large-scale analysis of thousands of samples using variety of available tools highlighted important issues with data quality, pre-analytic quality controls, software reproducibility and post-analytic quality controls. Existing data analysis pipelines and algorithms must be modified to accommodate extra-large amounts of short read sequences and combination of shorter and longer read technologies.

To analyze the deep sequencing data for genetic consistency evaluation of influenza vaccine viruses, we have used the corresponding viral reference sequences from NCBI GenBank as a template for alignment of individual sequencing reads. First, sequencing reads with low quality (Phred) score are removed from the data set, and the remaining sequences aligned with reference influenza virus sequence using custom software: The High-performance Integrated Virtual Environment (HIVE, https://hive.biochemistry.gwu.edu/dna.cgi?cmd=main) computer cluster [67, 68].

To create a quantifiable measure comparing the quality of the sequencing and mapping at different positions on a genome, we developed a metrics for assessing positional variant-call quality. To do that, first a histogram is built at every position of a genome where the number

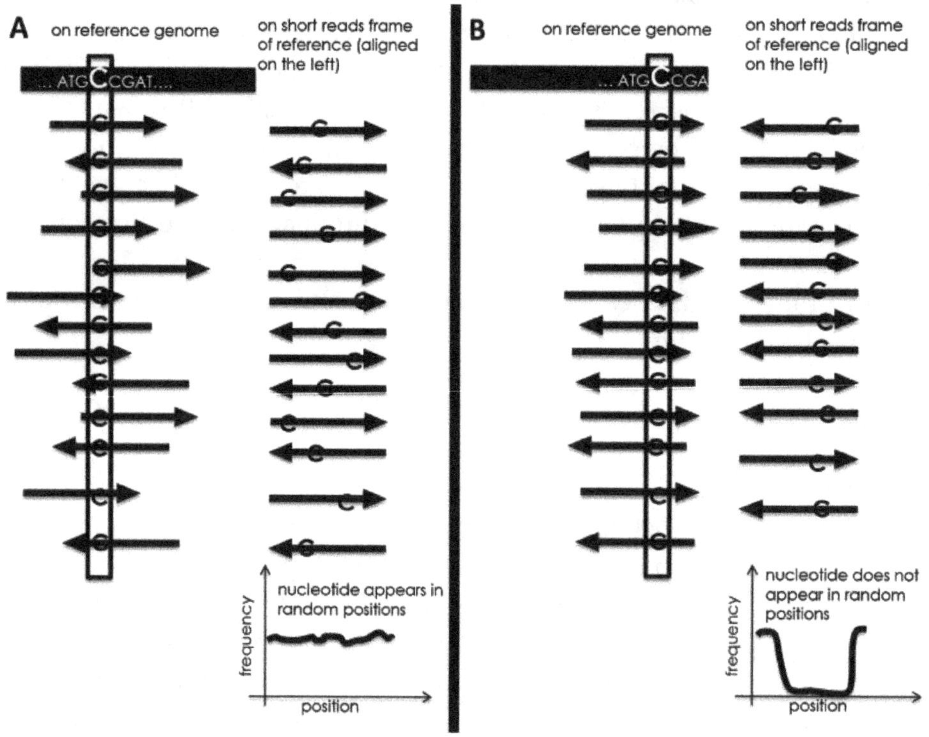

Figure 1. Explanation of entropy computation. For all bases aligned to a particular reference position, the coordinates on a read-frame are accumulated into a positional frequency histogram. For a non-biased position, such distribution is more or less uniform (A). For terminally biased base calls such frequency distribution is skewed towards ends (B) and the Shannon's entropy values drop closer to zero.

of times a base has occurred at a given read-position is accumulated. Additionally, positions of insertion and deletions are also collected in similar histogram. The underlying assumption of the next-generation sequencing method is that the DNA amplification and digestion procedure is random and the short sequences produced by DNA digestion are not strongly biased and not sequence dependent. The default assumption is that a particular variant call should be confirmed by different positions on many reads thus rendering the histogram distribution to be uniform along the entire length of sequence read.

Post-alignment quality control includes identification of mutations distributed non-randomly along individual sequencing reads, which may indicate artifacts in PCR amplification or DNA sequencing procedures (**Figure 1A** and **B**). Biased distribution of mutations along sequencing reads was revealed by calculating Shannon entropy values [69]. Low entropy value suggests that a mutation could be an artifact produced in sequencing procedures. This means that there is an abnormal bias in distribution of this mutation. This entropy-based post-alignment quality control value is calculated on the basis of the equation below. It is based on the normalized first order momentum of logarithmic probability distribution for a particular base (b) at a particular position (r) of reference genome:

$$Entropy(b,r) = -\frac{\sum_L p_i(b) \times log(p_i(b))}{\log(L^{-1})}$$

where L is the length of the longest read, p_i(b) is the frequency distribution of a base b in the reference frame of the reads mapped at the location r. The index i runs over all of the available positions from 1 to L. The denominator makes sure the Shannon's entropy is normalized to a unit value of 1 as the maximum value for entirely uniform distribution. In contrast singular value distribution would have a value for entropy equal to zero. This value is computed for all of the reference positions for every base.

Finally, aligned sequencing reads were used to compute SNP profiles for the entire viral genome.

5. The use of deep sequencing for evaluation of genetic consistency of influenza A vaccine viruses

Influenza A viruses are enveloped, single-stranded RNA viruses belonging to the Orthomyxoviridae family [70], which also contains four other viral species: influenza B virus, influenza C virus, thogotovirus, and isavirus. The segmented genome of influenza A virus is about 13.6 kb in size and encodes for at least 11 proteins. Its genome is highly variable due to the low fidelity of RNA polymerase and reassortment between co-infecting strains [71]. New virus mutants emerge continuously allowing viruses to survive in presence of the host immunity and cause repeated annual epidemics and occasionally pandemics. Because of this frequent change of the antigens, influenza vaccines must be frequently reformulated to include antigens of the currently circulating strains. Both live and inactivated influenza vaccines are produced mostly by reassortment with high-growth strains for vaccine production [72, 73]. As stated above, adaptation to growth in different cells can lead to changes in viral receptor-binding region, and also in protective epitopes. Therefore, it is desirable to monitor genetic stability of viruses used in vaccine manufacture to ensure that their antigenic structure remains unchanged.

Deep sequencing technology has opened up the possibility for the characterization of viral genomes directly from samples [74, 75]. The viral metagenome or "virome" refers to the collection of viruses found in a particular sample from humans, animals, plants or from a specific environmental sample. Virome studies can lead to the discovery of new viruses and/or to their association with known or novel diseases. Numerous viruses have been identified as part of the virome study, including influenza A viruses [2].

The deep sequencing technologies are a great tool to investigate genetically complex populations of influenza viruses and to detect minority mutant variants with clinical or epidemiological relevance. Deep sequencing-based methods have recently been applied for the assessment of influenza A viruses diversity and their dynamics of evolution [60, 76, 77]. Others have focused on the evolution of avian influenza strains with potential to become pandemic in humans [78–82], as well as the detection of virulence signatures [83] and reassortment patterns [84]. Other studies have investigated the transmission and adaptation of avian influenza viruses to humans, as part of preparedness for a potential influenza pandemic [12, 53, 85–98].

As it is crucial to study transmission and adaptation of avian influenza viruses, and swine strains for epidemics and pandemics in humans, many studies based on the use of deep sequencing techniques have described avian and swine influenza virus evolution [99–103]. Other studies have investigated the predominance and spread of different human influenza viruses in specific geographic areas [16, 104–106].

Study of drug escape variants is an important aspect of epidemiological and clinical virology. Sanger sequencing can only detect mutations present in around 20% of the viral population [37, 107–109], which excludes it for quantitation of low-level viral mutant variants. Using deep sequencing to detect low portion of mutant drug resistant variants at levels as low as 0.1% of the virus population has been demonstrated [110–116]. Other studies have focused on the use of deep sequencing for surveillance of drug resistance-associated mutations for both NA inhibitors and adamantanes [117–127]. Deep sequencing has also been used for the detection and subtyping of human influenza A viruses and reassortants [61, 84].

Recently, deep sequencing-based methods have been proposed for the assessment of influenza A viruses antigenic stability [128] using complete influenza A genomes and exploiting the ability to detect and quantify mutations in heterogeneous viral populations. Deep sequencing was used to study the evolution of influenza A viruses in the vaccinated pigs. The genetic diversity and evolution of the virus at an intra-host level was analyzed directly from nasal swabs collected during infection [129]. The obtained results demonstrated remarkable diversity of influenza A viruses, and rapid change of these viruses during infection of vaccinated pigs. These types of complex studies can be done only by high throughput sequence analysis.

To evaluate the genetic stability in influenza vaccine viruses, we have used a deep sequencing approach that was recently qualified for quantitation of all mutants in the entire genome including those that are present at low level in viral populations [59]. Recently, we explored the utility of deep sequencing methods for monitoring the consistency of influenza A vaccines [36, 60]. Also in the same study, we proposed new protocols for simultaneous amplification of all segments of influenza A genomes and new bioinformatic tools to analyze the data and to identify artifacts generated during PCR amplification and deep sequencing procedures. Amplification of the entire genome of influenza viruses presents a challenge because of the difference in size and sequence composition of the eight genomic segments.

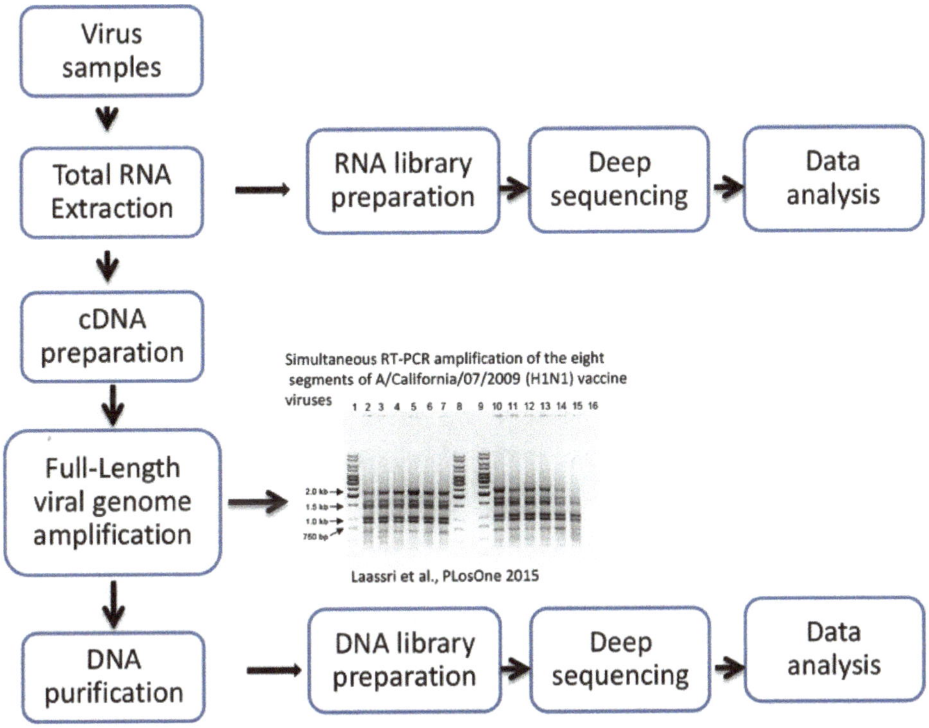

Figure 2. General steps followed for RNA/DNA libraries sequencing of influenza A/California/07/2009 (H1N1) vaccine viruses.

We described PCR conditions that allow to amplify all genomic segments of influenza A virus in one reaction [60] that was optimized subsequently during an analysis of the A/California/07/2009 (H1N1) vaccine viruses (derived from X-179A, X-181, 121XP viruses) [36]. We have used both the total RNA (without specific amplification of viral cDNA) and DNA amplicon, for RNA and DNA libraries preparation, respectively, and both protocols were compared for consistency in mutant variants quantitation.

The protocols for deep sequencing of viral DNA libraries and whole-RNA libraries used to determine quantitative profiles of mutations along the entire genome of viruses of influenza

A/California/07/2009 (H1N1) vaccine viruses were described [36]. The steps followed to perform the deep sequencing are presented in **Figure 2** and can be summarized as follows: The PCR product was purified by QIAquick PCR Purification Kit (Qiagen) and fragmented by an ultrasonicator (Covaris) to generate the optimal fragment sizes needed for Illumina sequencing, then the fragmented DNAs were used for library preparation with NEBNext® DNA Sample Prep Reagent Set 1 (New England BioLabs).

For preparation of Illumina sequencing libraries from total RNA, the NEBNext mRNA Sample Prep Master Mix Set 1 (New England BioLabs) was used. Briefly, total RNA (extracted as mentioned above) was fragmented as described above to generate the optimal fragment sizes. Double-stranded cDNA was prepared and ligated to the Illumina paired end adaptors. Finally, the libraries were amplified using 15 cycles of PCR with multiplex indexed primers and purified with magnetic beads using Agencourt Ampure Beads (Beckman Coulter). Deep sequencing was performed at Macrogen (Seoul, Korea) using HiSeq2000 (Illumina) or at our laboratory using MiSeq (Illumina).

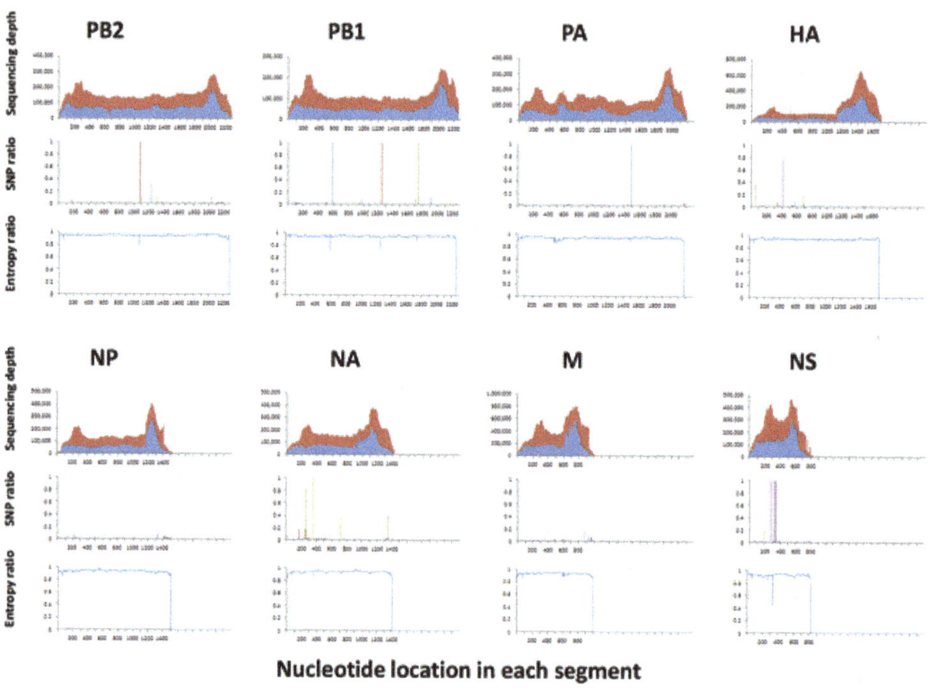

Figure 3. Sequencing analysis of the entire genome of the influenza A/California/07/2009 (H1N1) vaccine virus reassortant tenth passage in eggs sequenced by HiSeq (Macrogen) using 101 bp paired-end Illumina/Solexa sequencing technology. Computations were made by in-house custom software HIVE-align. For each segment, the charts of the depth of sequencing coverage distribution (the number of times every nucleotide was sequenced on ordinate plotted against the position on genome—abscissa), SNP profile (the ratio of mutants on ordinate plotted against the position on genome—abscissa), and entropy were built.

The sequencing data analysis was done using custom software, a highly integrated virtual environment (HIVE) computer cluster (https://hive.biochemistry.gwu.edu/dna.cgi?cmd=main) as described above. The RNA sequences of X-179A, X-181, 121XP, A/California/07/2009 (H1N1), and A/PR/08/34 viruses deposited in NCBI GenBank were used as references for alignment of the viral sequence reads. We analyzed the depth of sequencing, the single-nucleotide polymorphism profile, and entropy (that allow us to distinct between bias and true mutation) for each segment of influenza virus (see **Figure 3**, for example), the data analysis resulted also on generation of consensus sequences for each segment.

The deep sequencing results revealed several heterogeneities in most genomic segments, and several mutations led to amino acid changes. Deep sequencing of whole-RNA libraries was found to be more reproducible than sequencing of DNA libraries. This may be due to errors introduced during PCR amplification by DNA polymerase and non-specific alignment of primers [36].

The deep sequencing of the X-179A passaged viruses [36] identified several mutations in HA and NA genes. In HA two non-synonymous mutations; $Pro_{314}Gln$ (in 17% of the virus population) and $Asn_{146}Asp$ (in 78% of the virus population) were identified. The $Asn_{146}Asp$ mutation is found in the antigenic site Sa; it was detected at 11% in the A/California/07/2009 (H1N1) strain and as the dominant residue in the X-181 virus [36]. One X-179A stock contained the $Lys_{328}Thr$ mutation at a low level (9%). Viruses derived from X-179A were heterogeneous and contained some complete nucleotide substitutions in comparison to their published sequences in PB2, PB1, NP, and in NS segments [36]. The X-181 virus was developed from the X-179A seed lot by another round of reassortment, and also is subjected to several passages in eggs. Deep sequencing results [36] showed that the $G_{756}T$ ($Glu_{252}Asp$, present at 47%) mutation emerged in HA of the passaged X181 virus, and it is located in the conserved region of the antigenic site Ca [36].

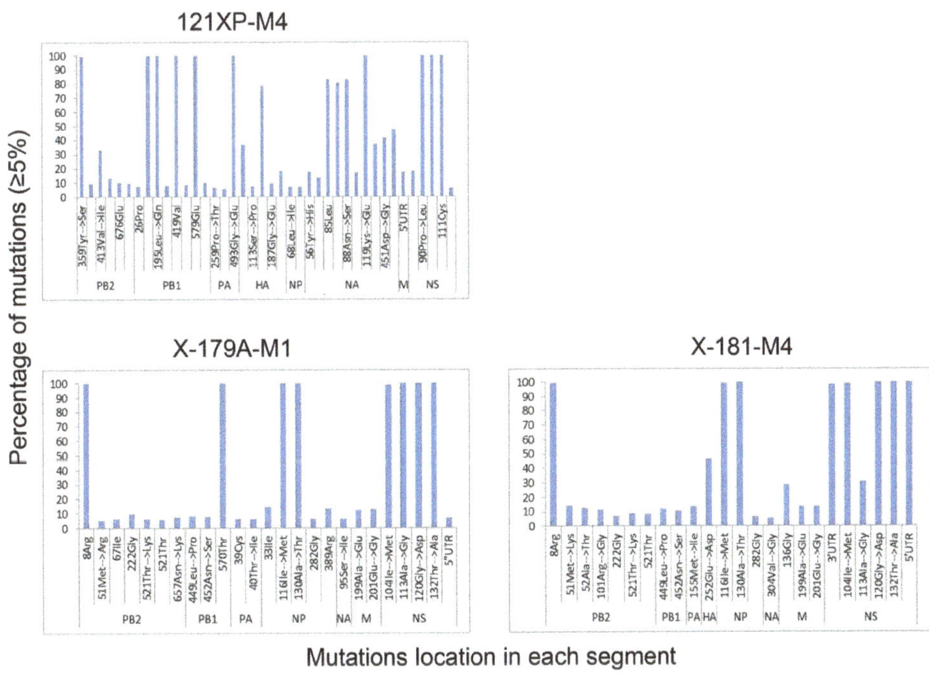

Figure 4. Percent of mutations (≥5%) emerged in X-179A-M1, X-181-M4, and 121XP-M4 viruses (derived from X-179A, X-181, and 121XP viruses, respectively) passaged 10 times in embryonated chicken eggs.

Unlike the X-179A and X-181 viruses, 121XP was developed by reverse genetics [130]. The deep sequencing of 121XP virus passaged 10 times in eggs (121XP-M4 virus) showed that this virus is more heterogenic than X-179A and X-181 viruses passaged 10 times in eggs (X-179A-M1 and X-181-M4 viruses respectively; **Figure 4**) [36]. In the passaged 121XP virus, the mutation $Lys_{226}Glu$ was emerged at low level (18%) in Ca antigenic site of HA, which is very close to the region that participates in the modulation of HA receptor specificity and that enables H3 influenza viruses to switch specificity from avian to human [131–133]; another mutation $Lys_{136}Asn$ was emerged at a high level (78%) close to the HA antigenic site Sa within the sialic acid-binding pocket [134]. Recently a similar deep sequencing approach was used to study the genetic and potential antigenic diversity of influenza viruses infecting humans, some of whom became infected despite recent vaccination [15].

We found that the deep sequencing approach based on RNA library preparation was effective and reproducible for detection of low quantities of mutants in the entire genome of influenza A vaccine viruses [36]. The deep sequencing approach revealed that the viruses derived from three pandemic A/Ca/07/2009 (H1N1) vaccine viruses have varying levels of sequence heterogeneities some of them in antigenic sites, which may affect their efficacy.

6. Conclusions

In the last few years, the use of deep sequencing has expanded largely to tackle problems in many fields of virology. The greatest benefit of deep sequencing is its ability to detect minor mutant variants, as low as 0.1% of virus population [36, 59, 60, 110, 111, 113, 114]. The deep sequencing approach based on RNA library preparation is effective and reproducible for detection of low quantities of mutants in the entire genome of influenza A vaccine viruses [36], and eliminates the need for full-length amplification. The deep sequencing platforms are improving continuously to combine low error rates with long reads and relatively low cost. It played a key role in the discovery of many new viruses, the characterization of virus populations in humans and the potential of their association with the pathogenesis of several diseases. As described here, there is no doubt that the deep sequencing is facilitating and accelerating the evaluation of the genetic consistency of vaccine viruses. It is an important tool for monitoring vaccine consistency during manufacture and after vaccination. Deep sequencing-based assays are already being implemented for the genetic consistency evaluation of oral polio vaccine and influenza A vaccine viruses [36, 59, 60]. The ability to quantify potentially undesirable mutations in vaccine batches makes this method suitable for quality control to ensure manufacture of safe and effective vaccines.

Acknowledgements

We thank Dr. Konstantin Chumakov and Dr. Christian Sauder for their critical review of this chapter. The contents of this chapter represent solely the opinion of authors and do not represent the official view of FDA.

Author details

Ewan Peter Plant, Tatiana Zagorodnyaya, Elvira Rodionova, Alin Voskanian-Kordi, Vahan Simonyan, Zhiping Ye and Majid Laassri*

*Address all correspondence to: majid.laassri@fda.hhs.gov

Center for Biologics Evaluation and Research, US Food and Drug Administration, Silver Spring, MD, USA

References

[1] Lamb, R.A. and R.M. Krug, Orthomyxoviridae: the viruses and their replication, in Fields virology, D.M.K. Bernard, N. Fields, P.M. Howley, Editor. 1996, Philadelphia: Lippincott-Raven Publishers, pp. 1353–96.

[2] Tong, S., et al., New world bats harbor diverse influenza A viruses. PLoS Pathog, 2013. 9(10): p. e1003657.

[3] Cheung, P.P., et al., Comparative mutational analyses of influenza A viruses. RNA, 2015. 21(1): pp. 36–47.

[4] Gutierrez, R.A., et al., Biased mutational pattern and quasispecies hypothesis in H5N1 virus. Infect Genet Evol, 2013. 15: pp. 69–76.

[5] Nobusawa, E. and K. Sato, Comparison of the mutation rates of human influenza A and B viruses. J Virol, 2006. 80(7): pp. 3675–8.

[6] Parvin, J.D., et al., Measurement of the mutation rates of animal viruses: influenza A virus and poliovirus type 1. J Virol, 1986. 59(2): pp. 377–83.

[7] Krasnitz, M., A.J. Levine, and R. Rabadan, Anomalies in the influenza virus genome database: new biology or laboratory errors? J Virol, 2008. 82(17): pp. 8947–50.

[8] Suarez, D.L., N. Chester, and J. Hatfield, Sequencing artifacts in the type A influenza databases and attempts to correct them. Influenza Other Respir Viruses, 2014. 8(4): pp. 499–505.

[9] Roedig, J.V., et al., Impact of host cell line adaptation on quasispecies composition and glycosylation of influenza A virus hemagglutinin. PLoS One, 2011. 6(12): p. e27989.

[10] Van den Hoecke, S., et al., Analysis of the genetic diversity of influenza A viruses using next-generation DNA sequencing. BMC Genomics, 2015. 16: p. 79.

[11] Wang, J., et al., MinION nanopore sequencing of an influenza genome. Front Microbiol, 2015. 6: p. 766.

[12] Watson, S.J., et al., Viral population analysis and minority-variant detection using short read next-generation sequencing. Philos Trans R Soc Lond B Biol Sci, 2013. 368(1614): p. 20120205.

[13] Zou, X.H., et al., Evaluation of a single-reaction method for whole genome sequencing of influenza A virus using next generation sequencing. Biomed Environ Sci, 2016. 29(1): pp. 41–6.

[14] Lee, H.K., et al., Comparison of mutation patterns in full-genome A/H3N2 influenza sequences obtained directly from clinical samples and the same samples after a single MDCK passage. PLoS One, 2013. 8(11): p. e79252.

[15] Dinis, J.M., et al., Deep sequencing reveals potential antigenic variants at low frequency in influenza A-infected humans. J Virol, 2016. 90(7): 3355–3365.

[16] Fordyce, S.L., et al., Genetic diversity among pandemic 2009 influenza viruses isolated from a transmission chain. Virol J, 2013. 10: p. 116.

[17] Nelson, M.I., et al., Evolutionary dynamics of influenza A viruses in US Exhibition Swine. J Infect Dis, 2016. 213(2): p. 173–82.

[18] Di Trani, L., et al., Serosurvey against H5 and H7 avian influenza viruses in Italian poultry workers. Avian Dis, 2012. 56(4 Suppl): pp. 1068–71.

[19] Heidari, A., et al., Serological evidence of H9N2 avian influenza virus exposure among poultry workers from Fars province of Iran. Virol J, 2016. 13(1): p. 16.

[20] Huang, S.Y., et al., Serological comparison of antibodies to avian influenza viruses, subtypes H5N2, H6N1, H7N3 and H7N9 between poultry workers and non-poultry workers in Taiwan in 2012. Epidemiol Infect, 2015. 143(14): pp. 2965–74.

[21] Broadbent, A.J., et al., Evaluation of the attenuation, immunogenicity, and efficacy of a live virus vaccine generated by codon-pair bias de-optimization of the 2009 pandemic H1N1 influenza virus, in ferrets. Vaccine, 2016. 34(4): pp. 563–70.

[22] Fan, R.L., et al., Generation of live attenuated influenza virus by using codon usage bias. J Virol, 2015. 89(21): pp. 10762–73.

[23] Kilbourne, E.D., Future influenza vaccines and the use of genetic recombinants. Bull World Health Organ, 1969. 41(3): pp. 643–5.

[24] Plant E.P. and Z. Ye., Gene constellation of influenza vaccine seed viruses in Current issues in molecular virology – viral genetics and biotechnological applications, V. Romanowski, Editor. 2013, InTech, pp 213–237.

[25] Buonagurio, D.A., et al., Genetic stability of live, cold-adapted influenza virus components of the FluMist/CAIV-T vaccine throughout the manufacturing process. Vaccine, 2006. 24(12): pp. 2151–60.

[26] Domingo, E., et al., The quasispecies (extremely heterogeneous) nature of viral RNA genome populations: biological relevance---a review. Gene, 1985. 40(1): pp. 1–8.

[27] Hansen, H., et al., Recombinant viruses obtained from co-infection in vitro with a live vaccinia-vectored influenza vaccine and a naturally occurring cowpox virus display different plaque phenotypes and loss of the transgene. Vaccine, 2004. 23(4): pp. 499–506.

[28] Xue, K.S., et al., Cooperation between distinct viral variants promotes growth of H3N2 influenza in cell culture. eLife 2016;5: p. e13974.

[29] Chumakov, K.M., Molecular consistency monitoring of oral poliovirus vaccine and other live viral vaccines. Dev Biol Stand, 1999. 100: pp. 67–74.

[30] Chumakov, K.M., et al., Correlation between amount of virus with altered nucleotide sequence and the monkey test for acceptability of oral poliovirus vaccine. Proc Natl Acad Sci U S A, 1991. 88(1): pp. 199–203.

[31] Bidzhieva, B., M. Laassri, and K. Chumakov, MAPREC assay for quantitation of mutants in a recombinant flavivirus vaccine strain using near-infrared fluorescent dyes. J Virol Methods, 2011. 175(1): pp. 14–9.

[32] Laassri, M., et al., Microarray hybridization for assessment of the genetic stability of chimeric West Nile/dengue 4 virus. J Med Virol, 2011. 83(5): pp. 910–20.

[33] Gambaryan, A.S., et al., Effects of host-dependent glycosylation of hemagglutinin on receptor-binding properties on H1N1 human influenza A virus grown in MDCK cells and in embryonated eggs. Virology, 1998. 247(2): pp. 170–7.

[34] Hughes, M.T., et al., Adaptation of influenza A viruses to cells expressing low levels of sialic acid leads to loss of neuraminidase activity. J Virol, 2001. 75(8): pp. 3766–70.

[35] Schild, G.C., et al., Evidence for host-cell selection of influenza virus antigenic variants. Nature, 1983. 303(5919): pp. 706–9.

[36] Laassri, M., et al., Deep sequencing for evaluation of genetic stability of influenza A/California/07/2009 (H1N1) vaccine viruses. PLoS One, 2015. 10(9): p. e0138650.

[37] Larder, B.A., et al., Quantitative detection of HIV-1 drug resistance mutations by automated DNA sequencing. Nature, 1993. 365(6447): pp. 671–3.

[38] Orita, M., et al., Detection of polymorphisms of human DNA by gel electrophoresis as single-strand conformation polymorphisms. Proc Natl Acad Sci U S A, 1989. 86(8): pp. 2766–70.

[39] Amexis, G., et al., Quantitative mutant analysis of viral quasispecies by chip-based matrix-assisted laser desorption/ionization time-of-flight mass spectrometry. Proc Natl Acad Sci U S A, 2001. 98(21): pp. 12097–102.

[40] Cherkasova, E., et al., Microarray analysis of evolution of RNA viruses: evidence of circulation of virulent highly divergent vaccine-derived polioviruses. Proc Natl Acad Sci U S A, 2003. 100(16): pp. 9398–403.

[41] Laassri, M., et al., Microarray techniques for evaluation of genetic stability of live viral vaccines, in Viral genomes – Molecular structure, diversity, gene expression mechanisms and host-virus interactions. Maria Laura Garcia Editor. 2012, InTech, pp. 181–94.

[42] Laassri, M., et al., Genomic analysis of vaccine-derived poliovirus strains in stool specimens by combination of full-length PCR and oligonucleotide microarray hybridization. J Clin Microbiol, 2005. 43(6): pp. 2886–94.

[43] Bidzhieva, B., M. Laassri, and K. Chumakov, Allele-specific PCR for quantitative analysis of mutants in live viral vaccines. J Virol Methods, 2014. 201: pp. 86–92.

[44] Shcherbik, S., et al., Application of real time RT-PCR for the genetic homogeneity and stability tests of the seed candidates for live attenuated influenza vaccine production. J Virol Methods, 2014. 195: pp. 18–25.

[45] Rogers, Y.H. and J.C. Venter, Genomics: massively parallel sequencing. Nature, 2005. 437(7057): pp. 326–7.

[46] Margulies, M., et al., Genome sequencing in microfabricated high-density picolitre reactors. Nature, 2005. 437(7057): pp. 376–80.

[47] Bentley, D.R., Whole-genome re-sequencing. Curr Opin Genet Dev, 2006. 16(6): pp. 545–52.

[48] Eid, J., et al., Real-time DNA sequencing from single polymerase molecules. Science, 2009. 323(5910): pp. 133–8.

[49] Victoria, J.G., et al., Metagenomic analyses of viruses in stool samples from children with acute flaccid paralysis. J Virol, 2009. 83(9): pp. 4642–51.

[50] Bainbridge, M.N., et al., Analysis of the prostate cancer cell line LNCaP transcriptome using a sequencing-by-synthesis approach. BMC Genomics, 2006. 7: p. 246.

[51] Cheval, J., et al., Evaluation of high-throughput sequencing for identifying known and unknown viruses in biological samples. J Clin Microbiol, 2011. 49(9): pp. 3268–75.

[52] Greninger, A.L., et al., A metagenomic analysis of pandemic influenza A (2009 H1N1) infection in patients from North America. PLoS One, 2010. 5(10): p. e13381.

[53] Kuroda, M., et al., Characterization of quasispecies of pandemic 2009 influenza A virus (A/H1N1/2009) by de novo sequencing using a next-generation DNA sequencer. PLoS One, 2010. 5(4): p. e10256.

[54] Nakamura, S., et al., Direct metagenomic detection of viral pathogens in nasal and fecal specimens using an unbiased high-throughput sequencing approach. PLoS One, 2009. 4(1): p. e4219.

[55] Pettersson, E., et al., Allelotyping by massively parallel pyrosequencing of SNP-carrying trinucleotide threads. Hum Mutat, 2008. 29(2): pp. 323–9.

[56] Satkoski, J.A., et al., Pyrosequencing as a method for SNP identification in the rhesus macaque (Macaca mulatta). BMC Genomics, 2008. 9: p. 256.

[57] Torres, T.T., et al., Gene expression profiling by massively parallel sequencing. Genome Res, 2008. 18(1): pp. 172–7.

[58] Wheeler, D.A., et al., The complete genome of an individual by massively parallel DNA sequencing. Nature, 2008. 452(7189): pp. 872–6.

[59] Neverov, A. and K. Chumakov, Massively parallel sequencing for monitoring genetic consistency and quality control of live viral vaccines. Proc Natl Acad Sci U S A, 2010. 107(46): pp. 20063–8.

[60] Bidzhieva, B., et al., Deep sequencing approach for genetic stability evaluation of influenza A viruses. J Virol Methods, 2014. 199: pp. 68–75.

[61] Seong, M.W., et al., Genotyping influenza virus by next-generation deep sequencing in clinical specimens. Ann Lab Med, 2016. 36(3): pp. 255–8.

[62] Kim, J.B., et al., Polony multiplex analysis of gene expression (PMAGE) in mouse hypertrophic cardiomyopathy. Science, 2007. 316(5830): pp. 1481–4.

[63] Leamon, J.H., et al., A massively parallel PicoTiterPlate based platform for discrete picoliter-scale polymerase chain reactions. Electrophoresis, 2003. 24(21): pp. 3769–77.

[64] Shendure, J., et al., Accurate multiplex polony sequencing of an evolved bacterial genome. Science, 2005. 309(5741): pp. 1728–32.

[65] Berka, J., et al., Bead emulsion nucleic acid amplification. 2005, Google Patents.

[66] Froehlich, T., D. Heindl, and A. Roesler, Miniaturized, high-throughput nucleic acid analysis. 2010, Google Patents.

[67] Simonyan, V. and R. Mazumder, High-performance integrated virtual environment (HIVE) tools and applications for big data analysis. Genes (Basel), 2014. 5(4): pp. 957–81.

[68] Wilson, C.A. and V. Simonyan, FDA's activities supporting regulatory application of "next gen" sequencing technologies. PDA J Pharm Sci Technol, 2014. 68(6): pp. 626–30.

[69] Shannon, C.E., A mathematical theory of communication. Bell Syst Technical J, 1948. 27(3): pp. 379–423.

[70] Lamb, R.A. and M.A. Krug, Orthomyxoviridae: the viruses and their replication, in Fields Virology, Howley P. M., Knipe D. M., Editor, 4th edition. 2007, Philadelphia: Lippincott Williams & Wilkins, pp. 1487–31.

[71] Steinhauer, D.A., E. Domingo, and J.J. Holland, Lack of evidence for proofreading mechanisms associated with an RNA virus polymerase. Gene, 1992. 122(2): pp. 281–8.

[72] Girard, M.P., et al., A review of vaccine research and development: human enteric infections. Vaccine, 2006. 24(15): pp. 2732–50.

[73] McCarthy, M.W. and D.R. Kockler, Trivalent intranasal influenza vaccine, live. Ann Pharmacother, 2004. 38(12): pp. 2086–93.

[74] Julian, T.R. and K.J. Schwab, Challenges in environmental detection of human viral pathogens. Curr Opin Virol, 2012. 2(1): pp. 78–83.

[75] Mokili, J.L., F. Rohwer, and B.E. Dutilh, Metagenomics and future perspectives in virus discovery. Curr Opin Virol, 2012. 2(1): pp. 63–77.

[76] Bhatt, S., E.C. Holmes, and O.G. Pybus, The genomic rate of molecular adaptation of the human influenza A virus. Mol Biol Evol, 2011. 28(9): pp. 2443–51.

[77] Tsai, K.N. and G.W. Chen, Influenza genome diversity and evolution. Microbes Infect, 2011. 13(5): pp. 479–88.

[78] Bourret, V., et al., Whole-genome, deep pyrosequencing analysis of a duck influenza A virus evolution in swine cells. Infect Genet Evol, 2013. 18: pp. 31–41.

[79] Crusat, M., et al., Changes in the hemagglutinin of H5N1 viruses during human infection--influence on receptor binding. Virology, 2013. 447(1–2): pp. 326–37.

[80] Hoper, D., et al., Highly pathogenic avian influenza virus subtype H5N1 escaping neutralization: more than HA variation. J Virol, 2012. 86(3): pp. 1394–404.

[81] Mertens, E., et al., Evaluation of phenotypic markers in full genome sequences of avian influenza isolates from California. Comp Immunol Microbiol Infect Dis, 2013. 36(5): pp. 521–36.

[82] Wilker, P.R., et al., Selection on haemagglutinin imposes a bottleneck during mammalian transmission of reassortant H5N1 influenza viruses. Nat Commun, 2013. 4: p. 2636.

[83] Waybright, N., et al., Detection of human virulence signatures in H5N1. J Virol Methods, 2008. 154(1–2): pp. 200–5.

[84] Deng, Y.M., N. Caldwell, and I.G. Barr, Rapid detection and subtyping of human influenza A viruses and reassortants by pyrosequencing. PLoS One, 2011. 6(8): p. e23400.

[85] Archer, J., et al., Analysis of high-depth sequence data for studying viral diversity: a comparison of next generation sequencing platforms using Segminator II. BMC Bioinformatics, 2012. 13: p. 47.

[86] Bartolini, B., et al., Assembly and characterization of pandemic influenza A H1N1 genome in nasopharyngeal swabs using high-throughput pyrosequencing. New Microbiol, 2011. 34(4): pp. 391–7.

[87] Deyde, V.M. and L.V. Gubareva, Influenza genome analysis using pyrosequencing method: current applications for a moving target. Expert Rev Mol Diagn, 2009. 9(5): pp. 493–509.

[88] Flaherty, P., et al., Ultrasensitive detection of rare mutations using next-generation targeted resequencing. Nucleic Acids Res, 2012. 40(1): p. e2.

[89] Hoper, D., B. Hoffmann, and M. Beer, Simple, sensitive, and swift sequencing of complete H5N1 avian influenza virus genomes. J Clin Microbiol, 2009. 47(3): pp. 674–9.

[90] Hoper, D., B. Hoffmann, and M. Beer, A comprehensive deep sequencing strategy for full-length genomes of influenza A. PLoS One, 2011. 6(4): p. e19075.

[91] Kampmann, M.L., et al., A simple method for the parallel deep sequencing of full influenza A genomes. J Virol Methods, 2011. 178(1–2): pp. 243–8.

[92] Levine, M., et al., Detection of hemagglutinin variants of the pandemic influenza A (H1N1) 2009 virus by pyrosequencing. J Clin Microbiol, 2011. 49(4): pp. 1307–12.

[93] Ren, X., et al., Full genome of influenza A (H7N9) virus derived by direct sequencing without culture. Emerg Infect Dis, 2013. 19(11): pp. 1881–4.

[94] Rutvisuttinunt, W., et al., Simultaneous and complete genome sequencing of influenza A and B with high coverage by Illumina MiSeq Platform. J Virol Methods, 2013. 193(2): pp. 394–404.

[95] Taubenberger, J.K., The virulence of the 1918 pandemic influenza virus: unraveling the enigma. Arch Virol Suppl, 2005(19): pp. 101–15.

[96] Taubenberger, J.K., et al., Characterization of the 1918 influenza virus polymerase genes. Nature, 2005. 437(7060): pp. 889–93.

[97] Tumpey, T.M., et al., Characterization of the reconstructed 1918 Spanish influenza pandemic virus. Science, 2005. 310(5745): pp. 77–80.

[98] Xiao, Y.L., et al., High-throughput RNA sequencing of a formalin-fixed, paraffin-embedded autopsy lung tissue sample from the 1918 influenza pandemic. J Pathol, 2013. 229(4): pp. 535–45.

[99] Clavijo, A., et al., Identification and analysis of the first 2009 pandemic H1N1 influenza virus from U.S. feral swine. Zoonoses Public Health, 2013. 60(5): pp. 327–35.

[100] Croville, G., et al., Field monitoring of avian influenza viruses: whole-genome sequencing and tracking of neuraminidase evolution using 454 pyrosequencing. J Clin Microbiol, 2012. 50(9): pp. 2881–7.

[101] Marchenko, V.Y., et al., Ecology of influenza virus in wild bird populations in Central Asia. Avian Dis, 2012. 56(1): pp. 234–7.

[102] Van Borm, S., et al., Phylogeographic analysis of avian influenza viruses isolated from Charadriiformes in Belgium confirms intercontinental reassortment in gulls. Arch Virol, 2012. 157(8): pp. 1509–22.

[103] Yu, X., et al., Influenza H7N9 and H9N2 viruses: coexistence in poultry linked to human H7N9 infection and genome characteristics. J Virol, 2014. 88(6): pp. 3423–31.

[104] Barrero, P.R., et al., Genetic and phylogenetic analyses of influenza A H1N1pdm virus in Buenos Aires, Argentina. J Virol, 2011. 85(2): pp. 1058–66.

[105] de la Rosa-Zamboni, D., et al., Molecular characterization of the predominant influenza A(H1N1)pdm09 virus in Mexico, December 2011-February 2012. PLoS One, 2012. 7(11): p. e50116.

[106] Lin, J., et al., Influenza seasonality and predominant subtypes of influenza virus in Guangdong, China, 2004-2012. J Thorac Dis, 2013. 5(Suppl 2): pp. S109–17.

[107] Church, J.D., et al., Sensitivity of the ViroSeq HIV-1 genotyping system for detection of the K103N resistance mutation in HIV-1 subtypes A, C, and D. J Mol Diagn, 2006. 8(4): pp. 430–2; quiz 527.

[108] Halvas, E.K., et al., Blinded, multicenter comparison of methods to detect a drug-resistant mutant of human immunodeficiency virus type 1 at low frequency. J Clin Microbiol, 2006. 44(7): pp. 2612–4.

[109] Leitner, T., et al., Analysis of heterogeneous viral populations by direct DNA sequencing. Biotechniques, 1993. 15(1): pp. 120–7.

[110] Archer, J., et al., Use of four next-generation sequencing platforms to determine HIV-1 coreceptor tropism. PLoS One, 2012. 7(11): p. e49602.

[111] Dudley, D.M., et al., Low-cost ultra-wide genotyping using Roche/454 pyrosequencing for surveillance of HIV drug resistance. PLoS One, 2012. 7(5): p. e36494.

[112] Fisher, R., et al., Deep sequencing reveals minor protease resistance mutations in patients failing a protease inhibitor regimen. J Virol, 2012. 86(11): pp. 6231–7.

[113] Gibson, R.M., et al., Sensitive deep-sequencing-based HIV-1 genotyping assay to simultaneously determine susceptibility to protease, reverse transcriptase, integrase, and maturation inhibitors, as well as HIV-1 coreceptor tropism. Antimicrob Agents Chemother, 2014. 58(4): pp. 2167–85.

[114] Shao, W., et al., Analysis of 454 sequencing error rate, error sources, and artifact recombination for detection of low-frequency drug resistance mutations in HIV-1 DNA. Retrovirology, 2013. 10: p. 18.

[115] Simen, B.B., et al., Low-abundance drug-resistant viral variants in chronically HIV-infected, antiretroviral treatment-naive patients significantly impact treatment outcomes. J Infect Dis, 2009. 199(5): pp. 693–701.

[116] Wang, C., et al., Characterization of mutation spectra with ultra-deep pyrosequencing: application to HIV-1 drug resistance. Genome Res, 2007. 17(8): pp. 1195–201.

[117] Arvia, R., et al., Monitoring the susceptibility to oseltamivir of Influenza A(H1N1) 2009 virus by nested-PCR and pyrosequencing during the pandemic and in the season 2010-2011. J Virol Methods, 2012. 184(1–2): pp. 113–6.

[118] Chen, L.F., et al., Cluster of oseltamivir-resistant 2009 pandemic influenza A (H1N1) virus infections on a hospital ward among immunocompromised patients--North Carolina, 2009. J Infect Dis, 2011. 203(6): pp. 838–46.

[119] Correia, V., et al., Antiviral drug profile of seasonal influenza viruses circulating in Portugal from 2004/2005 to 2008/2009 winter seasons. Antiviral Res, 2010. 86(2): pp. 128–36.

[120] Dharan, N.J., et al., Infections with oseltamivir-resistant influenza A(H1N1) virus in the United States. JAMA, 2009. 301(10): pp. 1034–41.

[121] Duwe, S.C., et al., Genotypic and phenotypic resistance of pandemic A/H1N1 influenza viruses circulating in Germany. Antiviral Res, 2011. 89(1): pp. 115–8.

[122] Pontoriero, A., et al., Virological surveillance and antiviral resistance of human influenza virus in Argentina, 2005-2008. Rev Panam Salud Publica, 2011. 30(6): pp. 634–40.

[123] Tellez-Sosa, J., et al., Using high-throughput sequencing to leverage surveillance of genetic diversity and oseltamivir resistance: a pilot study during the 2009 influenza A(H1N1) pandemic. PLoS One, 2013. 8(7): p. e67010.

[124] Bright, R.A., et al., Incidence of adamantane resistance among influenza A (H3N2) viruses isolated worldwide from 1994 to 2005: a cause for concern. Lancet, 2005. 366(9492): pp. 1175–81.

[125] Bright, R.A., et al., Adamantane resistance among influenza A viruses isolated early during the 2005-2006 influenza season in the United States. JAMA, 2006. 295(8): pp. 891–4.

[126] Deyde, V.M., et al., Surveillance of resistance to adamantanes among influenza A(H3N2) and A(H1N1) viruses isolated worldwide. J Infect Dis, 2007. 196(2): pp. 249–57.

[127] Higgins, R.R., et al., Differential patterns of amantadine-resistance in influenza A (H3N2) and (H1N1) isolates in Toronto, Canada. J Clin Virol, 2009. 44(1): pp. 91–3.

[128] Warren, S., et al., Extreme evolutionary conservation of functionally important regions in H1N1 influenza proteome. PLoS One, 2013. 8(11): p. e81027.

[129] Diaz, A., et al., Genome plasticity of triple-reassortant H1N1 influenza A virus during infection of vaccinated pigs. J Gen Virol, 2015. 96(10): pp. 2982–93.

[130] Robertson, J.S., et al., The development of vaccine viruses against pandemic A(H1N1) influenza. Vaccine, 2011. 29(9): pp. 1836–43.

[131] Connor, R.J., et al., Receptor specificity in human, avian, and equine H2 and H3 influenza virus isolates. Virology, 1994. 205(1): pp. 17–23.

[132] Matrosovich, M., et al., Early alterations of the receptor-binding properties of H1, H2, and H3 avian influenza virus hemagglutinins after their introduction into mammals. J Virol, 2000. 74(18): pp. 8502–12.

[133] Stevens, J., et al., Structure and receptor specificity of the hemagglutinin from an H5N1 influenza virus. Science, 2006. 312(5772): pp. 404–10.

[134] Varghese, J.N., et al., The structure of the complex between influenza virus neuraminidase and sialic acid, the viral receptor. Proteins, 1992. 14(3): pp. 327–32.

6

Development of Vaccines for Poultry Against H5 Avian Influenza Based on Turkey Herpesvirus Vector

Atsushi Yasuda, Motoyuki Esaki,
Kristi Moore Dorsey, Zoltan Penzes, Vilmos Palya,
Darrell R. Kapczynski and Yannick Gardin

Abstract

Avian influenza (AI) remains a major threat to public health as well as to the poultry industry. AI vaccines are considered a suitable tool to support AI control programs in combination with other control measures such as good biosecurity and monitoring programs. We constructed recombinant turkey herpesvirus (HVT) vector vaccines expressing the hemagglutinin gene of AI virus H5 subtype (rHVT-H5) and evaluated their characteristics and efficacy against AI. We found that the cytomegalovirus (CMV) promoter is the most suitable for expression of the hemagglutinin gene among three promoters we evaluated. The rHVT-H5 vaccine did not cause any adverse reactions and did not revert to virulence after passages in chicken. Finally, efficacy of the rHVT-H5 vaccine was evaluated. We demonstrated that it provided protection against diverse AI H5 viruses belonging to different clades and reduced virus shedding from the challenged chicken. We also proved that efficacy provided by the rHVT-H5 vaccine was not significantly affected by presence of maternally derived antibodies (MDA) against AI virus. Furthermore, the rHVT-H5 vaccine could be applicable to the differentiating infected from vaccinated animals (DIVA) strategy. In summary, we successfully developed a HVT vector AI vaccine that possesses features that could be beneficial to AI control.

Keywords: avian influenza, turkey herpesvirus, vector vaccines, DIVA, hemagglutinin gene

1. Introduction

Avian influenza (AI) is an important zoonotic disease and it remains a major threat to public health and to the poultry industry. The highly pathogenic (HP) H5N1 outbreaks were first reported in China in 1996 and then spread to other parts of the world. These HP avian influenza viruses (AIV) have become endemic in several countries including China, Indonesia, Vietnam, and Egypt [1]. Between 2003 and 2015, 846 confirmed human cases of AI (H5N1) have been reported and 449 of those human patients have died (WHO, 2016). Most recently, HP H5N2 and H5N8 viruses caused outbreaks in the United States from December 2014 to June 2015, which resulted in depopulation of more than 48 million chickens and turkeys. These outbreaks cost farmers, the government, and consumers in the United States billions of dollars. France has also been hit by HP H5 viruses since November 2015 and the outbreaks have caused significant damages to its poultry industry. These recent HP H5 AIV continued to evolve into various clades as defined by the World Health Organization (WHO)/World Organisation for Animal Health (OIE)/Food and Agriculture Organization (FAO) H5N1 Evolution Working Group according to phylogenetic topology based on *hemagglutinin* (HA) gene sequences [2]. Another significant event of AI is the series of human infections in China caused by H7N9 AIV since March 2013. Although these viruses are low pathogenic (LP) for poultry, 277 human deaths have been reported out of 693 confirmed cases (WHO, 2016). These cases emphasize importance of controlling AIV in poultry for the industry as well as for public health.

Control of HP AI in poultry has been achieved traditionally through (1) education, (2) biosecurity, (3) diagnostics and surveillance, and (4) elimination of infected poultry (stamping-out) [3]. Viruses were successfully eradicated through a combination of those measures in many countries affected by HP AIV. However, in endemically infected countries, viruses had spread widely before executing effective measures, and therefore, it was impossible to identify and eliminate all of infected birds. In such endemic situations, vaccines are considered suitable and powerful tools to support AI eradication or control programs in combination with other control measures such as good biosecurity and monitoring programs [4–6]. When used properly, vaccines for AI have been demonstrated to protect poultry against clinical signs and mortality, increase resistance to infection, and reduce virus shedding markedly, thus decreasing the possibility of virus spreading among birds [7]. Most frequently used AI vaccines have been oil-adjuvanted, inactivated whole-virus vaccines and fowlpox virus or Newcastle disease virus (NDV)-vectored vaccines are also available. However, efficacy of these vaccines is limited especially against antigenically distant viruses [8–10]. Also, efficacy of these vaccines is known to be severely impaired by maternally derived antibodies (MDA) [11, 12]. Furthermore, oil-adjuvanted, inactivated whole-virus vaccines impede virus surveillance programs based on serology because serological responses elicited by the inactivated whole-virus vaccines are indistinguishable to those elicited by live field viruses. Therefore, development of novel vaccines which are efficacious in the face of MDA and are compatible with so-called differentiate infected from vaccinated animals (DIVA) strategy is necessary.

Turkey herpesvirus (HVT), or the meleagrid herpesvirus 1, belongs to the family of *Herpesviridae*, the subfamily of *Alphaherpesvirinae*, and the genus *Mardivirus*. It is classified as part of the Marek's disease virus (MDV) group and designated as serotype 3 MDV. HVT is non-oncogenic and antigenically related to oncogenic serotype 1 MDV. The virus has been utilized extensively as a vaccine against Marek's disease for over 30 years and considered extremely safe [13, 14]. It is administered at hatcheries either to day-of-age chicks by subcutaneous (SQ) route or in ovo to chicken embryos at 18–19 days of incubation and is known to elicit strong cell-mediated immunity as well as humoral immunity [15–17]. Furthermore, since HVT becomes latent and persists in inoculated chickens [18], a longer period of protection is expected. Indeed, HVT-vectored Newcastle disease vaccine has been shown to be efficacious for 72 weeks after inoculation into day-of-age chicks [19]. For aforementioned reasons and also because of its large genome that can be potentially used for insertion of heterologous genes [20], HVT has been evaluated as vectors expressing protective antigen gene(s) of various poultry pathogens including NDV, infectious bursal disease virus (IBDV), and infectious laryngotracheitis virus (ILTV) [21–26]. These HVT vector vaccines have shown to be very safe and induce effective humoral and cellular immunity that is long lasting. Also, the efficacy of HVT vector vaccines does not appear to be excessively affected by the presence of MDA, probably because HVT replicates in a cell-associated manner [22]. Here, we intended to apply the HVT vector technology to develop an effective poultry vaccine against AI. Several HVT vector vaccines expressing *HA* gene of H5 AIV (rHVT-H5) were constructed and evaluated for their characteristics and efficacy against AI.

2. Construction of rHVT-H5 vaccines

2.1. Construction of recombinant viruses

A number of HVT vector vaccines have been constructed and evaluated for their characteristics and efficacy against avian pathogens [21–26]. There are three important elements in HVT vector vaccines that can impact efficacy of these vaccines in chicken: insertion sites, antigen genes, and promoters. Several insertion sites including US2, US10, UL39 [21], and an intergenic region between UL45 and UL46 (UL45/46) [24–26] have been evaluated. Out of these potential insertion sites, we demonstrated that insertion of extraneous genes at the UL45/46 site did not alter their capacity to replicate [26]. Furthermore, using the UL45/46 as the insertion site, we were successful in constructing HVT vector vaccines having antigen genes of NDV, IBDV, or ILTV that are highly efficacious against these pathogens [24–26]. Therefore, we decided to use the UL45/46 site for insertion of antigen genes of AIV.

Eight segments of genomic RNA of influenza A virus encode three membrane-associated proteins, HA, neuraminidase (NA), and Matrix (M) 2, five internal proteins, nucleoprotein (NP), PB1, PB2, PA, and M1, and two nonstructural (NS) proteins, NS1 and NS2. Out of these viral proteins, the HA surface glycoprotein is known to be the major antigen and elicits neutralizing antibodies that provide protection against the disease [27]. We used the *HA* gene cloned from LP A/turkey/Wisconsin/68 (H5N9) strain or HP A/Swan/Hungary/4999/2006

(H5N1) clade 2.2 strain. The cleavage site of the *HA* gene from A/Swan/Hungary/4999/2006 (H5N1) strain was altered to a typical cleavage site sequence of LP AIV strains.

Selection of promoters that control the expression of antigen genes is also an important factor. Tsukamoto et al. compared the cytomegalovirus (CMV) promoter and CMV/chicken β-actin chimera (Pec) promoter for expression of IBDV *VP2* gene in HVT vectors and found that the Pec promoter expressed more VP2 protein and provided superior protection against challenge with IBDV [24]. In MDV serotype 1 (MDV1) vectors expressing NDV *fusion* gene, less potent MDV glycoprotein B promoter gave better protection than the simian virus 40 (SV40) late promoter when tested in chickens with MDA [28]. Another group compared five different promoters for expression of the *HA* gene of AIV H9N2 subtype in MDV vectors and found that two MDV endogenous promoters (pp38 and gB) with relatively low expression activities provided better protection than the other three promoters (CMV, SV40, and p1.8 kb) [29]. In this experiment, to find the most appropriate promoter to express the *HA* gene of AIV H5 subtype in HVT vectors, we compared three different promoters: the CMV promoter, the chicken β-actin (Bac) promoter, and the Pec promoter.

To prepare for construction of recombinant HVT, HVT insertion site sequences (*UL45* and *UL46* genes) were isolated by polymerase chain reaction (PCR) and cloned into pUC18. Homology plasmids were then constructed by inserting the *HA* gene with the promoter into the insertion site (between *UL45* gene and *UL46* gene) of the HVT sequences. The homology plasmid along with HVT infectious genomic DNA was transfected into chicken embryo fibroblasts (CEF), where homologous recombination took place. Recombinant HVT with the inserted gene was identified by an in situ immunostaining assay called black plaque assay (BPA) using anti-HA (H5) antibodies. Recombinant HVT was purified from HVT parent through several rounds of screening process by the BPA.

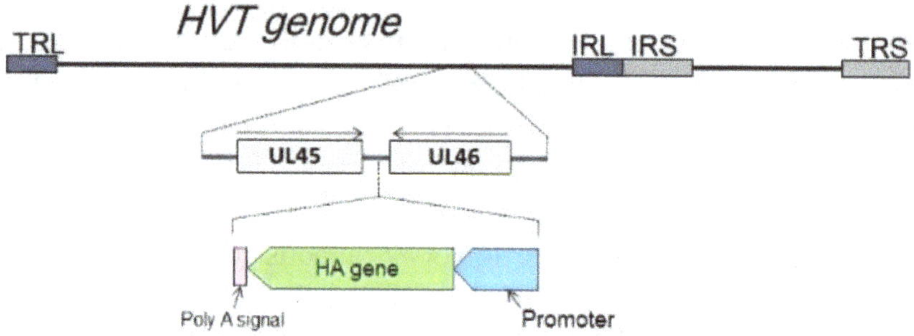

Figure 1. Genomic structure of rHVT-H5 vaccines.

2.2. In vitro characterization of rHVT-H5

Figure 1 shows genomic structures of the constructed rHVT-H5 vaccines. The genomic structures of the rHVT-H5 vaccines were confirmed by PCR assays with one primer binding to the insert sequence and the other primer binding to the HVT insertion site sequences (data not shown). The genomic structures were further confirmed by Southern blot analysis using

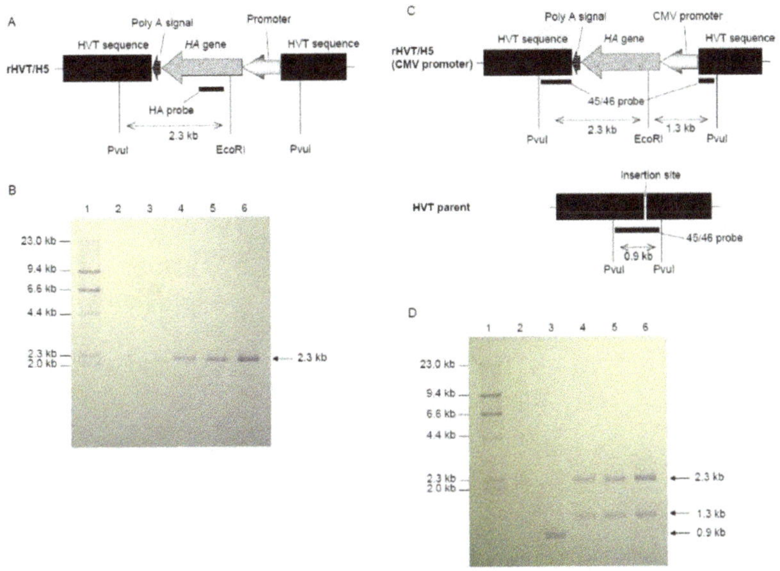

Figure 2. (A) Gene structure of rHVT/H5 and expected annealing site of the HA probe. (B) Result of Southern blot using the HA probe. Lane 1 = DNA molecular weight marker II, DIG-labeled (Roche); Lane 2 = uninoculated CEF control; Lane 3 = HVT parent; Lane 4 = rHVT/H5; Lane 5 = rHVT/H5 passage 5; Lane 6 = homology plasmid. (C) Gene structure of rHVT/H5 with CMV promoter and HVT parent and expected annealing site of the 45/46 probe. (D) Result of Southern blot using the 45/46 probe. Lane 1 = DNA molecular weight marker II, DIG-labeled (Roche); Lane 2 = uninoculated CEF control; Lane 3 = HVT parent; Lane 4 = rHVT/H5 with CMV promoter; Lane 5 = rHVT/H5 with CMV promoter passage 5; Lane 6 = homology plasmid.

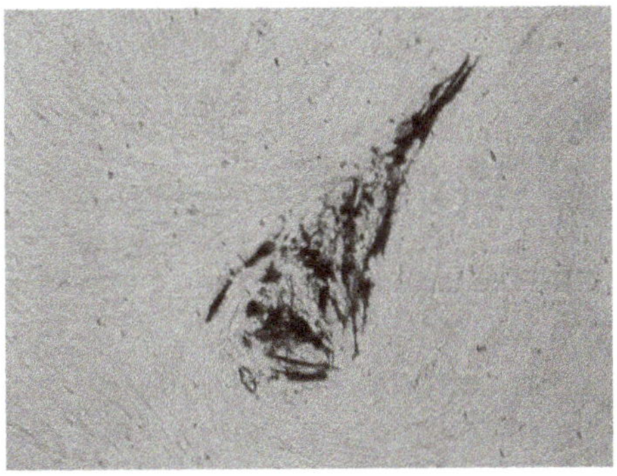

Figure 3. Black plaque assay on a rHVT/H5 plaque detecting expression of the HA protein of AIV H5 subtype. CEF monolayer infected with rHVT/H5 was incubated for 5 days and fixed with methanol:acetone. The monolayer with rHVT/H5 plaques was reacted with chicken anti-AIV HA serum, then with biotinylated anti-chicken IgG antibody and finally with streptavidin-alkaline phosphatase conjugates. Plaques expressing HA protein were stained by addition of BCIP/NBT solution.

digoxigenin-labeled probes specific to the *HA* gene or HVT insertion site sequences (**Figure 2**). Expression of the HA protein by the rHVT-H5 vaccines was confirmed by BPA using the chicken anti-HA serum (**Figure 3**). Western blot analysis using the chicken anti-HA serum detected a 75-kDa band with CEF infected with the rHVT-H5 (**Figure 4**). This band corresponds to non-cleaved HA protein that is produced by the rHVT-H5. Since the cleavage sites of the expressed HA proteins are those of LP AIV strains, the HA protein was not cleaved to HA1 and HA2 subunits in CEF.

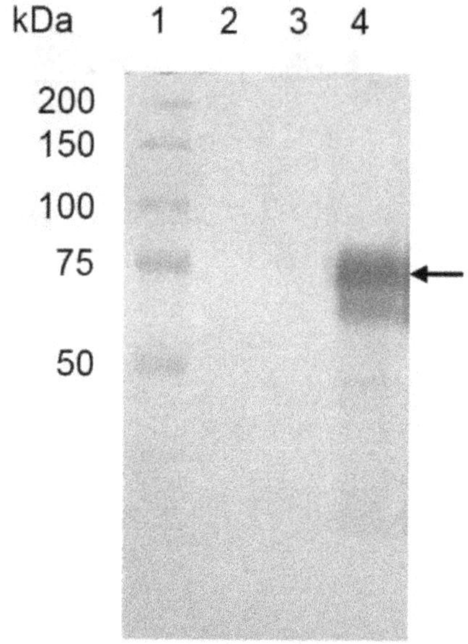

Figure 4. Western blot assay detecting expression of the HA protein by rHVT/H5. Lane 1 = Precision Plus Protein All Blue Standards (Bio-Rad Laboratories); Lane 2 = CEF control; Lane 3 = HVT FC126 parent strain; Lane 4 = rHVT/H5. An arrow indicates the HA protein with a molecular weight of 75 kDa.

In order to assess genetic and phenotypic stability of the rHVT-H5 vaccines, the viruses were passed in CEF 20 times. Viruses after the passages were characterized by PCR, Southern blot, BPA, and western blot. Results obtained with the passed viruses were identical to those obtained with the viruses before the passage (data not shown), and therefore, it was concluded that these viruses were genetically and phenotypically stable.

2.3. Evaluation of promoters for expression of HA gene

In order to identify the most suitable promoter among the CMV promoter, the Bac promoter, and the Pec promoter for expression of the *HA* gene, we compared three rHVT-H5 vaccines harboring the *HA* gene from A/turkey/Wisconsin/68 (H5N9) strain with one of these promoters. The rHVT-H5 vaccines with the CMV promoter, the Bac promoter, and the Pec promoter were designated as HVT-CMV-H5Wis68, HVT-Bac-H5Wis68, and HVT-Pec-H5Wis68, respectively.

One-day-old specific pathogen free (SPF) White Leghorn chicks were vaccinated subcutaneously with one of the rHVT-H5 vaccines. A group of chickens was held as a non-inoculated negative control group and another group of chickens was vaccinated subcutaneously with inactivated A/turkey/Wisconsin/68 (H5N9) vaccine at 3 weeks of age as an inactivated vaccine control group. Chickens in each group were bled each week between 3 and 7 weeks of age (6 and 7 weeks of age for the inactivated vaccine control group) and obtained sera were evaluated by the AIV hemagglutination inhibition (HI) test and AIV enzyme-linked immunosorbent assay (ELISA). The AIV HI tests were conducted using four hemagglutination units of an inactivated AIV homologous antigen of the A/turkey/Wisconsin/68 (H5N9) strain according to the standard procedure [30].

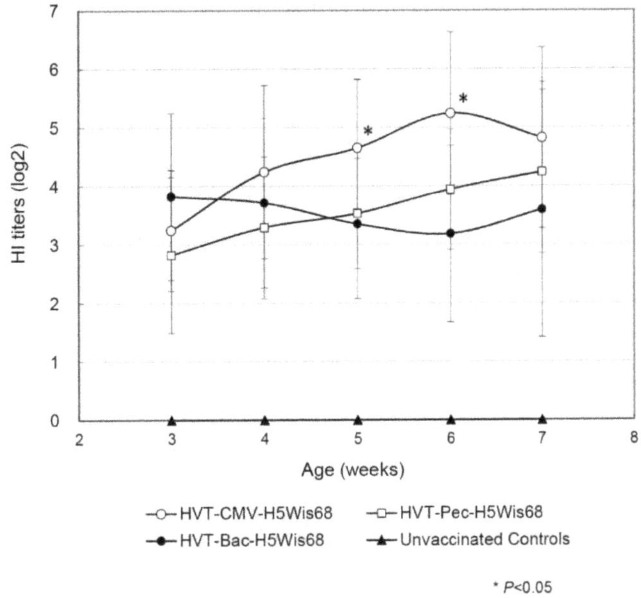

Figure 5. HI titers in chickens vaccinated with rHVT-H5 vaccines with different promoters.

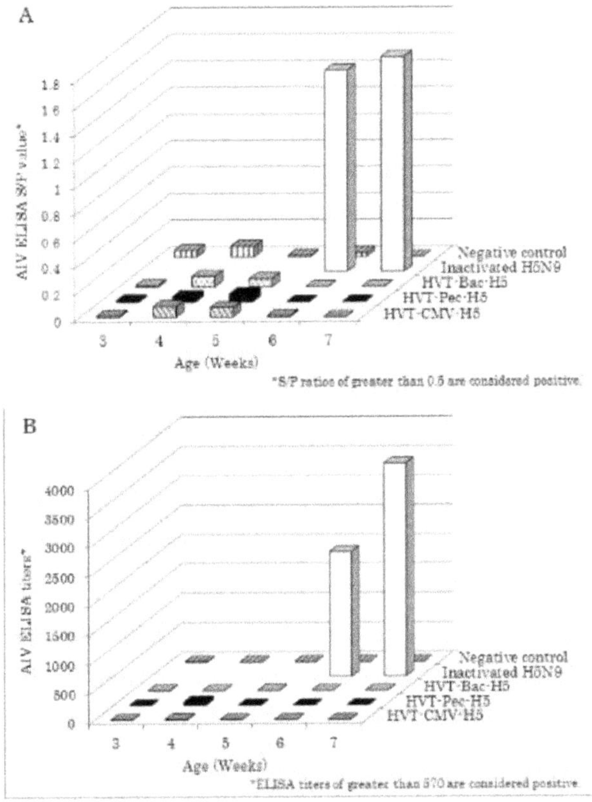

Figure 6. ELISA titers in chickens vaccinated with three rHVT-H5 vaccines using (A) FlockChek™ AIV Ab kit (Idexx Laboratories) and (B) ProFLOK® AIV Ab test kit (Zoetis).

As shown in **Figure 5**, the rHVT-H5 vaccines induced increased HI titers as early as 3 weeks of age and the increased titers were maintained through 7 weeks of age. Chickens vaccinated with HVT-CMV-H5Wis68 had higher mean HI titers than HVT-Pec-H5Wis68 and HVT-Bac-H5Wis68 vaccinated groups had between 4 and 7 weeks of age, with the differences statistically significant at 5 and 6 weeks of age. As expected, the inactivated A/turkey/Wisconsin/68 (H5N9) vaccine induced high HI titers at 6 and 7 weeks of age (3 and 4 weeks post-vaccination), confirming validity of the assay. When tested with the commercial AIV ELISA kits, Flock-Chek™ AIV Ab kit (Idexx Laboratories) and ProFLOK® AIV Ab test kit (Zoetis), sera collected from the rHVT-H5 vaccinated chickens were negative between 3 and 7 weeks of age, whereas sera collected from the inactivated vaccine control chickens showed highly positive ELISA titers with both kits (**Figure 6**).

This result demonstrated that the CMV promoter was the most suitable for expression of the *HA* gene in HVT vector vaccines. Furthermore, sera from the rHVT-H5 vaccinated chickens were found to be negative by the commercially available ELISA kits, although they were highly positive by the AIV HI test. This is most likely because these ELISA kits are designed to detect antibodies to more conserved internal protein, NP, of AIV, in order to detect antibodies to many different subtypes of AIV. This feature of the rHVT-H5 vaccines will be useful in differentiating chicken infected with field AIV viruses from vaccinated chicken (DIVA).

3. Safety of rHVT-H5 vaccine

Based on the results described above, the CMV promoter was selected for the expression of the *HA* gene. The rHVT-H5 vaccine with the CMV promoter attached to the *HA* gene from A/Swan/Hungary/4999/2006 (H5N1) strain (rHVT-H5h) was evaluated further for its safety and efficacy.

Safety of the rHVT-H5h vaccine was evaluated by an overdose study and a backpassage study. For the overdose study, SPF embryos at 18 days of incubation or day-of-age SPF chicks received rHVT-H5h at 10 times the typical field dose. In ovo application of rHVT-H5h at overdose did not affect hatchability and the vaccinated chickens remained free from any clinical signs or adverse reactions until 18 weeks of age. Chickens were necropsied at 18 weeks of age and no gross lesions were observed in any of the vaccinated chickens. Similarly, rHVT-H5h did not cause any clinical signs, adverse reactions, or gross lesions in other avian species such as turkeys, quail, pheasants, and pigeons.

For the backpassage study, to confirm that the rHVT-H5h vaccine will not revert to virulence, rHVT-H5h was passed five times in SPF chickens by using heparinized blood from chickens in the previous passage to inoculate a new set of SPF chicks. Chickens inoculated with the virus at the fifth passage, that is, inoculated with the heparinized blood from the fourth passage, were observed closely for any clinical signs for 45 days. Chickens were then necropsied and observed for grossly observable lesions. No chickens had any clinical signs, adverse reactions, or gross lesions. Therefore, it was concluded that rHVT-H5h did not revert to virulence after backpassages in chickens.

We conducted another study to evaluate the ability of the rHVT-H5h vaccine to transmit from vaccinated chickens to non-vaccinated chickens in contact. Day-of-age SPF chickens vaccinated in ovo with rHVT-H5h or parental HVT were commingled in isolators with non-vaccinated contact chickens. Virus isolation was attempted from the peripheral mononuclear blood lymphocytes collected from chickens at 10, 14, and 21 days of age. No virus was isolated from any of the contact chickens at any time points while the viruses were isolated from the vaccinated chickens, indicating that neither rHVT-H5h nor parental HVT spread from vaccinated chickens to non-vaccinated contact chickens. It appears that transmissibility of HVT parent and the rHVT-H5h vaccine between chickens is negligible.

In summary, similar to parent HVT vaccines and other HVT vector vaccines, the rHVT-H5h vaccine is extremely safe causing no adverse effects and does not revert to virulence after passages in chickens. The lack of transmission of the rHVT-H5h vaccine further strengthens the safety profile of this vaccine in terms of containment of the genetically modified organism.

4. Efficacy of rHVT-H5 vaccine

4.1. Efficacy against homologous challenge

Finally, efficacy of the rHVT-H5h vaccine was evaluated. After vaccination, humoral immune response was evaluated by the AIV HI tests. After challenge with HP AIV, vaccine efficacy was evaluated for (1) protection against mortality and clinical signs and (2) reduction of challenge virus shedding from challenged birds. Both the criteria are important for AI vaccines because these features will ensure that the vaccine will be beneficial as a measure to contain spread of field AI viruses as well as to reduce economical burdens in both endemic and emergent situations [4, 31].

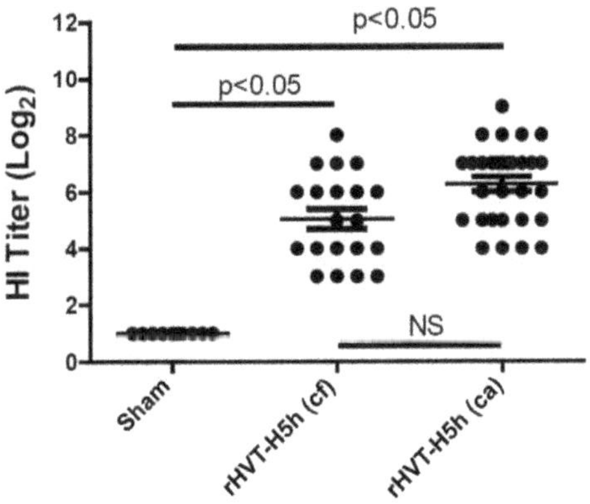

Figure 7. Individual HI titers (log_2) and standard error for bird groups at 5 weeks post-vaccination (prechallenge). Statistical significance between mean titers was determined with ANOVA using the Tukey's multiple comparison test ($p < 0.05$). NS = no significant difference. Modified from "Vaccine protection of chickens against antigenically diverse H5 highly pathogenic avian influenza isolates with a live HVT vector vaccine expressing the influenza hemagglutinin gene derived from a clade 2.2 avian influenza virus" by D.R. Kapczynski et al., 2015, Vaccine, 33, p1200.

Initial evaluation of the rHVT-H5h vaccine efficacy was conducted using homologous AIV as a challenge virus [32]. Day-of-age SPF chicks were vaccinated subcutaneously with either a frozen, cell-associated (ca) form or a lyophilized, cell-free (cf) form of the rHVT-H5h vaccine. At 5 weeks of age before challenge, increased HI titers were observed in all the rHVT-H5h vaccinated chicken with mean titers of $2^{6.3}$ for the ca group and $2^{5.1}$ for the cf group (**Figure 7**) when using homologous antigen.

Chickens were challenged with 10^6 mean embryo infectious dose (EID_{50}) HP H5N1 AIV A/Whooper Swan/Mongolia/3/2005 clade 2.2 strain at 6 weeks of age. The *HA* gene from the A/Whooper Swan/Mongolia/3/2005 strain has 100% gene homology with the A/Swan/Hungary/4999/2006 (H5N1) *HA* gene sequence. All chickens in the diluent-vaccinated, challenge control group died within 3 days. However, none of the rHVT-H5h vaccinated chickens succumbed to challenge and all the chickens were free from clinical signs of AI.

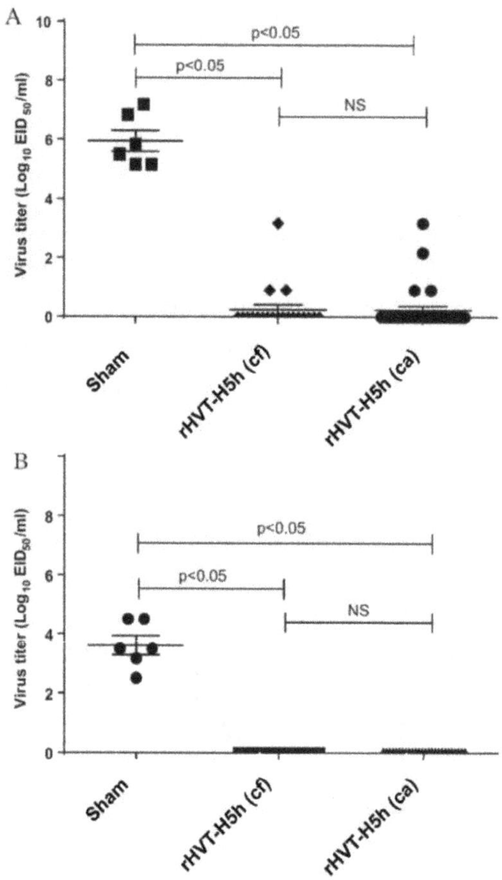

Figure 8. Viral titers from oral (A) and cloacal swabs (B) on day 2 post-challenge. Birds were vaccinated with a single dose rHVT-H5h in cell-associated (ca) or cell-free (cf) form at 1 day-of-age and challenge at 6 weeks with homologous HPAI H5N1. Viral titers are expressed as $log_{10}EID_{50}$ per milliliter. The lower limit of detection is 0.9 $log_{10}EID_{50}$ per milliliter. Statistical significance between mean titers was determined with ANOVA using Tukey's multiple comparison test ($p < 0.05$). NS = no significant difference. Modified from "Vaccine protection of chickens against antigenically diverse H5 highly pathogenic avian influenza isolates with a live HVT vector vaccine expressing the influenza hemagglutinin gene derived from a clade 2.2 avian influenza virus" by D.R. Kapczynski et al., 2015, Vaccine, 33, p1200.

We observed 3–6 $\log_{10}$ reduction of challenge virus shedding in the rHVT-H5h vaccinated chickens. From oropharyngeal swabs at 2 days post-challenge (dpc), only 4/30 (13%) chickens in the ca rHVT-H5h group and 3/20 (15%) chickens in the cf rHVT-H5h group shed virus with minimal virus titers (10^1–10^3 EID_{50}/ml), while all the challenge controls shed significant amounts (10^5–$10^7 EID_{50}$/ml) of virus (**Figure 8A**). From cloacal swabs, no virus was isolated from any of the rHVT-H5h vaccinated chickens at 2 dpc, while all the challenge controls shed virus at 10^2–$10^5 EID_{50}$/ml (**Figure 8B**).

These results demonstrated high potential of the rHVT-H5h vaccine as an excellent tool to support control of AI. Therefore, we proceeded to further evaluation of the rHVT-H5h, especially for protection against heterologous virus challenge and effects of MDA. Since the ca form appeared to provide slightly better immunogenicity than the cf form, the following evaluation was conducted using the ca form of the vaccine.

4.2. Efficacy against heterologous challenge

Since HP H5 viruses have become diverse and have evolved into various different clades, it is highly important that AI vaccines exert broad "cross-clade" efficacy against diverse AIV strains. Indeed, one of the limitations of conventional oil-adjuvanted, inactivated vaccines is that they are not as effective against heterologous viruses as homologous viruses [8–10]. Therefore, we tested efficacy of the rHVT-H5h vaccine against various AIV HP H5 strains.

Day-of-age SPF broiler chicks were vaccinated with the rHVT-H5h vaccine. A commercially available inactivated vaccine based on H5N2 Mexican strain (iH5N2) was used as a control and injected into birds at 10 days of age. Challenge was conducted at 4 weeks of age using the Indonesian A/chicken/WestJava Sbg/29/2007 H5N1 strain (CW07). The CW07 virus belongs to clade 2.1.3 and sequence similarity of the HA gene between the rHVT-H5h insert and the CW07 virus was 93%. After challenge, all chickens in the sham-vaccinated, challenge control group died within 2 days. In the group vaccinated with rHVT-H5h, 80% (16/20) of the chickens survived the challenge, while only one bird (5%) vaccinated with iH5N2 survived the challenge. When rHVT-H5h vaccinated chickens received boost with iH5N2 vaccine at 10 days of age, protection increased to 90% (18/20). Reduction in virus shedding up to 3 $\log_{10}$ was observed in rHVT-H5h vaccinated chickens compared to the challenge control. When the homologous antigen was used, rHVT-H5h, either with or without boost with iH5N2 vaccine, it induced average HI titers of 2^5–2^6 prior to challenge. HI titers were much lower with the heterologous CW07 antigen with average between 2^1 and 2^2. These results indicate that cell-mediated immunity as well as mucosal immunity provided by HVT vector vaccines might be involved in protective efficacy against heterologous CW07 strain.

In the next trial, another AIV HP H5 strain, A/Viet Nam/1203/04 (H5N1) (VN04), was used for challenge. The VN04 virus belongs to clade 1 and shares 96.5% HA gene similarity with the rHVT-H5h insert. Vaccination was conducted at the day of age to SPF layer chicks and challenge was conducted at 4 weeks of age. Protection was 85% (17/20) while all challenge control chickens died and reduction of virus shedding of 3 $\log_{10}$ was observed in the rHVT-H5h group.

Since these two trials using heterologous HP H5 strains demonstrated that the rHVT-H5h provided "cross-clade" efficacy, we went further and conducted another efficacy trial using Mexican H5N2 HP strain which shares only 82% HA gene similarity with the rHVT-H5h insert. Day-of-age chicks vaccinated with rHVT-H5h were challenged with A/chicken/Queretaro/14588-19/95 (H5N2) strain at 4 weeks of age. Nineteen out of 20 (95%) chickens survived the challenge, while all the challenge control died. This result demonstrated very broad cross-protective efficacy provided by rHVT-H5h.

We further evaluated efficacy of the rHVT-H5h vaccine against various HP AIV H5 isolates including several Egyptian isolates and a recent 2014 H5N8 isolate from Germany, as summarized in **Figure 9**. Protection in rHVT-H5h vaccinated chickens ranged between 60 and 100% with significant reduction in virus shedding, further strengthening evidence of very broad "cross-clade" efficacy provided by the rHVT-H5h vaccine. In one study where layer chickens were vaccinated and raised under field conditions in Egypt, a single rHVT-H5h vaccination at day of age conferred a high level of protection (60–73%) for a relatively extended period (up to 19 weeks of age) against an Egyptian isolate [33].

Type of bird	with MDA against:		HPAIV used for challenge			Challenge	% Protection		
	HVT	AIV	Strain	S.type	Clade	at:	Vaccinated	Not vaccinated	Reference
SPF CK	No	No	A/CK/Viet Nam/1203/2004	H5N1	1	4 woa	85%	0%	Perez D. 2012
COM BR	Yes	No	A/Duck/Hungary/11804/2006	H5N1	2.2	2 woa	90%	0%	De Vriese J. et al. 2009
COM BR	Yes	Yes (H5N2)	A/Duck/Hungary/11804/2006	H5N1	2.2	2 woa	100%	20%	De Vriese J. et al. 2009
COM BR	Yes	Yes (H5N2)	A/Duck/Hungary/11804/2006	H5N1	2.2	3 woa	90%	0%	De Vriese J. et al. 2009
SPF CK	No	No	A/CK/Egypt/1709-1 VIR08/2007	H5N1	2.2.1	3 woa	100%	0%	Rauw F. et al. 2011
SPF CK	No	No	A/CK/Egypt/1709-6/2008	H5N1	2.2.1.1	3 woa	100%	0%	Rauw F. et al. 2011
COM BR	Yes	No	A/CK/Egypt/1709-6/2008	H5N1	2.2.1.1	4 woa	90%	0%	Rauw F. et al. 2012
COM BR	Yes	Yes (H5N1)	A/CK/Egypt/1709-6/2008	H5N1	2.2.1.1	4 woa	100%	0%	Rauw F. et al. 2012
COM BR	Yes	Yes (H5N1)	A/CK/Egypt/1709-1 VIR08/2007	H5N1	2.2.1	4 woa	90%	0%	Rauw F. et al. 2012
COM BR	Yes	Yes (H5N1)	A/CK/Egypt/1709-6/2008	H5N1	2.2.1.1	4 woa	70%	0%	Rauw F. et al. 2012
COM BR	Yes	Yes (H5N1)	A/CK/West Java Subang/29/2007	H5N1	2.1.3	4 woa	80%	0%	Soejoedono R. D. et al. 2012
COM BR	Yes	Yes (H5N1)	A/CK/Puwakarta-Ciingga/142/2010	H5N1	2.1.3	4 woa	95%	0%	Soejoedono R. D. et al. 2012
SPF CK	No	No	A/Whooper Swan/Mongolia/3/2005	H5N1	2.2	6 woa	100%	0%	Kapczynski D.R. et al. 2015
SPF CK	No	No	A/CK/West Java Subang/29/2007	H5N1	2.1.3	4 woa	80%	0%	Kapczynski D.R. et al. 2015
SPF CK	No	No	A/CK/Queretaro/14588/1995	**H5N2**	-	4 woa	95%	0%	Kapczynski D.R. et al. 2015
SPF CK	No	No	A/CK/Egypt/1709-6/2008	H5N1	2.2.1.1	4 woa	100%	0%	Rauw F. et al. 2012
SPF CK	No	No	A/CK/Egypt/1709-6/2008	H5N1	2.2.1.1	8 woa	100%	0%	Rauw F. et al. 2012
COM BR	Yes	Yes (H5N1)	A/CK/Egypt/1709-6/2008	H5N1	2.2.1.1	4 woa	93%	0%	Kilany W. H. et al. 2012
COM BR	Yes	Yes (H5N1)	A/CK/Egypt-63/2010 "variant"	H5N1	2.2.1.1	5 woa	80%	0%	Kilany W. H. et al. 2012
SPF CK	No	No	A/CK/Germany/2014	**H5N8**	2.3.4.4	4 woa	100%	0%	Steensels M. et al. 2015
SPF CK	No	No	A/CK/Bangladesh/11RS1 984-33/2011	H5N1	2.3.2.1	4 woa	100%	0%	Bonfante F. et al. 2013
COM LY	Yes	Yes (H5N1)	A/CK/Egypt/128s/2012	H5N1	2.2.1	19 woa	73%	0%	Kilany W. H. et al. 2014
COM LY	Yes	Yes (H5N1)	A/CK/Egypt/128s/2012	H5N1	2.2.1	19 woa	60%	0%	Kilany W. H. et al. 2014
SPF TK	No	No	A/WS/Mongolia/2005	H5N1	2.2	4 woa	96%	0%	Kapczynski et al. 2012

SPF CK = SPF Chickens; SPF TK = SPF Turkeys; COM BR = Commercial broilers; COM LY = Commercial Layers; S.type = serotype; woa = weeks of age

Figure 9. Summary of challenge experiments conducted with the rHVT-H5 vaccine. Modified from "Experimental and field results regarding immunity induced by a recombinant HVT-H5 vector vaccine against H5N1 and other H5 Highly Pathogenic Avian Influenza Virus challenge." by Y. Gardin et al., 2016, Avian Dis, in press.

To see if cellular immunity indeed is involved in this broad protective efficacy, we conducted in vitro cytotoxicity assay. Splenic lymphocytes collected from chickens vaccinated with the rHVT-H5h vaccine were incubated with chicken lung cells infected with either H5N9, H6N2, H7N2, or H9N2 low pathogenic AIV. The highest level of lysis by splenic cytotoxic T cells was observed with H5-infected target cells. Lysis was also observed with other heterologous AIV (H6, H7, or H9), although to a lower degree. Negligible lysis was observed with naïve uninfected lung cells. These results indicated that the rHVT-H5h vaccine induced AIV-specific cytotoxic T-cell activity and it may contribute in part to broad protective immunity induced by the rHVT-H5h.

4.3. Efficacy of rHVT-H5 in chicken with maternally derived antibodies

In endemic countries, most breeders are vaccinated with AI vaccines and/or exposed to field AIV challenge and therefore, their progeny possess MDA against AIV. Efficacy of oil-adjuvanted, inactivated AIV vaccines and fowlpox-vectored AI vaccines has been shown to be significantly impaired in the presence of MDA. On the other hands, HVT vector vaccines have been shown not to be excessively affected by the presence of MDA against inserted antigens. Indeed, with the rHVT-H5h vaccine, several studies demonstrated lack of significant interference on its protective efficacy by the presence of MDA when administered to day-of-age chicks [10, 34].

4.4. DIVA

AI surveillance is conducted through serological assays including ELISA and HI. Except in endemic countries, positive serological response in those assays will lead to immediate and extreme actions including "stamping-out." Also, there are trade implications because many countries ban importation of poultry from AI-positive countries. Therefore, when AI vaccination is introduced, it is critical that AI vaccines do not interfere with the AI surveillance. It is highly favorable that serological responses elicited by AI vaccines may be distinguished from those elicited by infection of field AIV. Since conventional inactivated vaccines elicit humoral immune responses that lead to positive titers in both ELISA and HI tests, these vaccines do interfere with the surveillance [7].

The rHVT-H5h vaccine elicits antibodies against the HA protein and the antibody responses can be detected by the HI tests. However, those sera from vaccinated chickens were negative in commercial ELISA kits because the ELISA kits are designed to detect antibodies against more conserved internal protein (NP) in order to offer coverage over different subtypes of AIV. When we examined serological responses in chickens that were vaccinated with the rHVT-H5h and then challenged with HP AIV, we found positive ELISA titers in chickens that excreted challenge viruses. These results demonstrated that the rHVT-H5h vaccines may be applied to the DIVA strategy and do not interfere with AI surveillance.

5. Conclusions

Our studies demonstrated that the rHVT-H5h vaccine possesses characteristics that could be beneficial to control of AI in endemic countries and in emergency situations. Those characteristics are (1) broad "cross-clade" protective efficacy against diverse AIV H5 isolates, (2) lack of interference by MDA, (3) applicability to hatchery vaccination, and (4) applicability to DIVA. The rHVT-H5h vaccine has been approved by authorities in Egypt, Mexico, and Bangladesh and is in use in the field. An independent survey conducted by FAO, General Organization for Veterinary Services in Egypt, and Centre International de Recherche en Agriculture pour le Développement in France concluded that day-of-age vaccination utilizing the rHVT-H5h vaccine at hatcheries is more efficient than the program using the inactivated vaccines at farms and it would have a positive impact for disease control in Egypt [35].

It is clear that vaccines alone cannot solve all the problems associated with AI. However, we believe that in conjunction with active and efficient surveillance and strict biosecurity measures, the rHVT-H5h vaccine can contribute to disease control by increasing resistance against infection and decreasing the amount of virus shed to the environment. It would also remove economical burdens from farmers and consumers and improve animal welfare by protecting chickens from mortality and clinical signs. In conclusion, we successfully developed a HVT vector AI vaccine that possesses many features that could be beneficial to AI control. It remains to be seen whether this vaccine is truly useful in the field.

Author details

Atsushi Yasuda[1*], Motoyuki Esaki[1], Kristi Moore Dorsey[2], Zoltan Penzes[3], Vilmos Palya[3], Darrell R. Kapczynski[4] and Yannick Gardin[5]

*Address all correspondence to: atsushi.yasuda@ceva.com

1 Ceva Animal Health, Yokohama, Japan

2 Ceva Animal Health, Lenexa, Kansas, USA

3 Ceva Animal Health, Budapest, Hungary

4 Exotic and Emerging Avian Viral Disease Research Unit, Southeast Poultry Research Laboratory, U.S. National Poultry Research Center, Athens, Georgia, USA

5 Ceva Animal Health, Libourne, France

References

[1] Food and Agriculture Organization (FAO). Approaches to controlling, preventing and eliminating H5N1 highly pathogenic avian influenza in endemic countries. Rome; 2011.

[2] WHO/OIE/FAO H5N1 Evolution Working Group. Continued evolution of highly pathogenic avian influenza A (H5N1): updated nomenclature. Influenza and Other Respiratory Viruses. 2012;6:1–5.

[3] Swayne D.E., Suarez D.L., Sims L.D. Influenza. In: Swayne DE, Glisson JR, McDougald LR, Nair V, Nolan LK, Suarez DL, editors. Diseases of Poultry. 13th ed. Ames, IA: Wiley-Blackwell; 2013. pp. 181–218.

[4] Swayne D.E. The role of vaccines and vaccination in high pathogenicity avian influenza control and eradication. Expert Review of Vaccines. 2012;11:877–880.

[5] Capua I., Alexander D.J. Avian influenza vaccines and vaccination in birds. Vaccine. 2008;26:D70–D73.

[6] Sims L.D. Lessons learned from Asian H5N1 outbreak control. Avian Diseases. 2007;51:174–181.

[7] Swayne D.E. Vaccines for list A poultry diseases: Emphasis on avian influenza. Developmental Biology (Basel). 2003;114:201–212.

[8] Abdelwhab E.M., Grund.C, Aly M.M., Beer M., Harder T.C., Hafez H.M. Multiple dose vaccination with heterologous H5N2 vaccine: immune response and protection against variant clade 2.2.1 highly pathogenic avian influenza H5N1 in broiler breeder chickens. Vaccine. 2011;29:6219–6225.

[9] Swayne D.E., Kapczynski D. Strategies and challenges for eliciting immunity against avian influenza virus in birds. Immunolgical Reviews. 2008;225:314–331.

[10] Rauw F., Palya V., Gardin Y., Tatar-Kis T., Dorsey K.M., Lambrecht B. et al. Efficacy of rHVT-AI vector vaccine in broilers with passive immunity against challenge with two antigenically divergent Egyptian clade 2.2.1 HPAI H5N1 strains. Avian Diseases 2012;56:913–922.

[11] Abdelwhab E.M., Grund C., Aly M.M., Beer M., Harder T.C., Hafez H.M. Influence of maternal immunity on vaccine efficacy and susceptibility of one day old chicks against Egyptian highly pathogenic avian influenza H5N1. Veterinary Microbiology. 2012;155:13–20.

[12] De Vriese J., Steensels M., Palya V., Gardin Y., Dorsey K.M., Lambrecht B. et al. Passive protection afforded by maternally-derived antibodies in chickens and the antibodies' interference with the protection elicited by avian influenza-inactivated vaccines in progeny. Avian Diseases. 2010;54:246–252.

[13] Schat K.A., Nair V. Marek's disease. In: Swayne D.E., Glisson J.R., McDougald L.R., Nolan L.K., Suarez D.L., Nair V, editors. Diseases of Poultry. 13th ed. Hoboken, NJ: Wiley-Blackwell; 2013. pp. 515–552.

[14] Okazaki W., Purchase H.G., Burmester B.R. Protection against Marek's disease by vaccination with a herpesvirus of turkeys. Avian Diseases. 1970;14:413–429.

[15] Heller E. D., Schat K.A. Enhancement of natural killer cell activity by Marek's disease vaccines. Avian Pathology. 1987;16:51–60.

[16] Kitamoto N., Ikuta K., Kato S., Yamaguchi S. Cell-mediated cytotoxicity of lymphocytes from chickens inoculated with herpesvirus of turkey against a Marek's disease lymphoma cell line (MSB-1). Biken Journal. 1979;22:11–20.

[17] Rauw F., Gardin Y., Palya V., Anbari S., Lemaire S., Boschmans M. et al. Improved vaccination against Newcastle disease by an in ovo recombinant HVT-ND combined with an adjuvanted live vaccine at day-old. Vaccine. 2010;28:823–833.

[18] Witter R.L., Offenbecker L. Duration of vaccinal immunity against Marek's disease. Avian Diseases. 1978;22:396–407.

[19] Palya V., Tatár-Kis T., Mató T., Felföldi B., Kovács E., Gardin Y. Onset and long-term duration of immunity provided by asingle vaccination with a turkey herpesvirus vector ND vaccine in commercial layers. Veterinary Immunology and Immunopathology. 2014;158:105–115.

[20] Afonso C.L., Tulman E.R., Lu Z., Zsak L., Rock D.L., Kutish G.F. The genome of turkey herpesvirus. Journal of Virology. 2001;75:971–978.

[21] Darteil R., Bublot M., Laplace E., Bouquet J.F., Audonnet J.C., Rivière M. Herpesvirus of turkey recombinant viruses expressing infectious bursal disease virus (IBDV) VP2 immunogen induce protection against an IBDV virulent challenge in chickens. Virology. 1995;211:481–490.

[22] Morgan R.W., Gelb J. Jr, Schreurs C.S., Lütticken D., Rosenberger J.K., Sondermeijer P.J.. Protection of chickens from Newcastle and Marek's diseases with a recombinant herpesvirus of Turkeys vaccine expressing the Newcastle disease virus fusion protein. Avian Diseases. 1992;36:858–870.

[23] Ross L.J., Binns M.M., Tyers P., Pastorek J., Zelnik V., Scott S. Construction and properties of a turkey herpesvirus recombinant expressing the Marek's disease virus homologue of glycoprotein B of herpes simplex virus. Journal of General Virology. 1993;74:371–377.

[24] Tsukamoto K., Saito S., Saeki S., Sato T., Tanimura N., Isobe T. et al. Complete, long-lasting protection against lethal infectious bursal disease virus challenge by a single vaccination with an avian herpesvirus vector expressing VP2 antigens. Journal of Virology. 2002;76:5637–5645.

[25] Esaki M., Godoy A., Rosenberger J.K., Rosenberger S.C., Gardin Y., Yasuda A. et al. Protection and antibody response caused by turkey herpesvirus vector Newcastle disease vaccine. Avian Diseases. 2013;57:750–755.

[26] Esaki M., Noland L., Eddins T., Godoy A., Saeki S., Saitoh S. et al. Safety and efficacy of a turkey herpesvirus vector laryngotracheitis vaccine for chickens. Avian Diseases. 2013;57:192–198.

[27] Swayne D.E., Suarez D.L., Sims L.D. Influenza. In: Swayne D.E., Glisson J.R., McDougald L.R., Nolan L.K., Suarez D.L. and Nair V, editors. Diseases of Poultry. 13th ed. Hoboken, NJ: Wiley-Blackwell; 2013. pp. 181–218.

[28] Sonoda K., Sakaguchi M., Okamura H., Yokogawa K., Tokunaga E., Tokiyoshi S. et al. Development of an effective polyvalent vaccine against both Marek's and Newcastle diseases based on recombinant Marek's disease virus type 1 in commercial chickens with maternal antibodies. Journal of Virology. 2000;74:3217–3226.

[29] Ma C., Zhang Z., Zhao P., Duan L., Zhang Y., Zhang F. et al. Comparative transcriptional activity of five promoters in BAC-cloned MDV for the expression of the hemagglutinin gene of H9N2 avian influenza virus. Journal of Virological Methods. 2014;206:119–127.

[30] Pedersen J.C. Hemagglutination-Inhibition Test for Avian Influenza Virus Subtype Identification and the Detection and Quantitation of Serum Antibodies to the Avian Influenza Virus. Methods in Molecular Biology. 2008;436:53–66.

[31] Gardin Y., Palya V., Dorsey K.M., El-Attrache J., Bonfante F., de Wit S. et al. Experimental and field results regarding immunity induced by a rHVT-H5 vector vaccine against H5N1 and other H5 type highly pathogenic avian influenza viruses. Avian Diseases. Forthcoming. DOI: 10.1637/11144-050815-ResNote.1

[32] Kapczynski DR, Esaki M, Dorsey KM, Jiang H, Jackwood M, Moraes M, Gardin Y. Vaccine protection of chickens against antigenically diverse H5 highly pathogenic avian influenza isolates with a live HVT vector vaccine expressing the influenza hemagglutinin gene derived from a clade 2.2 avian influenza virus. Vaccine. 2015;33:1197–1205.

[33] Kilany W.H., Dauphin G., Selim A., Tripodi A., Samy M., Sobhy H. et al. Protection conferred by recombinant turkey herpesvirus avian influenza (rHVT-H5) vaccine in the rearing period in two commercial layer chicken breeds in Egypt. Avian Pathology. 2014;43:514–523.

[34] Kilany W.H., Hassan M.K., Safwat M., Mohammed S., Selim A., VonDobschuetz S. et al. Comparison of the effectiveness of rHVT-H5, inactivated H5 and rHVT-H5 with inactivated H5 prime/boost vaccination regimes in commercial broiler chickens carrying MDAs against HPAI H5N1 clade 2.2.1 virus. Avian Pathology. 2015;44:333–341.

[35] Peyre M., Choisy M., Sobhy H., Kilany W.H., Gély M., Tripodi A. et al. Added value of avian influenza (H5) day old chick vaccination for disease control in Egypt. Avian Diseases. Forthcoming. DOI: 10.1637/11131-050715-ResNote.1

7

Biosensors for Rapid Detection of Avian Influenza

Ronghui Wang and Yanbin Li

Abstract

The scope of this chapter was to review the advancements made in the area of biosensors for rapid detection of avian influenza viruses (AIVs). It is intended to provide general background about biosensor technology and to discuss important aspects for developing biosensors, such as selection of the suitable biological recognition elements (anti-AIV bioreceptors) as well as their immobilization strategies. A major concern of this chapter is also to critically review the biosensors' working principles and their applications in AIV detection. A table containing the types of biosensor, bioreceptors, target AIVs, methods, etc. is given in this chapter. A number of papers for the different types of biosensors give hints on the current trends in the field of biosensor research for its application on AIV detection. By discussing recent research and future trends based on many excellent publications and reviews, it is hoped to give the readers a comprehensive view on this fast-growing field.

Keywords: biosensor, avian influenza virus, rapid detection, bioreceptor, nanobiosensor

1. Introduction

Influenza viruses, which belong to the *Orthomyxoviridae* family, are classified as A, B, and C based on antigenic differences in their nucleoprotein (NP) and matrix (M_1) protein [1]. All avian influenza viruses (AIV) are classified as type A. Type A viruses are further subtyped on the basis of antigenic differences of the surface glycoproteins, the hemagglutinin (HA), and the neuraminidase (NA) proteins [2]. So far, seventeen HA (H1 through H17) and ten NA (N1 through N10) subtypes have been identified [3]. **Figure 1** presents a schematic diagram of influenza A virus, and **Figure 2** shows a transmission electron microscopy photograph. Influenza A virus is an enveloped RNA virus approximately 80–120 nm in diameter [1, 2]. There are two major surface glycoproteins (HA and NA) and a small number of M2 protein, which has ion channel activity. The ratio of HA and NA is approximately 4:1. The genome of type A virus consists of eight segments of negative-sense single-stranded RNA, which are associated with many NP and the transcriptase complex (RNA polymerase components PB1, PB2 and PA) to form ribonucleoproteins (RNPs). The matrix protein M1 has an interaction with the RNPs and is under the lipid bilayer. NS_1 is found only in infected cells and is not thought to be a structural component of the virus, but small amount of NS_2 are present in purified viruses.

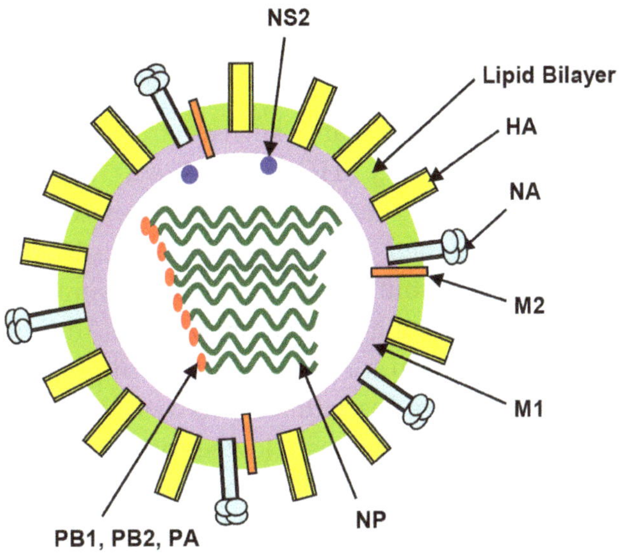

Figure 1. A schematic diagram of the structure of the influenza A virus particle.

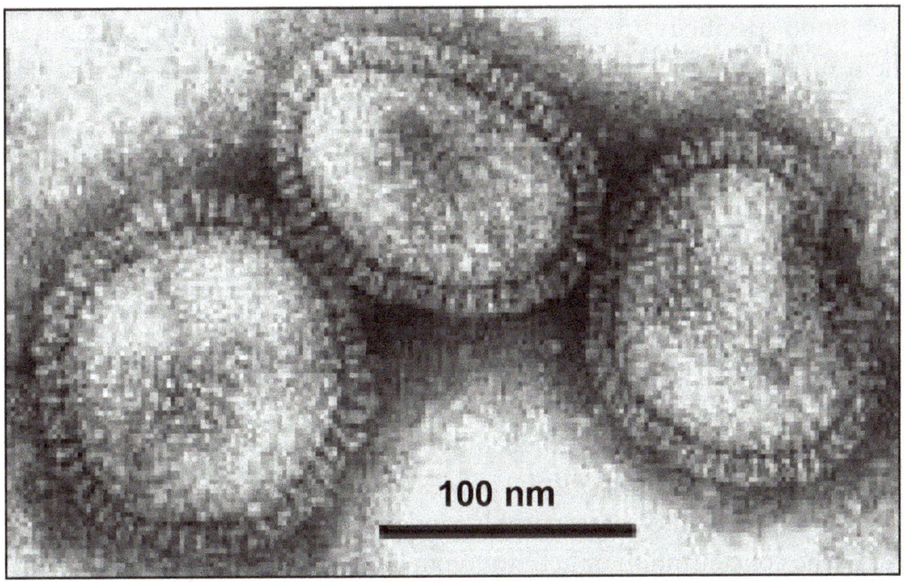

Figure 2. A transmission electron micrograph of influenza A virus particles.

AIVs have a large impact on the poultry each year and also represent a threat to human health. The highly pathogenic H5N1 avian influenza (HPAI H5N1), which originally emerged in Southeaster Asia in late 1990s, cost the poultry industry an estimated $10 billion between 1997 and 2008 [4]. HPAI H5N1 has also caused global concerns for public health and continues to spread throughout the world. Since 2003, a total of 62 countries (regions) have been affected by HPAI H5N1 and new human and animal cases are continuously being confirmed and reported [5]. The link between human and AI has raised concern among public health authorities and the scientific community about the prevalence and pandemic potential of AI virus. The H5N1 virus has caused 449 deaths of 846 people infected since 2003, according to the World Health Organization [5]. Therefore, advanced technologies for more rapid and sensitive AIV detection are needed for better surveillance and control of the outbreaks.

Current virus detection techniques are available, such as virus isolation, immunofluorescence antibody (FA) test, immunohistochemistry (IHC), and ELISA as well as rapid procedures based on molecular tools, such as polymerase chain reaction (PCR)-based assays, gene sequencing, and microarrays. Among these test methods, virus isolation has been the "gold standard" as its highest sensitivity and reliability, but it is a very time-consuming procedure (4–7 days). ELISA is a simple and rapid test in testing mass serum samples; thus, it is commonly used for serum antibody detection, but not used for virus detection in practice or diagnostics. Other immunoassays of FA or IHC can be used as a direct virus detection test from tissue specimens, but they either require labels or have limitations of low sensitivity and cross-reactions in certain circumstances. The molecular assays of RT-PCR and real-time RT-PCR methods have the advantages of high sensitivity and good specificity, but possess disadvantages of requiring expensive PCR equipment and reagents, and well-trained skillful technical personnel. Therefore, in order to minimize the social and economic costs, the development of rapid detection methods is essential. These rapid detection methods should meet the following requirements: (1) high throughput, (2) possibility of multiple target detection, (3) high sensitivity, (4) good specificity, (5) high speed, (6) simple operation, (7) suitability for on-site and/or in-field use, and (8) less cost. Biosensors have shown a great potential to meet such criteria.

The biosensor research began in the early 60 s of the twentieth century, when a glucose biosensor was proposed by Clark and Lyons [6] at Children's Hospital in Cincinnati. From then on, biosensor applications have expanded throughout the medical diagnosis field and also into the fields of environmental monitoring, agricultural production, food safety, pharmaceutical screening, and biodefense. A biosensor can be defined as a "compact analytical device or unit incorporating a biological or biologically derived sensitive recognition element integrated or associated with a physiochemical transducer" [7]. This device is composed of a biological recognition element (often called bioreceptor) and directly interfaced signal transducer (**Figure 3**). The selective and reversible process of interaction between the analyte and bioreceptor is transduced into a measurable signal, for example, electrical signal, which is proportional to the concentration or activity of an analyte in any type of samples. Biosensors can be classified based on the transduction element or the biological element. According to the basic principles of signal transduction, there are three main biosensor types, which have been studied for use in AIVs detection: piezoelectric, optical, and electrochemical biosensors. If we follow the types of biological element or bioreceptors, AIV biosensors can be classified into immunosensors, aptasensors, DNA or RNA-probe sensors, and more. In this chapter, we focus on these types of biosensors studied and developed recently for rapid detection of AIVs. It offers a survey of the principles, fabrication, operation, and the most popular types of biosensing devices in research or application today for AIVs detection. By discussing recent research and future trends based on many excellent publications and reviews, it is hoped to give the readers a comprehensive view on this fast-growing field.

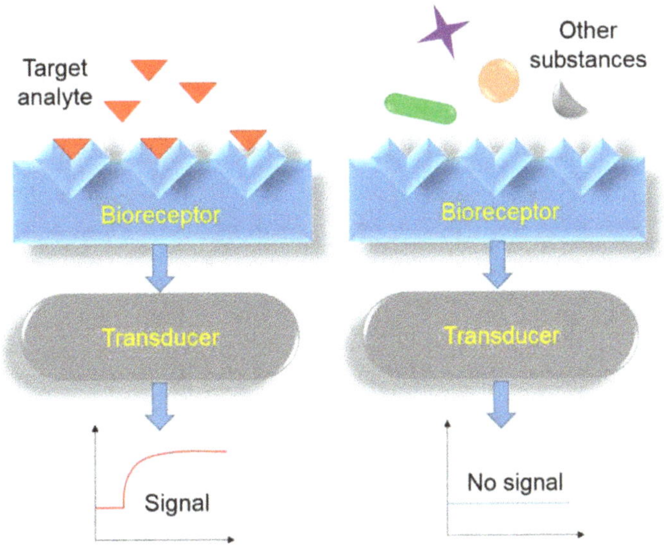

Figure 3. A schematic diagram of biorecognition and signal transduction in a typical biosensor.

2. Biosensors for detection of AIVs

As shown in **Figure 4**, the number of papers published in the field of biosensor research for detection of AI has kept increasing from year 2001 to 2015 based on PubMed. Biosensors offer the advantages of simple operation, rapid response, low cost, portability, automation, and easy to integrate with nanomaterials/nanostructure, Micro-Electro-Mechanical System(MEMS)/ Nano-Electro-Mechanical System(NEMS), biotechnology, Global Position System(GPS)/ wireless, and image technologies. One of the major requirements in developing a biosensor for AIVs is the need for a sensitive analytical device that can easily go down to very low detection levels without significant changes in selectivity. AIVs will spread rapidly through a community before any symptoms appear for the identification. A biosensor that can rapidly, sensitively and selectively detect target virus will be invaluable. In addition, a simple, robust, rapid, cost-effective, and potable biosensor, suitable for use in the field, is urgently needed. While a variety of biosensors have been developed for use in different applications, three types of biosensors have been mainly studied for AIV detection: piezoelectric, optical, and electrochemical biosensors.

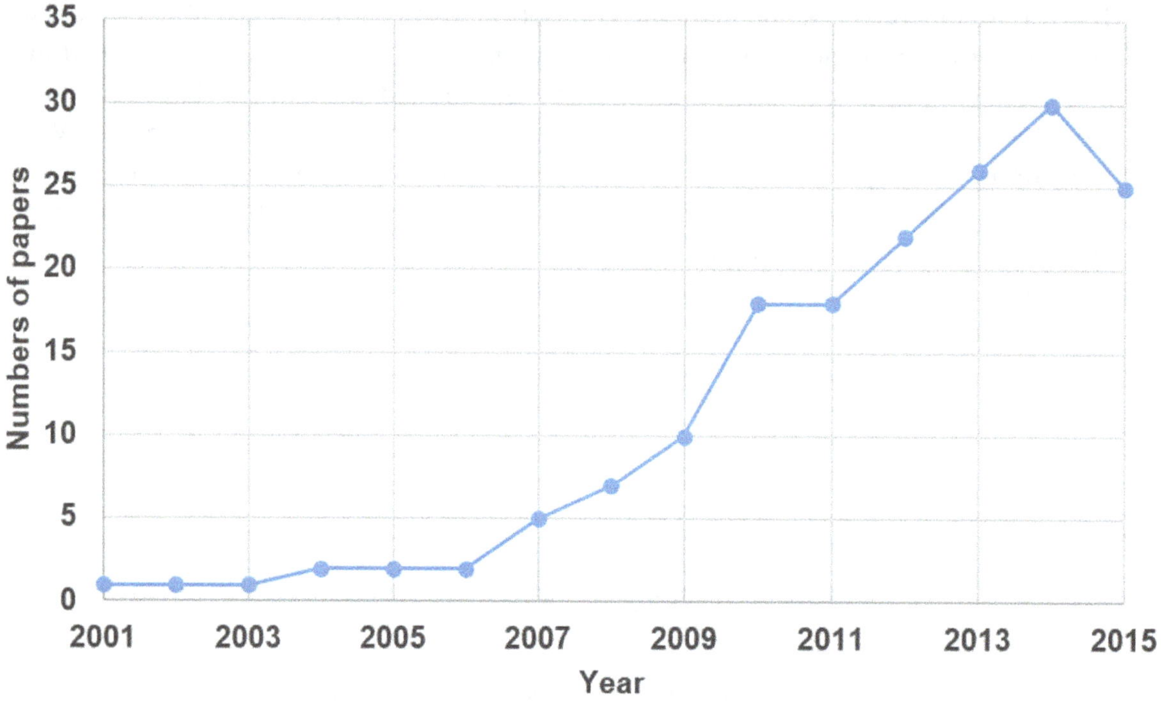

Figure 4. Numbers of papers published in the field of biosensor research for detection of AIVs between year 2001 and 2015.

2.1. Piezoelectric biosensors

Piezoelectric biosensors utilize crystals capable of generating a piezoelectric field to detect mass changes in the sensing environment [8]. The crystal is sandwiched between two excitation electrodes, which apply an electrical field that causes the crystal to undergo dimensional changes, or oscillations, at the crystals natural resonant frequency. An increase in the mass on the surface of the crystal, such as antibody immobilization or capture of antigen, decreases the resonant frequency. Piezoelectric biosensors are useful because they are low cost, label free, sensitive, and have extremely low detection levels [8]. The most intensively studied piezo-electric biosensor is the quartz crystal microbalance (QCM), which uses a thin wafer of quartz as the transducing crystal. Quartz crystals have the advantages of being widely available, relatively inexpensive, durable, direct detection, and real-time output. Other techniques are often coupled with QCM to increase the performance and capability of the biosensor. QCM biosensors have attracted interest in applications for AIVs detection. **Table 1** summarizes the main analytical features of QCM biosensors for detection of AIVs. Different studies used different concentration units for AIV. It would be helpful to know the comparable relationship between them. The common concentration units for AIV contain EID_{50} (50% egg infectious does), ELD_{50} (50% egg lethal does), PFU (plague-forming units), and HAU (hemagglutination unit). 1×10^3 EID_{50} ml^{-1} equals to ~0.0128 HAU/50 μl [9], $1 \times 10^{6.2}$ ELD_{50} ml^{-1} equals to 128 HAU/50 μl [10], and 1×10^5 PFU equals to 1 HAU [11].

Influenza subtype	Target	Bioreceptor	Sensitivity	Detection range	Detection time	Labelling method	Reference
H3N2	Virus	Antibody	4 virus particles/ml	0.02–3 HAU	–	Label-free	[12]
H1N1	Virus	Antibody	10^4 pfu/ml	10^3–10^7 pfu/ml	45 min	Label-free	[13]
			10^3 pfu/ml		105 min	Label with 13 nm gold nanoparticles	
H5N1	Virus	Antibody	0.0128 HAU	0.128–12.8 HAU	120 min	Label with 30 nm magnetic nanobeads	[14]
H5N1	Virus	Aptamer	1 HAU	1–4 HAU	60 min	Label with 30 nm magnetic nanobaeds	[22]
H5N1	Virus	Aptamer hydrogel	0.0128 HAU	0.0128–0.64 HAU	30 min	Label-free	[9]
H5N3	HA	Glycan	K_d 1.44 × 10^{-8} M	–	–	Label-free	[26]
H5N3	Virus	N-Acetylglucosamine (GlcNAc)	K_a 2.03 × 10^{10} M	–	–	Label-free	[27]
H5N1			K_a 4.35 × 10^{10} M				
H1N3			K_a 2.56 × 10^{12} M				

Table 1. QCM biosensors for detection of AIVs.

Antibodies are the most common bioreceptor of choice for sensing, and they are generated by immunizing an animal system with antigen. The interaction between antibody and antigen can be transduced into measurable signal changes. Early studies focused on the development of QCM immunosensor based on antibody-antigen interaction for influenza virus detection [12–14]. For example, the characterization of a QCM biosensor for the direct detection of influenza A viruses was reported by Owen et al. [12]. Self-assembled monolayers (SAMs) of mercaptoundecanoic acid (MUA) were formed on QCM gold electrodes for the immobilization of anti-influenza A antibodies, and the limit of detection was estimated to be 4 virus particles/ml. QCM immunosensor has been used also to detect avian influenza label free in nasal washings with a lower detection limit of 10^4 pfu/ml, although, with the addition of a gold nanoparticle conjugate, the detection limit was reduced to 10^3 pfu/ml, which is comparable to the sensitivity and specificity of viral isolation techniques [13]. Li et al. [14] reported a nanobeads amplified QCM immunosensor with polyclonal antibody as the recognition ligand for detection of AIV H5N1.

In recent years, aptamers have been investigated as an alternative of sensing elements, which have the potential to replace the antibodies. This is possible due to the unique features of aptamers (sensitivity, specificity, reusability, stability, nonimmunogenicity), which can be easily exploited in biosensor technology. Aptamers are single-stranded RNA or DNA oligonucleotides which rely on hydrogen bonding, electrostatic and hydrophobic interactions rather than Watson-Crick base pairing for recognition to their target. Aptamers can fold into distinct secondary and tertiary structures, bind to their targets with high affinity (dissociation constants on the order of nano- to picomolar), and recognize their targets with a specificity that challenges antibodies and other biological ligands. They are selected in vitro through systematic evolution of ligands by exponential enrichment (SELEX). The selection procedure involves the iterative isolation of ligands out of the random sequence pool with affinity for a defined target molecule and PCR-based amplification of the selected RNA or DNA oligonucleotides after each round of isolation. As biorecognition ligands, aptamers possess numerous advantages, including small size, rapid and reproducible synthesis, simple and controllable modification to fulfill different diagnostic and therapeutic purposes, slow degradation kinetics, nontoxicity, and a lack of immunogenicity.

The majority of aptamers developed for AIVs have focused on inhibition of the hemagglutinin protein preventing viral infection. For example, a DNA aptamer was developed by Jeon and co-workers [15]. RNA aptamers that inhibit membrane fusion of AIV H3N2 and influenza B virus hemagglutinin also were developed [16, 17]. DNA and RNA aptamers that target HA1 proteins of influenza virus hemagglutinin subtype H5 were investigated in two different studies [18, 19]. An aptamer that binds efficiently to the HA of highly pathogenic AIV H5N1 and H7N7 was studied by Suenaga and Kumar [20], which inhibits HA-glycan interactions. These aptamers were developed to inhibit function of the hemagglutinin protein and prevent or treat influenza infection. Based on the function and likely binding sites of these aptamers, it seems unlikely these aptamers would be optimal sequences to use in a biodetection assay. A DNA aptamer for avian influenza H5N1 was developed by Wang et al. [21] using a combination of protein and whole virus targets. It is unique in its binding affinity in that it specifically targets the H5N1 subtype, having no binding activity with other H5 or N1 subtype viruses. This suggests that the binding site be at an intersection of the H5 and N1 proteins.

Aptamer-based QCM biosensors, also called QCM aptasensors, have been developed for the detection of AIVs. Brockman et al. [22] studied a QCM aptasensor for detection of AIV H5N1 using magnetic nanobeads labels as mass amplifiers. The biosensor was found to have a lower detection limit of 1 HAU, although the detection time was reduced by half compared to a similar QCM biosensor using antibodies [14]. A hydrogel-based QCM aptasensor (**Figure 5**) was able to detect AIV H5N1 at 0.0128 HAU in 30 min [9]. The QCM aptasensor was based on swelling of the hydrogel after AIV H5N1 capture due to dissolution of the cross-linked aptamers and ssDNA in the hydrogel polymer. The developed aptasensor was both rapid and sensitive.

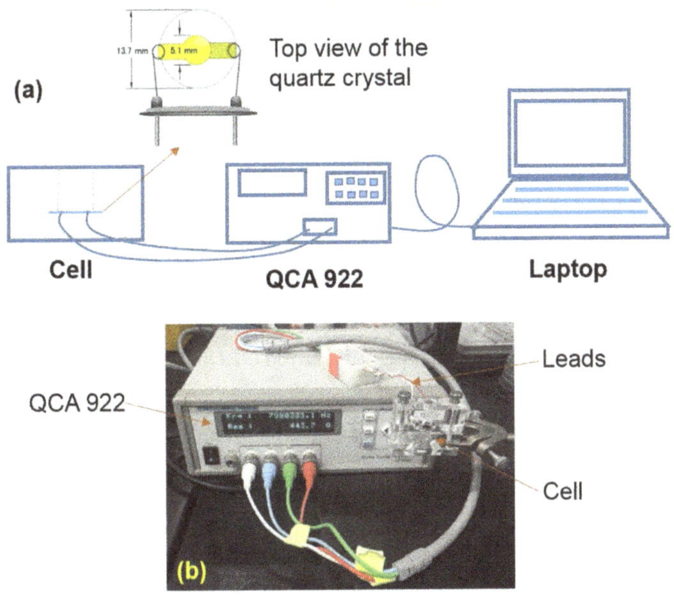

Figure 5. (a) Schematic of the QCM aptasensor; (b) a photograph of the QCM aptasensor setup. The aptamer hydrogel is immobilized on the gold electrode surface. The quartz in the electrode acts as a transducer, converting the mass and viscosity change to a frequency signal.

Influenza virus specificity for the host is mediated by the viral surface glycoprotein hemagglutinin (HA), which binds to receptors containing glycans with terminal sialic acids. This molecular recognition process leads to the host cell-virus adhesion stage [23]. The sialic acid receptor of various influenza virus strains differs in affinity to sialic acids terminally linked either in α(2,3) or α(2,6) position to the galactose (Gal) residues. Human influenza A viruses preferentially recognize the α(2,6)-linkage, while avian viruses have preference for the α(2,3)-linkage [24, 25]. Each monovalent sialic acid-binding site of HA is weak, with dissociation constants in the millimolar range, while the high virus-cell affinity is due to multivalency.

Takahashi and co-workers [26] demonstrated kinetics of HA binding to sulfatide and ganglioside GD1a by QCM analysis. QCM analysis showed that the HA bound with the K_d of 1.44×10^{-8} M to sulfatide immobilized on a sensor chip, which indicated that sulfatide directly binds to the ectodomain of HA with high affinity. N-Acetylglucosamine (GlcNAc) is a natural ligand and is part of the oligosaccharide ligand responsible for the influenza virus binding first step. In a report by Wangchareansak et al. [27], GlcNAc was employed as bioreceptor immobilized on QCM gold sensor surface for detection of influenza A virus (H5N3, H5N1, H1N3), which displayed high binding affinity with K_a values of 2.03×10^{10}, 4.35×10^{10}, and 2.56×10^{12} M, respectively.

QCM biosensor has advantages, such as simplicity, cost-effectiveness, real-time output, and direct detection. But there also exists some disadvantages, such as the lack of stability, difficulty with sensor surface regeneration, loss of the immobilized ligands after multiple washing and regeneration, nonspecific binding of other nontarget biomaterials, and relatively long incubation time. Further improvements are required to address these limitations before the QCM biosensor technology can be routinely employed for AIVs detection.

2.2. Optical biosensors

Optical biosensors rely on visual phenomena to detect the interaction between the biological element and the target analyte. Examples of optical biosensors include surface plasmon resonance (SPR), absorption, luminescence, and fluorescent sensors. Detection by optical biosensors can occur in two ways: by the analyte directly affecting the optical properties of the sensing environment, such as in SPR or absorption methods, or by the analyte being tagged with a label that produces an optical phenomenon, such as in fluorescence methods. Optical biosensors, which are sometimes referred to as "optodes," have received considerable interest in the detection of AIVs. The main analytical features of optical biosensors for detection of AIVs are summarized in **Table 2** [3, 28–38]. The target "virus" in **Table 2** is the entire virus particle and target "HA" is the HA protein or recombinant HA protein of virus.

Influenza subtype	Target	Bioreceptor	Sensitivity	Sensor	Labelling method	Reference
H1N1	Virus	Glycan	45.6×10^{-13} M	SPR	Label-free	[29]
H3N2	HA	Antibody	1 nM	Waveguide	Dye	[32]
H5N1	HA	Glycan	K_d 1.6×10^{-9} M	SPR	Label-free	[30]
H5N1	Virus	Aptamer	0.128 HAU	SPR	Label-free	[31]
H1N1	HA	Aptamer	K_d 67 fM	SPR	Label-free	[28]
H3N2	Virus	Antibody	0.2 HAU/ml	Prism-free SPR	Fluorescent	[33]
H3N2	Virus	Antibody	–	Waveguide	Gold nanoparticles	[3]
H9N2	Virus	Antibody	8.94 ng/ml	Nanobioprobe coupled with immunomagnetic beads, Fluorescent		[36]
H7 subtype	HA gene	Oligonucleotide probe	7 pM	Luminescence resonance energy transfer (LRET)		[37]
H1N1	Virus	Antibody	1.0×10^{-13} g/ml	Silver nanoparticles labeled antibodies with indirect fluorescence		[35]
H5N1	HA	Aptamer	2 ng/ml (buffer); 3.5 ng/ml (human serum)	Silver nanoparticles; Fluorescent		[34]
H1N1 H3N2	Virus	Antibody	0.1 pg/ml 50 pfu/ml	Gold nanoparticle-decorated carbon nanotubes; photoluminescence		[38]

Table 2. A list of optical biosensors reported for the detection of AIVs.

Various modes of optical measurement exist (i.e., absorption, reflection, fluorescence, chemiluminescence, and phosphorescence); however, biosensors based on surface plasmon resonance (SPR) and fluorescence principles are the most common and promising methods for AIVs detection.

The Kretschmann configuration [39] is the most popular optical setup for SPR applications. SPR biosensors measure the change in refractive index due to binding of biomolecules near the sensor surface. Refractive index is defined as the ratio of the speed of light in vacuum and the phase velocity of light in the medium. SPR is one of very few techniques that are able to provide noninvasive, real-time kinetic data on association, and dissociation rates, along with equilibrium binding constants for receptor or ligand systems. Estmer-Nilsson et al. [40] were able to utilize SPR to quantify influenza virus for vaccine production via an antibody inhibition assay using HA proteins immobilized on the sensor surface. Some research showed SPR biosensors for avian influenza DNA hybridization [41], adamantane binding sites in the influenza A M2 ion channel [42], influenza virus hemagglutinin monitoring [43], and binding kinetics study [44]. Studies by Gopinath et al. [28] revealed that SPR-based biosensor is a useful tool for detection of human and avian influenza viruses.

SPR-based Biacore technology has been designed to investigate biomolecular interactions, which was initiated in 1984. The commercial available systems include Biacore 1000, Biocore 3000, BIAlite, and Biacore T100. Biacore is the dominant SPR technique used for AIVs detection. The main advantage of this technology is its capacity to monitor weak macromolecular interactions that cannot be detected by other sensors and its subject ability to automation. SPR was used to evaluate the binding of influenza A virus H1N1 directly to a neomembrane of bovine brain lipid or an egg yolk lecithin fraction [29] and to monitor the interactions between influenza HA and glycan [30] or apatmers [28]. However, Biacore instruments are expensive and need proper maintenance. Bai and co-workers [31] have shown that a portable hand-held SPR-based biosensor (Spreeta™, Texas Instruments, Dallas, TX, USA) (**Figure 6**) can be employed for the detection of AIV H5N1. The fabrication of the SPR biosensor was based on the streptavidin-biotin binding. The streptavidin was directly adsorbed on the gold surface, and then, biotinylated ssDNA aptamers were immobilized. Target AIVs were captured by the immobilized aptamers and resulted in an increase in the refraction index. It was able to detect AIV H5N1 in poultry swab samples with a lower detection limit of 0.128 HAU in 1.5 h.

The working principle of a waveguide mode sensor is similar to that of a SPR sensor. The only difference is that the measurement is conducted using a waveguide mode rather than a surface mode [32]. Based on the properties of light-guiding and dimensions, there are two general classes, fiber optical waveguides and planar waveguides, which can be further divided into single mode and multimode [45]. Waveguide mode biosensors were developed using antibody as bioreceptor for the detection of HA from H3N2 [32] and H3N2 virus [3].

Of the optical methods requiring labels for detection, fluorescence is the most widely studied [34–36, 46, 47]. Fluorescence measurements are of particular interest in biosensor systems due to their high sensitivity. Commonly used labels in fluorescent biosensors are dyes, quantum dots (QDs), and fluorescent proteins, with the latter two becoming more popular as they are further researched [46]. A fluorescent aptasensor was developed by Pang and co-workers [34] for detection of AIV H5N1. The Ag@SiO_2 core-shell nanoparticles were coated with the anti-HA aptamers. The binding of aptamer-HA protein formed a G-quadruplex complex, which captured thiazole orange (TO) and reported the fluorescent signal of TO. Moreover, it caused a surface plasmon resonance enhancement and performed as a metal-enhanced fluorescence sensing. The detection of HA protein of the AIV H5N1 could be operated both in aqueous buffer and human serum with the detection limit of 2 and 3.5 ng/mL, respectively. The total detection time was only 30 min. Using antibodies as bioreceptors, Li et al. [35] developed a highly sensitive fluorescent immunosensor for detection of H1N1, which was based on Ag autocatalysis. It had a detection range of 1.0×10^{-12} to 1.0×10^{-8} g/ml with a detection limit of 10^{-13} g/ml.

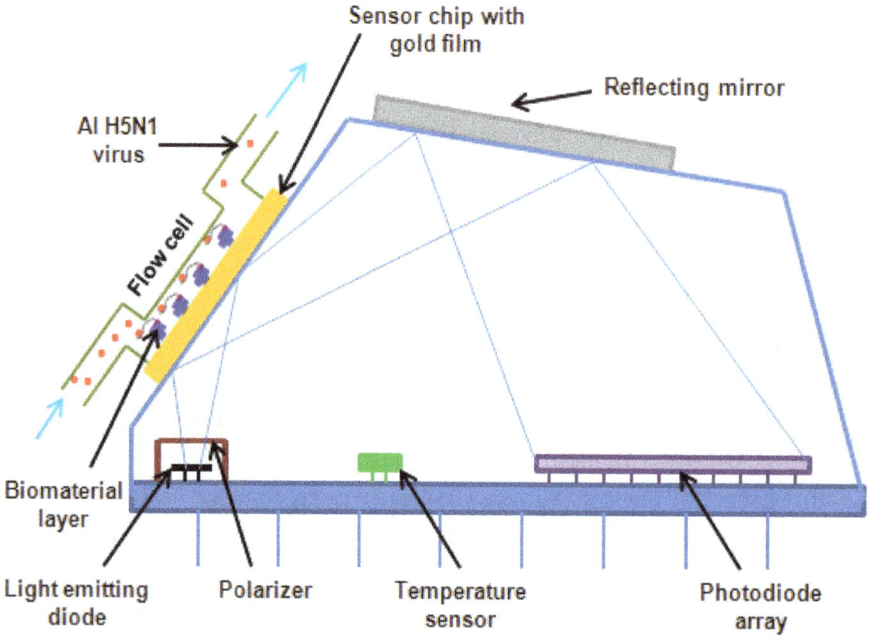

Figure 6. Configuration for measuring AIV H5N1using the portable SPR aptasensor (with permission from MDPI).

Fluorescence resonance energy transfer (FRET) is used in the design of a biosensor, which is based on the energy transfer between two light-sensitive molecules, a donor and an acceptor chromophore. In the nucleic acid-based FRET method, a reporter and a quencher are conjugated at the terminals of a nucleic acid probe. Without the target, the duplex is formed, bringing these two molecules in close proximity, which results in fluorescence quenching. The present of a target can cause the conformational change of the probe, which changes the position of the reporter and quencher and emits fluorescence. A QD-induced FRET system was developed by Chou and Huang [47] using two oligonucleotides. These two oligonucleotides were designed to specifically recognize two regions of the AIV H5 sequences and were employed as the capturing and reporter probes, respectively. They were conjugated to QD655 (donor) and Alexa Fluor 660 dye (acceptor), respectively. At target concentrations ranging from 0.5 nM to 1 μM, the QD emission decreased at 653 nm and dye emission increased at 690 nm. Another luminescence resonance energy transfer (LRET)-based biosensor was developed by Ye et al.

[37] for rapid and ultrasensitive detection of AIV H7 subtype. In this work, BaGdF5:Yb/Er upconversion nanoparticles (UCNPs) and gold nanoparticles (AuNPs) were used as the pair of donor and acceptor. The oligonucleotides with H7 HA gene sequence were conjugated with thiol and then were assembled on the AuNPs surfaces. The complementary sequence probes were modified with amino group and then were covalently bond to poly(ethylenimine) modified BaGdF5:Yb/Er UCNPs. The hybridization process brought these two molecules in close proximity, resulting in fluorescence quenching.

QDs are a type of semiconductor with a diameter typically between 2 and 10 nm whose excitons are confined in three spatial dimensions, giving them properties of both unconfined semiconductors and discrete molecules. In comparison with organic dyes and fluorescent proteins, QDs have unique optical and electronic properties including size-tunable light emission, improved signal brightness, high resistance against photobleaching, and simultaneous excitation of multiple fluorescence colors. QD-based bioconjugates used for optical sensing could dramatically increase the sensitivity that would permit simultaneous measurement of several targets. Lee and co-workers [38] developed a plasmon-assisted fluoro-immunosensor by the conjugation of antibody onto the surface of cadmium telluride QDs and the Au nanoparticle-decorated carbon nanotubes (AuCNTs) for the detection of H1N1 and H3N2. A detection limit of 0.1 pg/ml and 50 pfu/ml was obtained for H1N1 and H3N2, respectively.

Fluorescent biosensors are simple and show improved sensitivity and reduced detection time. But they have a drawback of requiring relatively expensive reagents. In order to apply the fluorescent biosensor for detection of real samples with complex background, such as tracheal and cloacal swabs from birds, further work would be required to combine an effective sample pretreatment method with the fluorescent biosensor for the detection of AIVs in the field.

2.3. Electrochemical biosensors

More than half of the biosensors used for the detection of AIVs are based on electrochemical transducers. Electrochemical biosensors use changes in the electrical properties caused by biochemical reactions to detect an analyte [48]. Electrochemical transducers offer several advantages: low cost, high sensitivity, ease of miniaturization, independence from solution turbidity, low power requirements, and simplicity of use [49]. These characteristics make electrochemical detection methods highly attractive for field monitoring of infectious diseases and biological warfare agents. Electrochemical biosensors can be divided by the electrical parameter that they measure: amperometric, potentiometric, conductimetric, and impedimetric. Amperometric biosensors work by applying a constant potential across an electrode and measuring the current associated with either the reduction or oxidation of an electroactive species created by the interaction of the biological element and the analyte. Amperometric biosensors are often used with an enzyme capable of catalyzing the production of an ionic product and increasing the selectivity and the sensitivity [50]. Potentiometric biosensors gather data by converting a biological reaction into a potential signal with the use of ion-selective electrodes [51]. Conductimetric biosensors simply measure the conductivity change in a medium caused by the analytes. Impedimetric biosensors measure a combination of the resistive and capacitive or inductive properties of a material in response to a small amplitude sinusoidal excitation signal [52].

A detailed review of the electrochemical biosensors for detection of AIVs before year 2014 can be found in the paper by Grabowska et al. [53], which covered the electrochemical genosensors and electrochemical immunosensors for detection of AIVs. A total of 69 references were cited in their review paper. Within the context of this chapter, the electrochemical biosensors reported prior to 2014 are referred to the review paper by Grabowska et al. and the electrochemical biosensors reported in the years 2014 and 2015 plus some impedance biosensors not mentioned by Grabowska et al. are reviewed in detail.

Impedance biosensors are a class of electrical biosensors that measure the electrical impedance of an interface in AC steady state with constant DC bias conditions. This is accomplished by imposing a sinusoidal voltage at a given frequency and measuring the current. This measurement can be done over a range of frequencies or at a given frequency [54]. Many impedance biosensors utilize a capture probe on the detecting surface to hold the target molecule, thereby stabilizing the point of detection. Due to the ease of miniaturization, low energy usage and relatively low cost, impedance biosensors show promise for AIVs applications. Impedance biosensors can use a variety of biological sensing elements but the most commonly used are antibodies. When using antibodies as the biological element the biosensor is often referred to as an impedance immunosensor. Impedance immunosensors rely on the interaction of the antibody and the antigen to generate a detectable signal for the transducing element. This allows the immunosensor to detect either indirect or direct impedance measurements. Direct impedance measurement, or label-free detection, is dependent on monitoring the changes in the electrical properties of the sensing environment caused by the antibody-antigen interaction. A label-free detection method has several advantages over an indirect detection method, including reduced detection time, lower cost, and simpler detection protocol.

There are two general classes of impedance biosensors, Faradic and non-Faradic impedance biosensor, which have been used for the detection of AIV H5N1 or subtype H5. A Faradic impedance biosensor was developed by Wang and co-workers [55] using an interdigitated array microelectrode. Polyclonal antibody against H5 was oriented immobilized on the gold surface through protein A to capture target virus, and red blood cells (RBCs) were used as biolabels for signal amplification. The biosensor had a lower detection limit of 10^3 EID_{50} ml^{-1}. Wang et al. [10] also reported a non-Faradic impedance biosensor for H5N2 avian influenza detection, which was based on the combination of an immunomagnetic nanobeads separation and a microfluidic chip with an interdigitated array microelectrode. A lower detection limit of 10^3 EID_{50} ml^{-1} was achieved with detection time less than 1 h. Then, Lum et al. [56] further improved the non-Faradic impedance biosensor for H5N1 detection by a combination of immunomagnetic nanoparticles, a microfluidic chip, an interdigitated array microelectrode, and RBCs for signal amplification. The specificity of the biosensor was improved due to the use of anti-H5 as a capture antibody and anti-N1 as a detection antibody.

A miniaturized biosensor was developed by Diouani et al. [57] for the detection of H7N1. Polyclonal antibodies against AIV H7N1 were attached to a gold electrode using a self-assembled monolayer. The impedance measurement was carried out in the presence of a redox probe and inside a Faraday cage. The lower detection limit of this biosensor was determined to be 5 μg/ml of specific antigen. Hassen et al. [58] developed an impedance biosensor capable of quantifying influenza A virus in a media comprised of numerous other proteins and viruses. The biosensor had a lower detection limit of 8 ng/ml, even in the presence of nonspecific viruses and proteins.

In **Table 3**, the electrochemical biosensors developed for the detection of AIVs in year 2014 and 2015 are summarized [59–79].

Influenza subtype	Target	Bioreceptor	Sensitivity	Detection range	Reference
H1N1	Virus	Antibody	1 pfu/ml	1–10^4 pfu/ml	[65]
H5N1	HA	Antibody	2.2 pg/ml	4–20 pg/ml	[66]
H1N1	PB1-F2 protein	Antibody	0.42 nM (monomeric); 16 nM (oligomeric)	5 nM–1.5 μM (monomeric); 5 nM–0.5 μM (oligomeric)	[60]
H5N1	Virus	Antibody	2^{-15} HAU/50 μl	2^{-15}–2^{-8} HAU/50 μl	[67]
H5N2, H7N1, H1N1	M1 protein	Antibody	20 pg/ml (80–100 virus/μl)	–	[59]
H1N1	PB1-F2 protein	Antibody	0.42 nM	5 nM–1.5 μM	[61]
H5N1	Antibody	HA	2.1 pg/ml	4–20 pg/ml	[63]
H5N1	Antibody	HA	2.4 pg/ml	4–100 pg/ml	[64]
H7N9	Virus	Antibody	6.8 pg/ml	0.01–20 ng/ml	[68]
H5N1	Virus	Antibody	2^{-1} HAU/50 μl	2^{-1}–2^{4} HAU/50 μl	[62]
H5N1	Complementary DNA (20-mer); RNA (280-mer)	Complementary sequences probe	73 pM (DNA 20-mer); 0.87 pM (RNA 280-mer)	–	[71]
H5N1	Full length H5 gene	DNA probe	fM level	–	[69]
H5N1	Full length H5 gene	DNA probe	0.03 fM (20-mer ssDNA); 0.08 fM (ds DNA)	–	[70]
H7N9	A fragment of the HA gene sequence	DNA probe	100 fM	–	[72]
H7N9	A fragment of the HA	Primer and DNAzyme	9.4 fM	50 fM–100 pM	[73]

Influenza subtype	Target	Bioreceptor	Sensitivity	Detection range	Reference
	gene sequence				
H5N1	Virus	Aptamer	8×10^{-4} HAU/ 200 μl	0.001–1 HAU	[74]
H5N1	Virus	Aptamer	0.0128 HAU	0.0128–12.8 HAU	[78]
H5N1	Viral proteins	Aptamer-antibody pair	100 fM	100 fM–10 pM	[75]
H5N1	Virus	Aptamer	2^{-9} HAU	0.001–4 HAU	[77]
H5N1	HA	Glycan	–	–	[76]
H5N1	HA	Glycan	aM level	140 aM–14 nM	[79]

Table 3. A list of electrochemical biosensors reported in 2014 and 2015 for the detection of AIVs.

For the past two years, the immunosensors have been the dominant electrochemical biosensors for detection of AIVs [59–68]. For example, universal anti-M1 antibodies, which allow detection of all serotypes of influenza A virus, were used for the development of an universal immunosensor for detection of the influenza A virus. It showed similar sensitivity (80–100 virus particles/μl) to molecular methods [59]. Miodek and co-workers [60, 61] developed an electrochemical immunosensor, which was based on conductive polypyrrole modified with ferrocenyl groups as a redox marker for the detection of PB1-F2, a nonstructural accessory protein of influenza A virus. Lin et al. [62] demonstrated that an impedance immunosensor, which was based on low-cost microelectrodes and specific monoclonal antibodies for rapid detection of AIV H5N1 in chicken swabs. Studies by Jarocka and co-workers [63, 64] revealed that the immobilization of the recombinant His-tagged HA was able to detect antibodies against AIV H5N1 in hen serum.

Although electrochemical biosensors for avian influenza detection have mostly been investigated for whole virus or virus protein detection, some groups have developed biosensors for the detection of avian influenza nucleic acid sequences [69–73]. These biosensors are based on the use of nucleic acid probes, which bind to specific sequence in the influenza genome. Several genosensors have been studied for the detection of the full length H5 gene of AIV H5N1. In the study of genosensors by Grabowska et al. [69, 70], redox active compounds (such as cobalt porphyrins or 3-iron bis(dicarbollide) were conjugated with the DNA probes, which were very close to the electrode surface. These developed genosensors showed a sensitivity in the fM range. Malecka and co-workers [71] reported an AET/Phen-Epoxy/Fe(III)/(Phen-Epoxy-NH2-NC3)2 genosensor, which has a working principle similar to this already reported by Grabowska et al. [69]. The hybridization process caused the formation of the duplex structure on the electrode surface, which resulted in the thickness changes of the double layer at the interface between the electrode and solution.

A new trend in the development of biosensors is the use of nanomaterials which exhibit unique and attractive chemical, physical, and electronic properties. Various nanomaterials have been used as an electrode platform in highly sophisticated electroanalytical biosensing devices. The working electrodes (actual physical transducers) upon modification with these materials gain large effective surface area, high catalytic capabilities, and high conductivity. Thus, these transducers could act as effective mediators and facilitate electron transfer between an active site on the receptor and the electrode surface. Nanoparticles [74, 75], carbon nanotubes [65], magnetic nanobeads [68, 74], or quantum dots [76] enhance sensitivity and selectivity of the electrochemical detection. Among the variety of metal nanoparticles, gold nanoparticles (GNPs) have been extensively utilized in recent years, mainly because of their nanoscopic size, good conductivity, and biocompatibility. One of the most commonly used is single-walled (SW) or multiwalled (MW) carbon nanotubes (CNTs) as well as graphene and graphene nanosheets. Thanks to their fast electron transfer ability, mechanical strength, chemical stability, catalysis effect, and thermal and electrical conductivity, they are attracting greater interest than other applied technologies.

A magnetic nanobeads-based impedance aptasensor was designed and developed by Fu and co-workers [74] (**Figure 7**). Briefly, H5N1 aptamers were coated on the magnetic nanobeads (MBs) for specifically capturing target AIV H5N1. Then, bionanocomposites (BNCs) were added using Au nanoparticles (AuNPs) as carriers, which were conjugated with concanavalin A (ConA) and glucose oxidase (GOx). The BNCs attached on the captured target virus through ConA-glycan interaction formed a sandwich complex. Finally, the sandwich complex was transferred to a glucose solution, resulting in an efficient enzymatic reaction and the impedance decreased correspondingly on a screen-printed interdigitated array electrode. This method took advantages of the high efficiency of enzymatic catalysis and the high susceptibility of electrochemical impedance on the ion strength and endowed the aptasensor with high sensitivity.

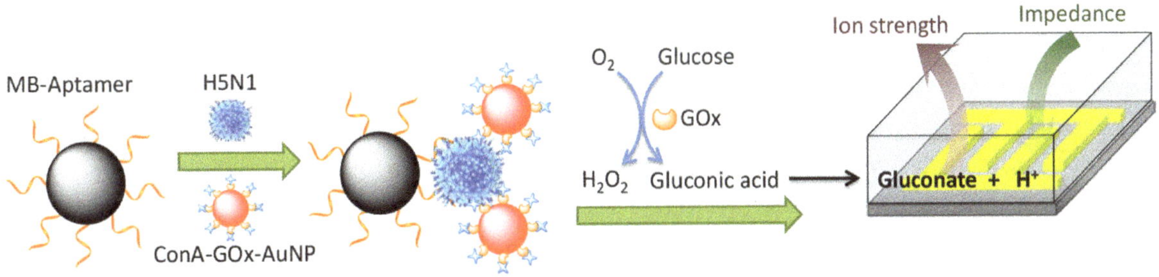

Figure 7. Illustration of the aptasensing mechanism and construction of the aptasensor (with permission from ACS).

Wang and co-workers [77] developed an aptamer-based bifunctional bionanogate, which could selectively respond to target molecules and control enzymatic reaction for electrochemical measurements (**Figure 8**). A nanoporous gold film with a pore size of ~20 nm was prepared by a metallic corrosion method and then was functionalized with two types of thiol-modified single-stranded oligos (SH-ssDNAs) by means of Au–thiolate bonding. The bases of the two immobilized SH-ssDNAs were selected to be partly complementary to that of the two ends of an aptamer, respectively. Then, aptamers were added and hybridized with the two immobilized SH-ssDNAs, resulting in the nanopore covered with aptamers, a "closed" bionanogate. Finally, the aptamer covered nanopore film was placed onto an enzyme precoated glassy carbon electrode to form an aptasensor. The working principle of the bionanogate-based aptasensor for detection of AIV H5N1 is illustrated in **Figure 8**. Initially, without the target AIV, the bionanogate was kept "closed," which isolated coenzymes and substrates in the testing solution from the enzymes immobilized on the electrode so that the enzymatic reaction was restricted (**Figure 8a**). Upon the target virus binding, the aptamers dissociated into solution from their ssDNAs and formed aptamer–virus complexes, which triggered the bionanogate "open" (**Figure 8b**). This "open" state allowed coenzymes and substrates to diffuse freely through the opened nanopore and to create contact with the immobilized enzymes, resulting in an efficient enzymatic reaction (**Figure 8c**).

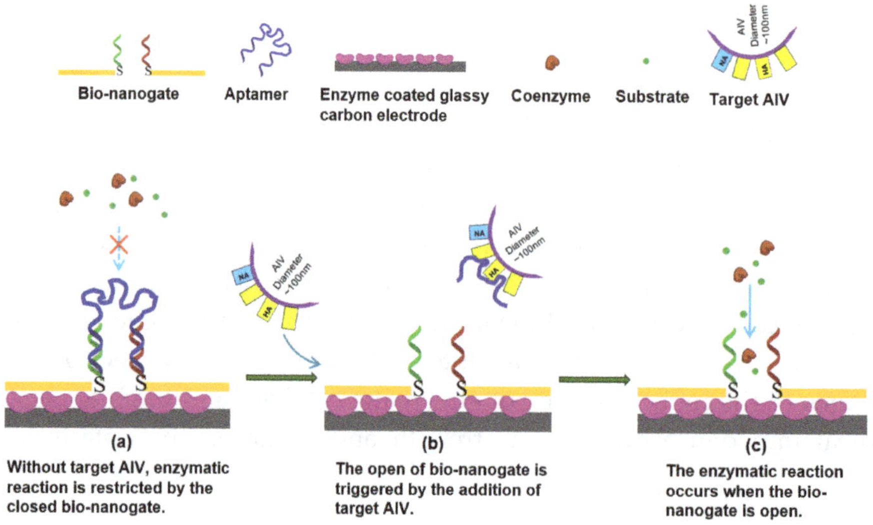

Figure 8. Principle of the bionanogate-based aptasensor for detection of AIV H5N1 (with permission from Elsevier).

Despite the remarkable sensitivity, rapid response, miniaturization capability, and low cost of the electrochemical biosensors for AIV detection, there are still problems with long-term stability and selectivity in real samples with complex background. Obviously, further work would be required to demonstrate that the electrochemical biosensors do not suffer from stability and selectivity problems when handling real samples in the field.

3. Conclusion

Biosensors have attracted tremendous interest in AIVs detection. They are characterized by good selectivity and sensitivity with a wide dynamic range from subfemtomolar to nanomolar, easy and rapid experimental protocol, reasonable cost, and usage of the sample volume in a μl range. Rapid development of nanotechnology has opened a new way for design and construction of biosensors with even better features. However, many contributions to the field of biosensors for AIVs detection still are at the "proof-of-concept" stage. Thus, authors hope that this chapter will promote lively and valuable discussions in order to generate new ideas and make new approaches toward the development of innovative biosensors for applications in AIVs detection.

Author details

Ronghui Wang[1,2] and Yanbin Li[1,2,3*]

*Address all correspondence to: yanbinli@uark.edu

1 College of Biosystems Engineering and Food Science, Zhejiang University, Hangzhou, China

2 Department of Biological and Agricultural Engineering, University of Arkansas, Fayetteville, AR, USA

3 Center of Excellence for Poultry Science, University of Arkansas, Fayetteville, AR, USA

References

[1] Murphy BR, Webster RG. Orthomyxoviruses. In: Fields, B.N., Knipe, D.M., Howley, P.M. editors. In Fields Virology. 3rd ed. Philadelphia, PA: Lippincott-Raven; 1996. p. 1397–1445.

[2] Lamb RA, Krug RM. Orthomyxoviridae. In: Knipe, D.M., Howley, P.M., editors. In Field Virology. Philadelphia, PA: Lippincott William & Wilkins Publisher; 2001. p. 1487–1531.

[3] Gopinath SC, Awazu K, Fujimaki M, Shimizu K. Evaluation of anti-A/Udorn/307/1972 antibody specificity to influenza A/H3N2 viruses using an evanescent-field coupled waveguide-mode sensor. PLoS One 2013;8(12):e81396. doi:10.1371/journal.pone.0081396

[4] Burns A, van der Mensbrugghe D, Timmer H. Evaluating the economic consequences of avian influenza. World Bank report [Internet]. 2008. Available from: http://siteresources.worldbank.org/EXTAVIANFLU/Resources/EvaluatingAHIeconomics_2008.pdf [Accessed: 2016-03-26]

[5] WHO. Cumulative number of confirmed human cases of avian influenza A (H5N1) reported to WHO, 2003–2015 [Internet]. 2016. Available from: http://www.who.int/influenza/human_animal_interface/2016_01_20_tableH5N1.pdf [Accessed: 2016-03-31]

[6] Clark LC, Jr., Lyons C. Electrode systems for continuous monitoring in cardiovascular surgery. Ann N Y Acad Sci 1962;102:29–45. doi:10.1111/j.1749-6632.1962.tb13623.x

[7] Turner AP. Biosensors-sense and sensitivity. Science 2000;290:1315–1317. doi:10.1126/science.290.5495.1315

[8] Amano Y, Cheng Q. Detection of influenza virus: traditional approaches and development of biosensors. Anal Bioanal Chem 2005;381(1):156–164. doi:10.1007/s00216-004-2927-0

[9] Wang R, Li Y. Hydrogel based QCM aptasensor for detection of avian influenza virus. Biosens Bioelectron 2013;42:148–155. doi:10.1016/j.bios.2012.10.038

[10] Wang R, Lin J, Lassiter K, Srinivasan B, Lin L, Lu H, Tung S, Hargis B, Bottje W, Berghman L, Li Y. Evaluation study of a portable impedance biosensor for detection of avian influenza virus. J Virol Methods 2011;178(1–2):52–58. doi:10.1016/j.jviromet.2011.08.011

[11] Jian YR, Chang SY, Lin PY, Yang YH, Chuang YH. Inactivated influenza virus vaccine is efficient and reduces IL-4 and IL-6 in allergic asthma mice. Influenza Other Respir Viruses 2013;7(6):1210–1217. doi:10.1111/irv.12150

[12] Owen TW, Al-Kaysi RO, Bardeen CJ, Cheng Q. Microgravimetric immunosensor for direct detection of aerosolized influenza A virus particles. Sens Actuators B Chem 2007;126:691–699. doi:10.1016/j.snb.2007.04.028

[13] Peduru-Hewa TM, Tannock GA, Mainwaring DE, Harrison S, Fecondo JV. The detection of influenza A and B viruses in clinical specimens using a quartz crystal microbalance. J Virol Methods 2009;162(1–2):14–21. doi:10.1016/j.jviromet.2009.07.001

[14] Li D, Wang J, Wang R, Li Y, Abi-Ghanem D, Berghman L, Hargis B, Lu H. A nanobeads amplified QCM immunosensor for the detection of avian influenza virus H5N1. Biosens Bioelectron 2011;26(10):4146–4154. doi:10.1016/j.bios.2011.04.010

[15] Jeon SH, Kayhan B, Ben-Yedidia T, Arnon R. A DNA aptamer prevents influenza infection by blocking the receptor binding region of the viral hemagglutinin. J Biol Chem 2004;279:48410–48419. doi:10.1074/jbc.M409059200

[16] Gopinath SC, Misono TS, Kawasaki K, Mizuno T, Imai M, Odagiri T, et al. An RNA aptamer that distinguishes between closely related human influenza viruses and inhibits haemagglutinin-mediated membrane fusion. J Gen Virol 2006;87(Pt 3):479–487. doi:10.1099/vir.0.81508-0

[17] Gopinath SC, Sakamaki Y, Kawasaki K, Kumar PK. An efficient RNA aptamer against human influenza B virus hemagglutinin. J Biochem 2006;139(5):837–846. doi:10.1093/jb/mvj095

[18] Cheng C, Dong J, Yao L, Chen A, Jia R, Huan L, et al. Potent inhibition of human influenza H5N1 virus by oligonucleotides derived by SELEX. Biochem Biophys Res Commun 2008;366(3):670–674. doi:10.1016/j.bbrc.2007.11.183

[19] Park SY, Kim S, Yoon H, Kim KB, Kalme SS, Oh S, et al. Selection of an antiviral RNA aptamer against hemagglutinin of the subtype H5 avian influenza virus. Nucleic Acid Ther 2011;21(6):395–402. doi:10.1089/nat.2011.0321

[20] Suenaga E, Kumar PK. An aptamer that binds efficiently to the hemagglutinins of highly pathogenic avian influenza viruses (H5N1 and H7N7) and inhibits hemagglutinin-glycan interactions. Acta Biomater 2014;10(3):1314–1323. doi:10.1016/j.actbio.2013.12.034

[21] Wang R, Zhao J, Jiang T, Kwon YM, Lu H, Jiao P, et al. Selection and characterization of DNA aptamers for use in detection of avian influenza virus H5N1. J Virol Methods 2013;189(2):362–369. doi:10.1016/j.jviromet.2013.03.006

[22] Brockman, L., Wang, R., Lum, L., Li, Y. QCM aptasensor for rapid and specific detection of avian influenza virus. O J Appl Biosens 2013;2:97–103. doi:10.4236/ojab.2013.24013

[23] Paulson JC. The Receptors. In: Conn M., editor. Orlando, FL: Academic Press; 1985. p. 131–219.

[24] Rogers GN, Paulson JC, Daniels RS, Skehel JJ, Wilson IA, Wiley DC. Single amino acid substitutions in influenza haemagglutinin change receptor binding specificity. Nature 1983;304(5921):76–78. doi:10.1038/304076a0

[25] Rogers GN, Paulson JC. Receptor determinants of human and animal influenza virus isolates: differences in receptor specificity of the H3 hemagglutinin based on species of origin. Virology 1983;127(2):361–373. doi:10.1016/0042-6822(83)90150-2

[26] Takahashi T, Kawagishi S, Masuda M, Suzuki T. Binding kinetics of sulfatide with influenza A virus hemagglutinin. Glycoconj J 2013;30(7):709–716. doi:10.1007/s10719-013-9477-7

[27] Wangchareansak T, Sangma C, Ngernmeesri P, Thitithanyanont A, Lieberzeit PA. Self-assembled glucosamine monolayers as biomimetic receptors for detecting WGA lectin and influenza virus with a quartz crystal microbalance. Anal Bioanal Chem 2013;405(20):6471–6478. doi:10.1007/s00216-013-7057-0

[28] Gopinath SC, Kumar PK. Aptamers that bind to the hemagglutinin of the recent pandemic influenza virus H1N1 and efficiently inhibit agglutination. Acta Biomater 2013;9(11):8932–8941. doi:10.1016/j.actbio.2013.06.016

[29] Critchley P, Dimmock NJ. Binding of an influenza A virus to a neomembrane measured by surface plasmon resonance. Bioorg Med Chem 2004;12:2773–2780. doi:10.1016/j.bmc.2004.02.042

[30] Suenaga E, Mizuno H, Penmetcha KK. Monitoring influenza hemagglutinin and glycan interactions using surface plasmon resonance. Biosens Bioelectron 2012;32(1):195–201. doi:10.1016/j.bios.2011.12.003

[31] Bai H, Wang R, Hargis B, Lu H, Li Y. A SPR aptasensor for detection of avian influenza virus H5N1. Sensors (Basel) 2012;12(9):12506–12518. doi:10.3390/s120912506

[32] Gopinath SC, Awazu K, Fujimaki M. Detection of influenza viruses by a waveguide-mode sensor. Anal Methods 2010;2:1880–1884. doi:10.1039/C0AY00491J

[33] Nomura K, Gopinath SC, Lakshmipriya T, Fukuda N, Wang X, Fujimaki M. An angular fluidic channel for prism-free surface-plasmon-assisted fluorescence capturing. Nat Commun 2013;4:2855. doi:10.1038/ncomms3855

[34] Pang Y, Rong Z, Wang J, Xiao R, Wang S. A fluorescent aptasensor for H5N1 influenza virus detection based-on the core-shell nanoparticles metal-enhanced fluorescence (MEF). Biosens Bioelectron 2015;66:527–532. doi:10.1016/j.bios.2014.10.052

[35] Li Y, Hong M, Qiu B, Lin Z, Chen Y, Cai Z, et al. Highly sensitive fluorescent immunosensor for detection of influenza virus based on Ag autocatalysis. Biosens Bioelectron 2014;54:358–364. doi:10.1016/j.bios.2013.10.045

[36] Xiong LH, Cui R, Zhang ZL, Yu X, Xie Z, Shi YB, et al. Uniform fluorescent nanobioprobes for pathogen detection. ACS Nano 2014;8(5):5116–5124. doi:10.1021/nn501174g

[37] Ye WW, Tsang MK, Liu X, Yang M, Hao J. Upconversion luminescence resonance energy transfer (LRET)-based biosensor for rapid and ultrasensitive detection of avian influenza virus H7 subtype. Small 2014;10(12):2390–2397. doi:10.1002/smll.201303766

[38] Lee J, Ahmed SR, Oh S, Kim J, Suzuki T, Parmar K, Park SS, Lee J, Park EY. A plasmon-assisted fluoro-immunoassay using gold nanoparticle-decorated carbon nanotubes for monitoring the influenza virus. Biosens Bioelectron 2015;64:311–317. doi:10.1016/j.bios. 2014.09.021

[39] Kretschmann E. The determination of the optical constants of metals by excitation of surface plasmons. Z Phys 1971;241:313–337.

[40] Estmer-Nilsson C, Abbas S, Bennemo M, Larsson A, Hämäläinen MD, Frostell-Karlsson Å. A novel assay for influenza virus quantification using surface plasmon resonance. Vaccine 2010;28:759–766. doi:10.1016/j.vaccine.2009

[41] Kim SA, Byun KM, Kim K, Jang SM, Ma K, Oh Y, et al. Surface-enhanced localized surface plasmon resonance biosensing of avian influenza DNA hybridization using subwavelength metallic nanoarrays. Nanotechnology 2010;21(35):355503. doi: 10.1088/0957-4484/21/35/355503

[42] Rosenberg MR, Casarotto MG. Coexistence of two adamantane binding sites in the influenza A M2 ion channel. Proc Natl Acad Sci USA 2010;107(31):13866–13871. doi: 10.1073/pnas.1002051107

[43] Mandenius CF, Wang R, Alden A, Bergstrom G, Thebault S, Lutsch C, et al. Monitoring of influenza virus hemagglutinin in process samples using weak affinity ligands and

surface plasmon resonance. Anal Chim Acta 2008;623(1):66–75. doi:10.1016/j.aca.2008.06.005

[44] Hidari KI, Shimada S, Suzuki Y, Suzuki T. Binding kinetics of influenza viruses to sialic acid-containing carbohydrates. Glycoconj J 2007;24(9):583–590. doi:10.1007/s10719-007-9055-y

[45] Schmitt K, Hoffmann C. Optical guided-wave chemical and biosensors I. In: Zourob, M., Lakhtakia, A., editors. Springer Series on Chemical Sensors and Biosensors. Berlin Heidelberg. Springer-Verlag; 2010. p. 21.

[46] Medintz IL, Uyeda HT, Goldman ER, Mattoussi H. Quantum dot bioconjugates for imaging, labelling and sensing. Nat Mater 2005;4(6):435–446. doi:10.1038/nmat1390

[47] Chou CC, Huang YH. Nucleic acid sandwich hybridization assay with quantum dot-induced fluorescence resonance energy transfer for pathogen detection. Sensors (Basel) 2012;12(12):16660–16672. doi:10.3390/s121216660

[48] Grieshaber D, MacKenzie R, Vörös J, Reimhult E. Electrochemical biosensors – sensor principles and architectures. Sensors 2008;8:1400–1458. doi:10.3390/s8031400

[49] Pejcic B, De Marco R, Parkinson G. The role of biosensors in the detection of emerging infectious diseases. Analyst 2006;131(10):1079–1090. doi:10.1039/b603402k

[50] Lojou E, Bianco P. Application of the electrochemical concepts and techniques to amperometric biosensor devices. J Electroceramics 2006;16:79–91. doi:10.1007/s10832-006-2365-9

[51] Koncki R. Recent developments in potentiometric biosensors for biomedical analysis. Anal Chim Acta 2007;599(1):7–15. doi:10.1016/j.aca.2007.08.003

[52] Varshney M, Li Y. Interdigitated array microelectrodes based impedance biosensors for detection of bacterial cells. Biosens Bioelectron 2009;24(10):2951–2960. doi:10.1016/j.bios.2008.10.001

[53] Grabowska I, Malecka K, Jarocka U, Radecki J, Radecka H. Electrochemical biosensors for detection of avian influenza virus-current status and future trends. Acta Biochim Pol 2014;61(3):471–478.

[54] Daniels JS, Pourmand N. Label-free impedance biosensors: opportunities and challenges. Electroanalysis 2007;19(12):1239–1257. doi:10.1002/elan.200603855

[55] Wang R, Wang Y, Lassiter K, Li Y, Hargis B, Tung S, et al. Interdigitated array microelectrode based impedance immunosensor for detection of avian influenza virus H5N1. Talanta 2009;79(2):159–164. doi:10.1016/j.talanta.2009.03.017

[56] Lum J, Wang R, Lassiter K, Srinivasan B, Abi-Ghanem D, Berghman L, et al. Rapid detection of avian influenza H5N1 virus using impedance measurement of immunoreaction coupled with RBC amplification. Biosens Bioelectron 2012;38(1):67–73. doi:10.1016/j.bios.2012.04.047

[57] Diouani MF, Helali S, Hafaid I, Hassen WM, Snoussi MA, Ghram A, Jaffrezic-Renault N, Abdelghani A. Miniaturized biosensor for avian influenza virus detection. Materials Sci Engr C 2008;28:580–583. doi:10.1016/j.msec.2007.10.043

[58] Hassen WM, Duplan V, Frost E, Dubowski JJ. Quantitation of influenza A virus in the presence of extraneous protein using electrochemical impedance spectroscopy. Electrochim Acta 2011;56:8325–8328. doi:10.1016/j.electacta.2011.07.009

[59] Nidzworski D, Pranszke P, Grudniewska M, Krol E, Gromadzka B. Universal biosensor for detection of influenza virus. Biosens Bioelectron 2014;59:239–242. doi:10.1016/j.bios.2014.03.050

[60] Miodek A, Vidic J, Sauriat-Dorizon H, Richard CA, Le Goffic R, Korri-Youssoufi H, et al. Electrochemical detection of the oligomerization of PB1-F2 influenza A virus protein in infected cells. Anal Chem 2014;86(18):9098–9105. doi:10.1021/ac5018056

[61] Miodek A, Sauriat-Dorizon H, Chevalier C, Delmas B, Vidic J, Korri-Youssoufi H. Direct electrochemical detection of PB1-F2 protein of influenza A virus in infected cells. Biosens Bioelectron 2014;59:6–13. doi:10.1016/j.bios.2014.02.037

[62] Lin J, Wang R, Jiao P, Li Y, Li Y, Liao M, et al. An impedance immunosensor based on low-cost microelectrodes and specific monoclonal antibodies for rapid detection of avian influenza virus H5N1 in chicken swabs. Biosens Bioelectron 2015;67:546–552. doi: 10.1016/j.bios.2014.09.037

[63] Jarocka U, Sawicka R, Góra-Sochacka A, Sirko A, Zagórski-Ostoja W, Radecki J, Radecka H. Electrochemical immunosensor for detection of antibodies against influenza A virus H5N1 in hen serum. Biosens Bioelectron 2014;55:301–306. doi: 10.1016/j.bios.2013.12.030

[64] Jarocka U, Sawicka R, Stachyra A, Gora-Sochacka A, Sirko A, Zagorski-Ostoja W, et al. A biosensor based on electroactive dipyrromethene-Cu(II) layer deposited onto gold electrodes for the detection of antibodies against avian influenza virus type H5N1 in hen sera. Anal Bioanal Chem 2015;407(25):7807–7814. doi:10.1007/s00216-015-8949-y

[65] Singh R, Sharma A, Hong S, Jang J. Electrical immunosensor based on dielectrophoretically-deposited carbon nanotubes for detection of influenza virus H1N1. Analyst 2014;139(21):5415–5421. doi:10.1039/c4an01335b

[66] Jarocka U, Sawicka R, Gora-Sochacka A, Sirko A, Zagorski-Ostoja W, Radecki J, et al. An immunosensor based on antibody binding fragments attached to gold nanoparticles for the detection of peptides derived from avian influenza hemagglutinin H5. Sensors (Basel) 2014;14(9):15714–15728. doi:10.3390/s140915714

[67] Xie Z, Huang J, Luo S, Xie Z, Xie L, Liu J, et al. Ultrasensitive electrochemical immunoassay for avian influenza subtype H5 using nanocomposite. PLoS One 2014;9(4):e94685. doi:10.1371/journal.pone.0094685

[68] Wu Z, Zhou CH, Chen JJ, Xiong C, Chen Z, Pang DW, Zhang ZL. Bifunctional magnetic nanobeads for sensitive detection of avian influenza A (H7N9) virus based on immu-

nomagnetic separation and enzyme-induced metallization. Biosens Bioelectron 2015;68:586–592. doi:10.1016/j.bios.2015.01.051

[69] Grabowska I, Singleton DG, Stachyra A, Gora-Sochacka A, Sirko A, Zagorski-Ostoja W, et al. A highly sensitive electrochemical genosensor based on Co-porphyrin-labelled DNA. Chem Commun (Camb) 2014;50(32):4196–4199. doi:10.1039/c4cc00172a

[70] Grabowska I, Stachyra A, Gora-Sochacka A, Sirko A, Olejniczak AB, Lesnikowski ZJ, et al. DNA probe modified with 3-iron bis(dicarbollide) for electrochemical determination of DNA sequence of Avian Influenza Virus H5N1. Biosens Bioelectron 2014;51:170–176. doi:10.1016/j.bios.2013.07.026

[71] Malecka K, Stachyra A, Gora-Sochacka A, Sirko A, Zagorski-Ostoja W, Dehaen W, et al. New redox-active layer create via epoxy-amine reaction—the base of genosensor for the detection of specific DNA and RNA sequences of avian influenza virus H5N1. Biosens Bioelectron 2014;65C:427–434. doi:10.1016/j.bios.2014.10.069

[72] Dong S, Zhao R, Zhu J, Lu X, Li Y, Qiu S, Jia L, Jiao X, Song S, Fan C, Hao R, Song H. Electrochemical DNA biosensor based on a tetrahedral nanostructure probe for the detection of avian influenza A (H7N9) virus. ACS Appl Mater Interfaces 2015;7(16): 8834–8842. doi:10.1021/acsami.5b01438

[73] Yu Y, Chen Z, Jian W, Sun D, Zhang B, Li X, Yao M. Ultrasensitive electrochemical detection of avian influenza A (H7N9) virus DNA based on isothermal exponential amplification coupled with hybridization chain reaction of DNAzyme nanowires. Biosens Bioelectron 2015;64:566–571. doi:10.1016/j.bios.2014.09.080

[74] Fu Y, Callaway Z, Lum J, Wang R, Lin J, Li Y. Exploiting enzyme catalysis in ultra-low ion strength media for impedance biosensing of avian influenza virus using a bare interdigitated electrode. Anal Chem 2014;86(4):1965–1971. doi:10.1021/ac402550f

[75] Diba FS, Kim S, Lee HJ. Amperometric bioaffinity sensing platform for avian influenza virus proteins with aptamer modified gold nanoparticles on carbon chips. Biosens Bioelectron 2015;72:355–361. doi:10.1016/j.bios.2015.05.020

[76] KrejcovaL,NejdlL,RodrigoMA,ZurekM,MatousekM,HynekD,etal.3Dprintedchipfor electrochemical detection of influenza virus labeled with CdS quantum dots. Biosens Bioelectron2014;54:421–427.doi:10.1016/j.bios.2013.10.031

[77] Wang R, Xu L, Li Y. Bio-nanogate controlled enzymatic reaction for virus sensing. Biosens Bioelectron 2015;67:400–407. doi:10.1016/j.bios.2014.08.071

[78] Lum J, Wang R, Hargis B, Tung S, Bottje W, Lu H, et al. An impedance aptasensor with microfluidic chips for specific detection of H5N1 avian influenza virus. Sensors (Basel) 2015;15(8):18565–18578.doi:10.3390/s150818565

[79] Hushegyi A, Bertok T, Damborsky P, Katrlik J, Tkac J. An ultrasensitive impedimetric glycan biosensor with controlled glycan density for detection of lectins and influenza hemagglutinins.ChemCommun(Camb)2015;51(35):7474–7477.doi:10.1039/c5cc00922g

8

The Impact of Adjuvanted and Non-Adjuvanted Influenza Vaccines on the Innate and Adaptive Immunity Effectors

Mikhail Petrovich Kostinov,
Nelli Kimovna Akhmatova,
Ekaterina Alexandrovna Khromova,
Svetlana Anatolyevna Skhodova,
Vera Nikolaevna Stolpnikova,
Alexander Petrovich Cherdantsev and
Anna Egorovna Vlasenko

Abstract

To date, the advantage of adjuvanted over non-adjuvanted vaccines in the specific antibodies formation is proved. However, cellular mechanisms, including parameters of the innate immunity, involved in the vaccine-induced immune response are not well studied. The human study of inactivated vaccines showed that both subunit vaccine and split vaccine induced cellular immune response, but adjuvanted vaccine containing Polyoxidonium had the greatest potential. Despite the fact that influenza vaccines must activate endosomal receptors, they cause non-specific activation of the surface TLRs. They can trigger intracellular signals leading to the induction of antiviral mechanisms and to the activation of the body's protective resources against microbial infections. To assess the immunological efficacy of adjuvanted vaccines and humoral reactions to vaccination it is necessary to evaluate activation of cellular mechanisms of innate and adaptive immunity.

Keywords: influenza vaccines, adjuvanted influenza vaccine, lymphocyte subpopulations, toll-like receptors

1. Introduction

Vaccination is the most effective means of preventing influenza and consequently reducing incidence and severity of complications. Modern influenza vaccines include a live attenuated, inactivated (whole-virion, split-virion and subunit) vaccines. Currently, inactivated split and subunit vaccines are used for influenza prevention as the safest ones and stimulating the production of a protective level of strain-specific virus-neutralizing antibodies to the globular domain of hemagglutinin protein and neuraminidase protein of contemporary serotypes of the influenza virus. These vaccines protect against infection with the appropriate antigenic variants of influenza virus. Not all inactivated vaccines have been reported to be effective enough for certain categories of vaccinated people [1–7]. Some of them are not able to protect against drift variants of influenza virus [8–11].

Due to the continuous antigenic drift of influenza viruses and the emergence of pandemic influenza viruses, the study of influenza vaccines causing broader protective immunity is of great interest [12]. In this regard, before influenza pandemic of 2009–2010 vaccination with adjuvanted vaccines began, aiming to enhance the synthesis of specific antibodies. In addition, given poor population health in the modern era, there is the need to enhance the efficacy of vaccines meant to activate all the components of the immune system. According to the literature data, adjuvanted vaccines seem to have such effect. However, a small number of human studies to investigate, how adjuvanted vaccine influence cellular immunity and activate of not only adaptive, but also innate immunity, have been conducted. In addition, unlike foreign adjuvanted influenza vaccines developed in 2009–2010, the National Immunization Calendar of the Russian Federation for more than 20 years applies polymer-subunit influenza vaccine containing immunomodulator PO as the adjuvant. Furthermore, immunomodulators have long been used in vaccination practice for immunocompromised patients in the Russian Federation. Immunomodulator use to support the vaccination was shown to promptly enhance the synthesis of specific antibodies and significantly decrease the incidence of respiratory infections in the postvaccinal period [13–15].

To date, the vaccine immunogenicity is assessed according to the requirements of the European Committee for influenza vaccines [16], and must meet at least one of the three criteria:

- seroconversion (percentage of subjects with a fourfold increase in antibody titers after vaccination)—at least 40%;
- seroprotection (percentage of subjects with a protective antibody titers before and 21–28 days after vaccination)—at least 70% and
- multiplicity factor for the increase of antibody titers compared to baseline—at least 2.5.

Taking into account a new type of vaccine (adjuvanted), not only humoral, but also cellular immune response is important for the evaluation of immunological efficacy. The activation of cellular immunity parameters, important to the formation of immunological memory, may differ from that of non-adjuvanted vaccines.

The aim of the study was to examine the effect of immunoadjuvant-containing and non-adjuvanted influenza vaccines on the immunophenotype of healthy donor lymphocytes and the number of cells with toll-like receptor expression *in vitro.*

2. Materials and methods

2.1. Clinical characteristics of patients

An open-label non-randomized monocenter study enrolled 27 healthy women of childbearing potential (aged 18–40 years) without co-morbidities who were not influenza-vaccinated within the previous 3 years and acquired no influenza or influenza-like illnesses within the previous 6 months.

2.2. Legal basis of the study

Once the signed informed consent for study participation was obtained, venous blood samples were drawn from volunteers with all applied aseptic and antiseptic techniques met and in accordance with the Study Protocol approved in 2015 by the Ethics Committee at the Mechnikov Research Institute of Vaccines and Sera. The study was conducted at the certified laboratory of the Mechnikov Research Institute of Vaccines and Sera (Moscow) using modern reagents and equipment.

2.3. Distribution pattern of lymphocyte subpopulations

The distribution pattern of peripheral blood lymphocyte subpopulations *in vitro* in healthy women exposed to influenza vaccine was tested by flow cytometer FC-500 (Beckman Coulter, USA), using anti-CD45/CD3, anti-CD45/CD3/CD4, anti-CD45/CD3/CD8, anti-CD16/56, anti-CD3/CD16/56, anti-CD45/CD20, anti-CD8/HLA-DR, anti-CD3/HLA-DR, anti-CD45/CD25, and anti-CD4/CD25/Foxp3 FITC- and PE-labeled monoclonal antibodies mAbs (Beckman Coulter, USA).

2.4. Toll-like receptors

The concentration of granulocytes with TLR expression was evaluated by flow cytometer FC-500 (Beckman Coulter, USA) using anti-TLR2, anti-TLR 3, anti-TLR4, anti-TLR6, anti-TLR8, and anti-TLR9 mAbs (eBioscience, USA).

Mononuclear WBCs were isolated from the whole blood using Ficoll-Urografin density gradients. We incubated 10^6 cells/mL in RPMI-1640 complete growth medium (PanEco, Russia) with 10% FBS (PanEco, Russia) and antibiotic (streptomycin) in the presence of 10 μL of a corresponding vaccine for 72 hours.

2.5. Study vaccines

Influvac ("Abbott biologicals" B.V., Netherlands) – inactivated subunit influenza vaccine, Vaxigrip ("Sanofi Pasteur", France)– inactivated split-virion influenza vaccine for influenza prevention. These vaccines contain hemagglutinin of the influenza virus type A subtypes A/H1N1 и A/H3N2 (15 μg each) and hemagglutinin of the influenza virus type B (15 μg). Grippol plus (LLC "NPO Petrovax Pharm," Russia) – trivalent polymer subunit inactivated influenza vaccine. It contains hemagglutinin of the influenza virus type A subtypes A/H1N1 и A/H3N2 and hemagglutinin of the influenza virus type B (5 μg each), and immunoadjuvant Polyoxidonium (500 μg). All the vaccines contained current influenza virus strains for epidemiological seasons 2015–2016 and 2016–2017.

Anti-influenza virus A/H1N1/California/07/09, p.149, A/H3N2/Switzerland/9715293/13 (subunit antigen), B/Phuket/3073/13, p. 25 (season 2015–2016); A/H1N1/California/07/09 p.124 till 01.17, A/H3N2/Hong Kong/4801/14 p.200, and B/Brisbane/60/08 p. 27 (season 2016–2017) **baseline serum antibody levels** were studied in volunteers using the standard method (MU 3.3.2 1758–03) for HAI assay. The 4+ system was applied to HAI assay: an antigen titer, i.e., 1 HAU, was highest antigen dilution giving complete hemagglutination of RBCs (3+ or 4+). In HAI assay the antigen working dose was the antigen dilution containing 4 hemagglutination units (4 HAU) in 0.2 mL.

2.6. Statistical analysis

Cell percentage difference between test groups was measured by a robust dispersion analysis of repeated measures (R Statistical Software, WRS2 package, rmanova function) with subsequent pairwise comparisons (R Statistical Software, WRS2 package, rmmcp function), the obtained significance level was corrected by Holm method [17]. Benjamini-Hochberg method was used to account for multiple comparison (false discovery rate control) [18]. The obtained data were described with the median and interquartile range.

3. Study results

First, we estimated vaccine effect on distribution pattern of lymphocyte subpopulations in PBMC cultures. Volunteers were divided into three groups according to the baseline antibody (AB) titers against the hemagglutin of the influenza virus A/H1N1, A/H3N2, and B: low AB titers (20–40 U) in the first group, medium AB titers (80–160 U) in the second group, and high AB titers (≥320 U) in the third group. Such differences in AB level indicate that influenza infection in the unvaccinated volunteers could have been masked under the guise of another infection, as all volunteers did not report previous influenza infection.

Immunophenotypic analysis showed changes in the number of T lymphocytes (CD45+/CD3+), NK cells (CD16+/56+), NKT cells (CD3 + CD16/56+), B lymphocytes (CD45+/CD20+), and activated cells (**Table 1**).

There were statistically significant differences ($F = 8.00$, $p < 0.001$, $q = 0.001$) in T lymphocytes (CD3+) distribution after incubation with different types of vaccines (**Figure 1**). It should be noted that regardless of the AB level vaccines did not have a significant effect on T lymphocyte number except subunit vaccine, which caused a decrease in the percent of T lymphocytes compared to control (PBMC culture without vaccine) while the absolute number did not change. These results may indicate a shift in the number of cells due to an increase in the number of other subpopulations.

Lymphocyte subpopulations	N	% in comparison groups – Me(Q1–Q3)				F	p	q
		Control	Subunit V	Adjuvanted V	Split-product V			
T lymphocytes (CD45/CD3+)	18	79.85 (74.17–83.35)	71.25 (64.7–79.75)	74.6 (66.38–79.17)	73.91 (66.92–78.22)	8.00	<0.001	0.001
Helper T cells (CD45/CD3/CD4+)	21	43.5 (41–49.8)	37.5 (32.7–43.8)	40.2 (31.8–46.5)	41.9 (35.6–47.7)	2.50	0.071	0.107
Cytotoxic T lymphocytes, CTL (CD45/CD3/CD8+)	21	23.5 (17.3–24.7)	21.2 (17.4–23.6)	22.5 (16.9–26.9)	21.5 (18.4–5.8)	0.64	0.533	0.601
Natural killer cells, NK cells (CD16/56+)	24	4.85 (4.175–5.9)	13.2 (11.15–14.85)	17.25 (15.93–18.25)	15 (13.8–16.25)	180.28	<0.001	<0.001
Natural killer T cells, NKT (CD3/CD16/56+)	24	1.6 (1.3–2.25)	3.6 (2.775–5.825)	7.5 (6.675–8.225)	5 (4.625–6.75)	57.52	<0.001	0.00001
B lymphocytes (CD45/CD20+)	24	5.15 (4.475–6.725)	16.36 (15.47–17.7)	21.15 (18.93–22.9)	18.1 (15.88–19.62)	167.44	<0.001	<0.001
Activated cytotoxic T lymphocytes, CTL(CD8/HLA-DR+)	20	0.4 (0.275–0.5)	0.7 (0.3–1.2)	1.6 (1.2–2.4)	1.35 (0.4875–1.975)	13.36	<0.001	<0.001
Activated T lymphocytes (CD3/HLA-DR+)	12	1.05 (0.65–1.65)	2.7 (1.875–3.375)	4.95 (3.775–7.1)	2.6 (1.9–3.575)	8.92	<0.001	0.002
Activated lymphocytes (CD45/CD25+)	16	1.45 (1–1.775)	3.7 (2.6–4.85)	4.15 (3.2–9.075)	4.15 (3.075–5.275)	12.94	<0.001	0.001
Regulatory T cells, Tregs (CD4/CD25/Foxp3+)	13	2.7 (1.7–2.9)	3.5 (3.2–4.9)	3.7 (3.2–5.5)	4.2 (2.2–4.5)	4.27	0.017	0.032
IRI (CD4/CD8)	20	1.825 (1.5–3.275)	1.85 (1.45–2.325)	1.85 (1.4–2.5)	1.65 (1.475–.525)	1.26	0.300	0.389

Note. Aliquots of 10 μL vaccines were added to cell suspensions (PBMC, 10^6 cells/mL). Cells were incubated for 72 hours at 37°C in 5% CO_2. The cells were then washed with RPMI-1640 at 1500 g for 10 min. Monoclonal antibodies against studied cell receptors were added in accordance with the manufacturer's instructions. The number of cells (%) in each sample was determined by flow cytometry.

Table 1. Distribution pattern of peripheral blood lymphocyte subpopulations incubated with influenza vaccines.

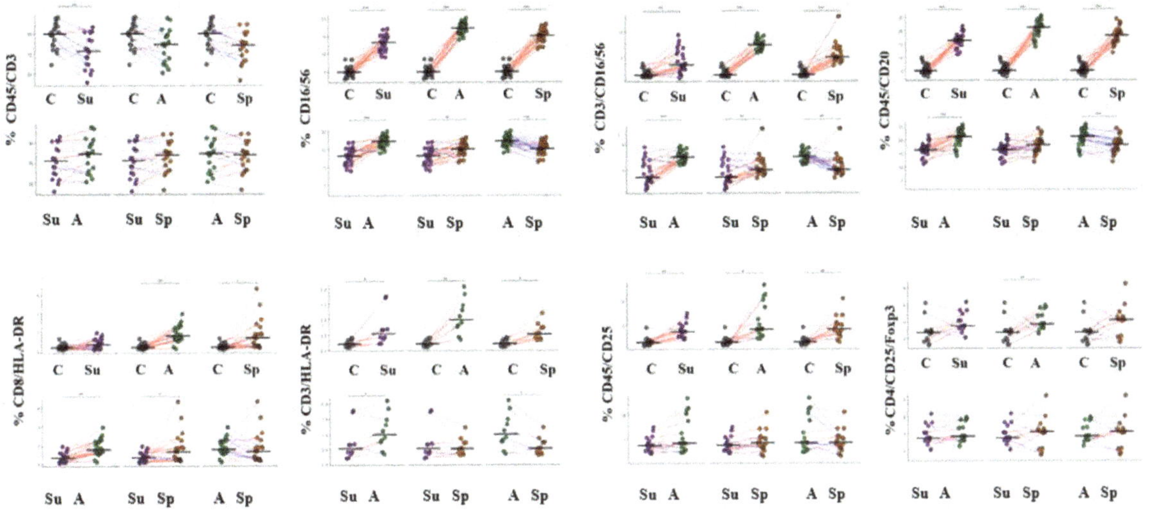

Figure 1. Lymphocyte count in PBMC culture after incubation with influenza vaccines. C = control; Su = inactivated subunit influenza vaccine; A = trivalent inactivated polymer-subunit influenza vaccine; Sp = inactivated split-product influenza vaccine.

The comparison of the T lymphocyte count between vaccines showed a significant decrease in the number of cells after incubation with subunit vaccine only (71.2% vs. 79.8% in control, $p = 0.008$) (**Figure 1**). However, the changes in the T lymphocyte (CD3+) number after incubation with different types of vaccines were observed only in women with medium AB level ($F = 6.40$, $p = 0.004$, $q = 0.007$). In this group, statistically significant differences were found for subunit vaccine (72 vs. 82.6% in control, $p = 0.022$) and split-product vaccine (74.8 vs. 82.6% in control, $p = 0.022$) (**Figure 2**).

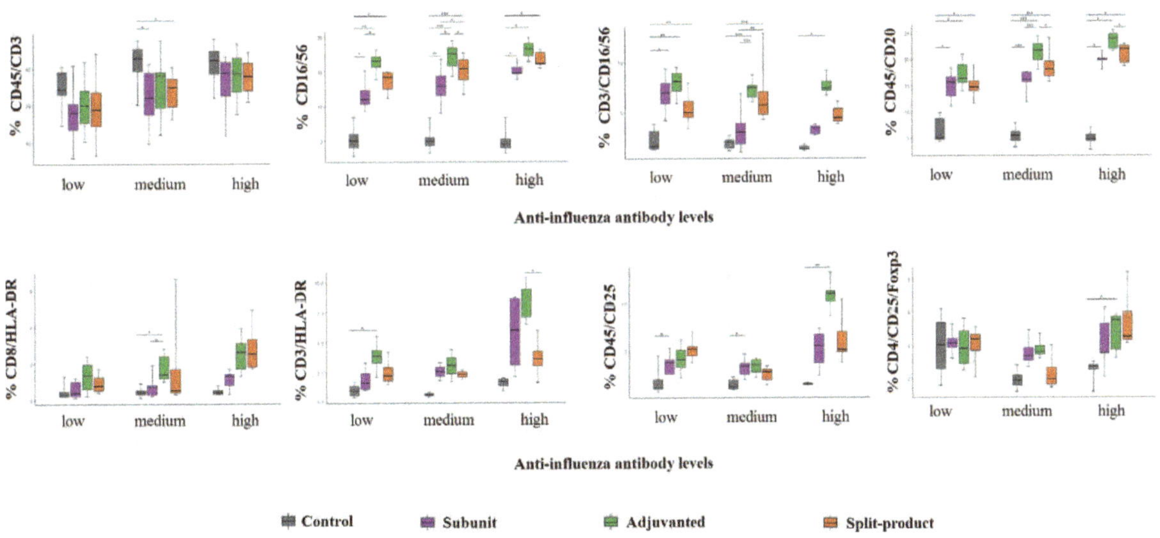

Figure 2. The impact of influenza vaccines on the lymphocyte count in PBMC cultures from volunteers with different antibody titers against the hemagglutinin of the influenza virus a/H1N1, a/H3N2, and B. Significant differences: *** $p < 0.001$, ** $p < 0.01$, * $p < 0.05$.

Analysis revealed significant changes ($F = 180.28$, $p < 0.001$, $q < 0.001$) in percent of natural killer cells (NK, CD16/56+) after incubation with different types of vaccines (**Table 1**, **Figure 1**). Regardless of the AB level there was an increase in number of NK cells from 4.8 (control) to 13.2% (subunit vaccine), 17.2% (adjuvanted vaccine), and 15% (split vaccine). There were statistically significant differences for subunit (13.2 vs. 4.8%, $p < 0.001$), adjuvanted (17.2 vs. 4.8%, $p < 0.001$), and split vaccines (15 vs. 4.8%, $p < 0.001$) compared to control, for subunit vaccine compared to adjuvanted (13.2% vs. 17.2%, $p < 0.001$) and split vaccines (13.2 vs. 15%, $p = 0.003$), and for adjuvanted vaccine compared to split vaccine (17.2 vs. 15%, $p < 0.001$). That means that incubation with influenza vaccines increased the number of NK cells in all cultures.

However, the changes in number of NK cells (CD16/56+) after incubation of PBMC with different types of vaccines were observed in all groups of volunteers, regardless of the baseline anti-influenza AB level ($F = 48.88$, $p < 0.001$, $q < 0.001$ – low AB level, $F = 103.04$, $p < 0.001$, $q < 0.001$ – medium AB level, $F = 89.09$, $p < 0.001$, $q < 0.001$ – high AB level) (**Figure 2**).In women with low anti-influenza AB level, percent of NK cells (CD16/56+) was significantly higher after incubation with subunit (11 vs. 5%, $p = 0.045$), adjuvanted (16.5% vs. 5%, $p = 0.001$), and split vaccines (14.2 vs. 5%, $p = 0.01$) compared to control. Immunoadjuvant-containing vaccine had a higher potential for elevation of NK cell number (3.3-fold increase) compared with subunit vaccine (2.2-fold increase) ($p = 0.017$).

In women with medium anti-influenza AB level, percent of NK cells (CD16/56+) was significantly higher after incubation with subunit (12.8 vs. 4.8%, $p = 0.001$), adjuvanted (17.5 vs. 4.8%, $p < 0.001$), and split vaccines (15.3 vs. 4.8%, $p < 0.001$) compared to control. This corresponds to a 2.6- to 3.6-fold increase. Immunoadjuvant-containing vaccine produced more pronounced increase compared to subunit vaccine (17.5 vs. 12.8%, $p = 0.029$) and split vaccine (17.5 vs. 15.3%, $p = 0.011$), and number of NK cells was significantly higher after incubation with split vaccine compared to subunit vaccine (15.3 vs.12.8%, $p = 0.029$).

In women with high anti-influenza AB level, percent of NK cells (CD16/56+) was significantly higher after incubation with subunit (14.8 vs. 4.4%, $p = 0.023$), adjuvanted (18.2 vs. 4.4%, $p = 0.046$), and split vaccines (16.1 vs. 4.4%, $p = 0.035$) compared to control. This corresponds to a 3.3-, 4.1-, and 3.6-fold increase, respectively. There were no statistically significant differences between various types of vaccines.

For NKT cells (natural killer T cells, CD3 + CD16/56+), following findings were revealed. Regardless of the AB level there were statistically significant changes ($F = 57.52$, $p < 0.001$, $q < 0.001$) in NKT cells distribution after incubation with different types of vaccines: for subunit (3.6 vs. 1.6%, $p = 0.006$), adjuvanted (7.5 vs. 1.6%, $p < 0.001$), and split vaccines (5 vs. 1.6%, $p < 0.001$) compared to control, for subunit vaccine compared to adjuvanted (3.6 vs. 7.5%, $p < 0.001$) and split vaccines (3.6 vs. 5%, $p = 0.007$), and for adjuvanted vaccine compared to split vaccine (7.5 vs. 5%, $p = 0.006$). Therefore, subunit vaccine caused a 2.2-fold increase in NKT cell number, adjuvanted vaccine caused a 4.6-fold increase, and split vaccine caused a 3.1-fold increase compared to control (**Table 1**, **Figure 1**).

An increase of NKT cell (CD3 + CD16/56+) number in all cultures was dependent of baseline anti-influenza AB level ($F = 22.08$, $p < 0.001$, $q < 0.001$ – low AB level, $F = 20.02$, $p < 0.001$, $q < 0.001$ – medium AB level, $F = 65.92$, $p < 0.001$, $q < 0.001$ – high AB level) (**Figure 2**).

In women with low anti-influenza AB level, NKT cell (CD16/56+) number was significantly higher after *in vitro* incubation with subunit (7 vs. 1.6%, $p = 0.033$), adjuvanted (8.1 vs. 1.6%, $p = 0.007$), and split vaccines (5 vs. 1.6%, $p = 0.005$) compared to control. There were no statistically significant differences between various types of vaccines.

In women with medium anti-influenza AB level, NKT cell number in PBMC cultures was significantly higher after incubation with adjuvanted vaccine compared to control (7.4 vs. 1.3%, $p < 0.001$) and subunit vaccine (7.4 vs. 3%, $p < 0.001$) (5.7- and 2.48-fold increase, respectively) and after incubation with split vaccine compared to control (4.4 vs. 1.3%, $p < 0.001$) and subunit vaccine (4.4 vs. 3%, $p = 0.009$) (3.38- and 1.46-fold increase, respectively).

In women with high anti-influenza AB level, percent of NKT cells (CD3 + CD16/56+) was significantly (4.6-fold) higher after incubation with adjuvanted vaccine compared to control (7.4 vs. 1.6%, $p = 0.043$).

Analysis also revealed statistically significant differences ($F = 167.44$, $p < 0.001$, $q < 0.001$) in B lymphocytes (CD45/CD20+) distribution after incubation of PBMC with different types of vaccines (regardless of the AB level): for subunit (16.3 vs. 5.1%, 3.1-fold increase, $p < 0.001$), adjuvanted (21.1 vs. 5.1%, 4.1-fold increase, $p < 0.001$), and split vaccines (18.1 vs. 5.1%, 3.5-fold increase, $p < 0.001$) compared to control, and for adjuvanted vaccine compared to subunit (21.1 vs. 16.3%, 1.3-fold increase, $p < 0.001$) and split vaccines (21.1 vs. 18.1%, 1.1-fold increase, $p < 0.001$). Therefore, adjuvanted vaccine was the most effective (**Table 1**, **Figure 1**).

Regardless of the AB level there was a significant increase in B lymphocyte number after incubation with different types of vaccines ($F = 24.09$, $p < 0.001$, $q < 0.001$ – low AB level, $F = 181.14$, $p < 0.001$, $q < 0.001$ – medium AB level, $F = 150.61$, $p < 0.001$, $q < 0.001$ – high AB level) (**Figure 2**). In women with low anti-influenza AB level, percent of B lymphocytes (CD20+) was significantly higher after incubation with subunit (15.6 vs. 5%, $p = 0.017$), adjuvanted (16.3 vs. 5%, $p = 0.046$), and split vaccines (14.7 vs. 5%, $p = 0.014$) compared to control. There were no statistically significant differences between various types of vaccines.

In women with medium anti-influenza AB level, percent of B lymphocytes (CD20+) was also significantly higher after incubation with all types of vaccines: subunit (16.2 vs. 5.3%, $p < 0.001$), adjuvanted (21.6 vs. 5.3%, $p < 0.001$), and split vaccines (18.1 vs. 5.3%, $p < 0.001$) compared to control. Immunoadjuvant-containing vaccine had the greatest potential for elevation of B lymphocyte number (21.6%) compared with subunit vaccine (16.2%, 1.3-fold increase) ($p < 0.001$) and split vaccine (18.1%, 1.2-fold increase) ($p = 0.013$).

In women with high anti-influenza AB level, there was a significant increase in B lymphocyte number after incubation with subunit (20 vs. 4.7%, $p = 0.021$), adjuvanted (23.6 vs. 4.7%, $p = 0.030$), and split vaccines (21.9 vs. 4.7%, $p = 0.030$) compared to control. Immunoadjuvant-containing vaccine induced higher (fivefold) increase of B lymphocyte number than split vaccine (4.6-fold, $p = 0.011$).

Analysis revealed statistically significant differences ($F = 13.36$, $p < 0.001$, $q < 0.001$) in the distribution of activated cytotoxic T lymphocytes (CD8/HLA-DR+) after incubation of PBMC with different types of vaccines (regardless of the AB level) (**Table 1**, **Figure 1**).

Immunoadjuvant-containing and split vaccines more effectively increased the number of this type of cells. There were statistically significant changes for subunit (1.6 vs. 0.4%, $p < 0.001$), adjuvanted (1.3 vs. 0.4%, $p = 0.050$), and split vaccines (1.6 vs. 0.7%, $p = 0.002$) compared to control, for adjuvanted vaccine compared to subunit vaccine (1.3 vs. 0.7%, respectively, $p = 0.046$), and for adjuvanted vaccine compared to split vaccine (4.9 vs. 2.6%, respectively, $p = 0.044$).

However, changes in the number of activated cytotoxic T lymphocytes *in vitro* between vaccine types were significant only in women with medium anti-influenza AB level ($F = 5.16$, $p = 0.020$, $q = 0.035$) (**Figure 2**). Incubation with adjuvanted vaccine caused significant increase of the number of activated cytotoxic T lymphocytes compared to control (1.4 vs. 0.4%, $p = 0.049$) and subunit vaccine (1.4 vs. 0.7%, $p = 0.047$).

Regardless of the AB level there were significant changes in the number of T lymphocytes with late activation marker (CD3/HLA-DR+) after incubation with different types of vaccines ($F = 8.92$, $p < 0.001$, $q = 0.002$) (**Table 1**, **Figure 1**). There were statistically significant changes for subunit (2.7 vs. 1%, $p < 0.044$), adjuvanted (4.9 vs. 1%, $p = 0.006$), and split vaccines (2.6 vs. 1%, $p = 0.010$) compared to control, and for adjuvanted vaccine compared to subunit (4.9 vs. 2.7%, $p = 0.015$) and split vaccines (4.9 vs. 2.6%, $p = 0.044$).

Statistically significant changes in the number of this type of cells were demonstrated only in women with low ($F = 30.17$, $p < 0.001$, $q < 0.001$) and high ($F = 12.49$, $p = 0.001$, $q = 0.003$) anti-influenza AB level (**Figure 2**). In women with low serum AB level, analysis of activated T lymphocytes showed significant activation by adjuvanted vaccine compared to control (3.8 vs. 0.9%, $p = 0.047$). In women with high serum AB level, the number of activated T lymphocytes was significantly higher after incubation with adjuvanted vaccine compared to split vaccine (8.2 vs. 3.5%, $p = 0.027$) (**Figure 2**).

For lymphocytes with early activation marker (CD45/CD25+), there was statistically significant increase ($F = 12.94$, $p < 0.001$, $q = 0.001$) after incubation of PBMC with different types of vaccines, regardless of the AB level (**Table 1**, **Figure 1**).All types of vaccines increased number of cells with early activation marker. Furthermore, there were statistically significant changes for subunit (3.7 vs. 1.4%, $p = 0.007$), adjuvanted (4.1 vs. 1.45%, $p = 0.049$), and split-product vaccines (4.1 vs. 1.4%, $p = 0.003$) compared to control. There were no statistically significant differences between various types of vaccines.

Regardless of the AB level there was a significant changes in the number of activated CD45/CD25+ lymphocytes. It was dependent of the vaccine type in all groups of volunteers ($F = 9.96$, $p = 0.002$, $q = 0.006$ – low AB level, $F = 7.92$, $p = 0.002$, $q = 0.005$ – medium AB level, $F = 25.89$, $p < 0.001$, $q < 0.001$ – high AB level) (**Figure 2**).

In women with low and medium AB level, percent of T lymphocytes with early activation marker (CD45/CD25+) was significantly increased after incubation of PBMC with subunit vaccine (3.8 and 3.3%, respectively) compared to control (1.1 and 1.2%, respectively) ($p = 0.024$ and $p = 0.036$). At the same time, in women with high AB level, the number of these cells was increased after incubation of PBMC with adjuvanted vaccine (11%) compared to control (1.5%) ($p = 0.009$).

Analysis also revealed significant changes (F = 4.27, p = 0.017, q = 0.032) in regulatory T cell (T-regs) number with CD4/CD25/Foxp3+ phenotype after incubation of PBMC with different types of vaccines, regardless of the AB level (**Table 1**, **Figure 1**). Immunoadjuvant-containing vaccine increased T-regs number compared to control (3.7 vs. 2.7%, 1.3-fold increase, p = 0.005). Other types of vaccines did not have a significant effect on these cells.

Significant changes in the number of T-regs between vaccine types were noted only in women with high AB level against influenza viruses A/H1N1, A/H3N2, and B (F = 8.15, p = 0.003, q = 0.006) (**Figure 2**).Incubation of PBMC with adjuvanted vaccine induced significant increase of T-regs count (CD25/CD4/Foxp3+) compared to control (5.5 vs. 2.7%, p = 0.049).

At the next step of the study we evaluated number of TLR-expressing granulocytes in PBMC cultures incubated with influenza vaccines.

All types of vaccines had immunostimulating effect on TLR-expressing cells by increasing the number of granulocytes expressing TLR 2,3,4,6,8, and 9, as shown in **Table 2**.

We found significant differences (F = 270.16, p < 0.001, q < 0.001) in the percent of granulocytes expressing TLR2 (**Table 2**, **Figure 3**) after incubation of PBMC with different types of vaccines, regardless of the AB level against the hemagglutinin of the influenza virus A/H1N1, A/H3N2 and B.. Subunit vaccine increased number of TLR2+ cells in PBMC culture from 16.6 (in control) to 38.2% (p < 0.001), adjuvanted vaccine—to 39.8% (p < 0.001), and split vaccine—to 37.5% (p < 0.001). However, there were no significant differences in TLR2 cell number between vaccine types.

Incubation of cell culture in the presence of influenza vaccines induced an increase in the number of TLR2+ granulocytes regardless of the baseline anti-influenza AB level (F = 53.25, p < 0.001, q < 0.001 – low AB level, F = 169.63, p < 0.001, q < 0.001 – medium AB level, F = 103.89, p < 0.001, q < 0.001 – high AB level) (**Figure 4**). In women with low AB level, the number

TLR	N	TLR-expressing granulocytes, %, Me (Q1-Q3)				F	p	q
		Control	Subunit	Adjuvanted	Split			
2	24	16.6 (14.2–18.38)	38.2 (36.45–40.05)	39.35 (37.73–42.4)	37.5 (35.38–39.27)	270.16	<0.001	<0.001
4	24	22.3 (19.75–25.4)	26.85 (25.23–29.43)	24.45 (22.15–26.9)	23.35 (21.5–25.35)	10.62	<0.001	<0.001
3	24	20.2 (18.23–22.95)	20 (18.02–24.05)	21.7 (19.5–23.05)	24.15 (21.95–25.95)	6.90	<0.001	<0.001
9	24	11.95 (9.825–12.85)	19.85 (17.95–25.2)	25.45 (24–26.32)	26.4 (24.48–28.23)	86.57	<0.001	<0.001
8	24	20.6 (18.68–22.4)	32.7 (30.12–35)	42.5 (37–45.1)	34.4 (29–37)	138.59	<0.001	<0.001
6	23	4.3 (4.05–5.15)	6.5 (5.95–7)	5.7 (5.2–6.9)	6.9 (5.95–7.55)	18.04	<0.001	<0.001

Table 2. Number of TLR-expressing granulocytes after incubation with influenza vaccines.

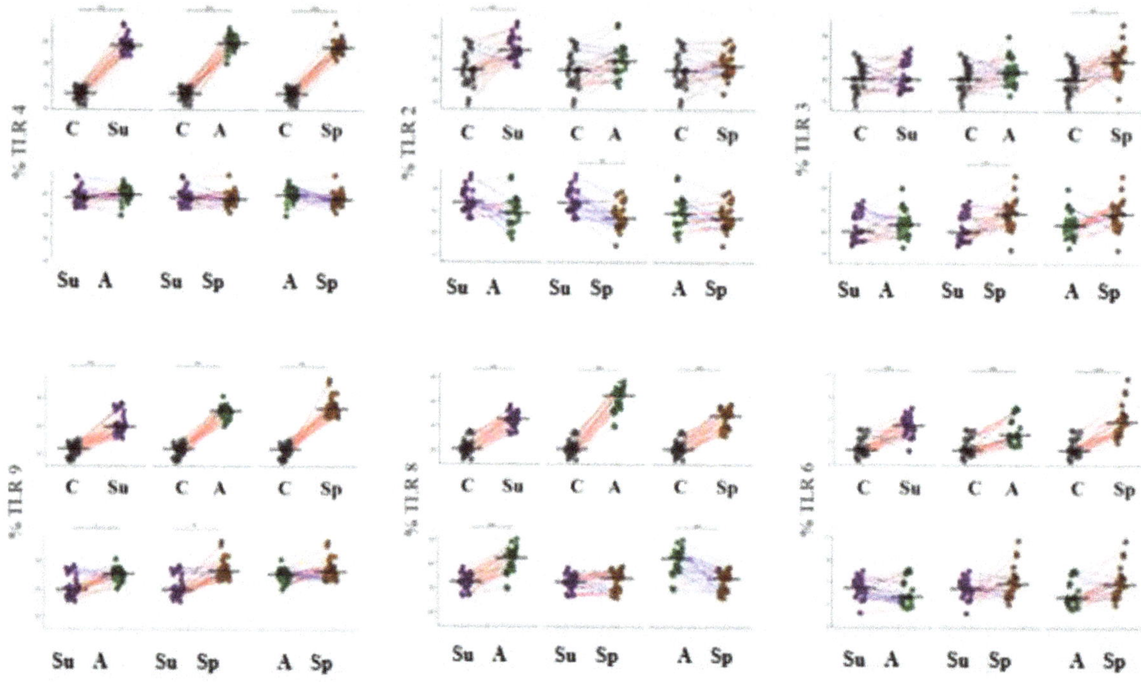

Figure 3. Number of TLR-expressing granulocytes in PBMC cultures incubated with influenza vaccines. C = control; Su = inactivated subunit influenza vaccine; A = trivalent inactivated polymer-subunit influenza vaccine; Sp = inactivated split-product influenza vaccine.

of TLR2-expressing granulocytes increased 2.4-fold after incubation with subunit vaccine ($p_h = 0.019$), 2.3-fold after incubation with adjuvanted vaccine ($p_h = 0.019$), and 2.2-fold after incubation with split vaccine ($p_h = 0.003$) compared with control.

In women with medium AB level, there was similar increase in the number of these cells: 2.3-fold for subunit and split vaccines ($p_h < 0.001$), and 2.4-fold for adjuvanted vaccine ($p_h = 0.001$) compared with control.

In women with high AB level, the number of TLR2-expressing granulocytes increased 2.6-fold after incubation with subunit vaccine ($p_h = 0.031$), 2.8-fold after incubation with adjuvanted vaccine ($p_h = 0.029$), and 2.7-fold after incubation with split vaccine ($p_h = 0.029$) compared with control.

Analysis revealed significant differences ($F = 10.62$, $p < 0.001$, $q < 0.001$) in the percent of granulocytes expressing TLR4 after incubation of PBMC with different types of vaccines, regardless of the AB level against the hemagglutinin of the influenza virus (**Table 2, Figure 3**). Subunit vaccine increased number of TLR4+ cells 1.2-fold compared to control ($p < 0.001$) and 1.1-fold compared to split vaccine ($p < 0.001$).

Statistically significant changes in the number of TLR4+ cells (**Figure 4**) between vaccine types were demonstrated only in women with medium AB level ($F = 5.24$, $p = 0.008$, $q = 0.010$): the number of these cells increased 1.1-fold after incubation with subunit vaccine compared to control ($p_h = 0.047$) and 1.2-fold compared to split vaccine ($p = 0.007$).

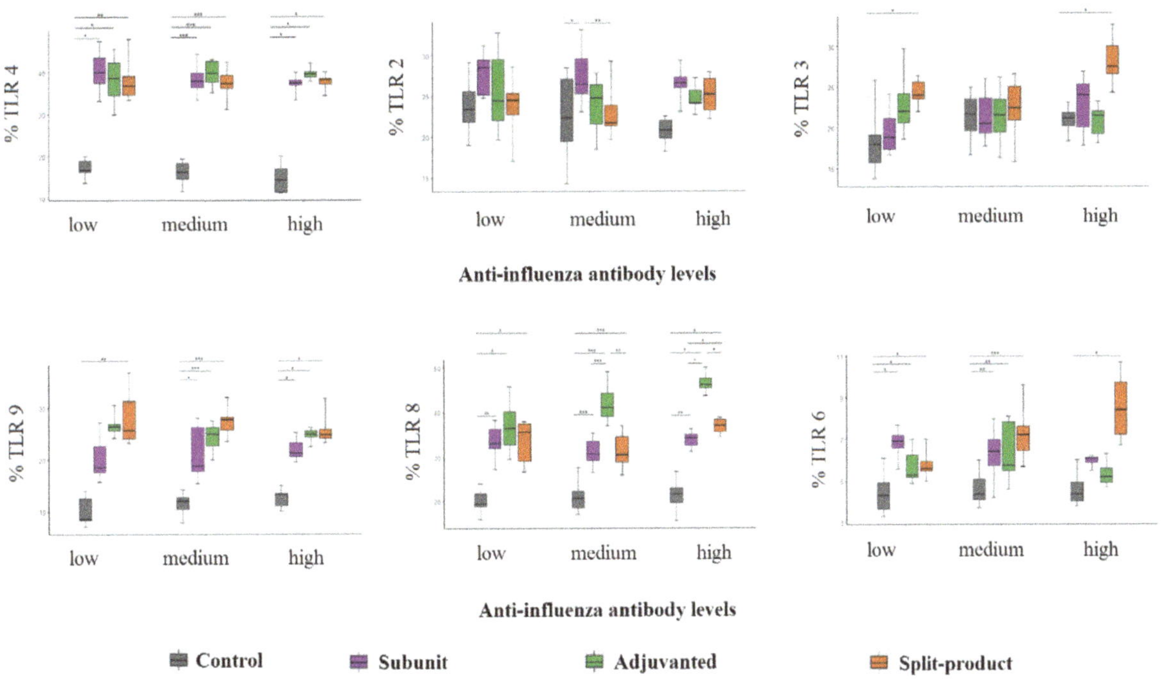

Figure 4. The impact of influenza vaccines on TLR-expressing granulocytes in PBMC cultures from volunteers with different AB titers against the hemagglutinin of the influenza virus A/H1N1, A/H3N2 and B.

Analysis of TLR3-expressing granulocytes (**Table 2**, **Figure 3**) revealed significant differences (F = 6.90, p < 0.001, q < 0.001) between groups, meaning that activation of the innate immunity effectors was dependent of the vaccine type, but not baseline AB level. There were significant differences for split vaccines compared to control (1.2-fold increase, p = 0.001) and subunit vaccine (1.2-fold increase, p = 0.008). That means that split vaccine had higher activity.

In women with low and high AB level, there were significant changes in the number of TLR3-expressing cells (**Figure 4**). The significance of differences was (F = 6.05, p = 0.025, q = 0.030) for low AB level and (F = 6.45, p = 0.008, q = 0.010) for high AB level. In women with low and high AB level, percent of TLR3-expressing granulocytes significantly increased after incubation with split vaccine (1.3-fold, $p_h = 0.042$ and $p_h = 0.050$, respectively) compared to control.

Analysis also revealed (**Table 2, Figure 3**) that different vaccines influenced (F = 86.57, p < 0.001, q < 0.001) the number of TLR9-positive cells regardless of the AB level. All types of vaccines increased the number of TLR9-expressing granulocytes in PBMC culture. Subunit vaccine caused 1.6-fold increase (p < 0.001), adjuvanted vaccine caused 2.1-fold increase (p < 0.001), and split vaccine caused 2.2-fold increase (p < 0.001) compared to control. Subunit vaccine was 1.2-fold less effective than adjuvanted vaccine (p = 0.012) and 1.3-fold less effective than split vaccine (p = 0.003).

Analysis showed that effect of different types of vaccines on TLR9-positive cells depended on the baseline AB level (F = 26.93, p < 0.001, q < 0.001 – low AB level; F = 39.81, p < 0.001, q < 0.001 – medium AB level; F = 29.41, p < 0.001, q < 0.001 – high AB level) (**Figure 4**). In women with low AB level, split vaccine induced threefold increase in the number of TLR9+ granulocytes compared to PBMC culture without stimulation ($p_h = 0.002$). However, in women with medium and high AB level, other types of vaccines stimulated TLR9+ granulocytes. There were following differences between vaccine types: subunit vaccine caused 1.6-fold increase ($p_h = 0.017$, $p_h = 0.050$), adjuvanted vaccine caused 2- and 1.8-fold increase ($p_h < 0.001$, $p_h = 0.040$), and split vaccine caused 2.3- and 1.8-fold increase ($p_h < 0.001$, $p_h = 0.050$) compared to control, respectively, in women with medium and high AB level.

Analysis of TLR8-expressing cells showed interesting results (**Table 2**, **Figure 3**). This receptor plays important role in recognition of viral single-stranded RNA. Analysis revealed a significant increase in the number of these cells in PBMC culture dependent on vaccine type ($F = 138.59$, $p < 0.001$, $q < 0.001$). All vaccines induced increase in the number of TLR8-positive granulocytes. This parameter increased 1.6-fold after incubation with subunit vaccine ($p < 0.001$), twofold after incubation with adjuvanted vaccine ($p < 0.001$), and 1.7-fold after incubation with split vaccine ($p < 0.001$) compared to control. Adjuvanted vaccine was 1.3-fold more effective than subunit vaccine ($p < 0.001$) and 1.2-fold more effective than split vaccine ($p < 0.001$).

Differences in the number of TLR8+ cells dependent on vaccine type were detected in all groups of volunteers, regardless of the baseline anti-influenza AB level ($F = 35.99$, $p < 0.001$, $q < 0.001$ – low AB level, $F = 76.10$, $p < 0.001$, $q < 0.001$ – medium AB level, $F = 116.13$, $p < 0.001$, $q < 0.001$ – high AB level) (**Figure 4**). In women with low, medium and high serum AB level, subunit vaccine induced 1.7-fold ($p_h < 0.001$), 1.5-fold ($p_h < 0.001$), and 1.6-fold ($p_h = 0.002$) increase, respectively, adjuvanted vaccine caused 1.9-fold ($p_h < 0.014$), twofold ($p_h < 0.001$), and 2.1-fold ($p_h = 0.014$) increase, respectively, and split vaccine caused 1.8-fold ($p_h < 0.029$), 1.5-fold ($p_h < 0.001$), and 1.7-fold ($p_h = 0.042$) increase of TLR8-expressing granulocyte number, respectively, compared to control. In women with medium and high serum AB level, immunoadjuvant-containing vaccine was, respectively, 1.3- and 1.2-fold more effective than split vaccine ($p_h = 0.002$ and $p_h = 0.042$), and 1.3-fold more effective than subunit vaccine ($p_h < 0.001$ и $p_h = 0.042$). In women with medium and high serum AB level, immunoadjuvant-containing vaccine was, respectively, 1.3- and 1.2-fold more effective than split vaccine ($p_h = 0.002$ and $p_h = 0.042$), and 1.3-fold more effective than subunit vaccine ($p_h < 0.001$ и $p_h = 0.042$).

Changes in the distribution of TLR6-expressing granulocytes were similar (**Table 2**, **Figure 3**). Analysis showed significant increase in the number of these cells in PBMC cultures dependent on vaccine type ($F = 18.04$, $p < 0.001$, $q < 0.001$). TLR6-expressing granulocyte number increased 1.5-fold after incubation with subunit vaccine, 1.3-fold after incubation with adjuvanted vaccine, and 1.6-fold after incubation with split vaccine compared to control ($p < 0.001$). However, there were no statistically significant differences between various types of vaccines.

Analysis also showed that effect of different types of vaccines on TLR6-positive cells depended on the baseline AB level ($F = 26.38$, $p < 0.001$, $q < 0.001$ – low AB level; $F = 11.71$, $p < 0.001$, $q < 0.001$ – medium AB level; $F = 16.57$, $p = 0.001$, $q = 0.001$ – high AB level) (**Figure 4**). In women with low and medium serum AB level, subunit vaccine induced 1.6-fold ($p_h = 0.043$) and 1.5-fold ($p_h = 0.004$) increase, respectively, adjuvanted vaccine caused 1.2-fold ($p_h = 0.032$) and 1.3-fold ($p_h = 0.004$) increase, respectively, and split vaccine caused 1.3-fold ($p_h = 0.027$) and 1.6-fold ($p_h < 0.001$) increase of TLR6-expressing granulocyte number, respectively, compared to control.

In women with high serum AB level, the number of TLR6-expressing granulocytes increased only after incubation with split vaccine ($p_h = 0.050$).

4. Discussion

Considering that inactivated influenza vaccines have a number of drawbacks (lack of efficacy in certain patients [1–7], no protection against drift influenza viruses [8–11]), there is a need for next generation vaccines to be developed. Besides, the effect many influenza vaccines have on the cellular and molecular immunologic mechanisms remains poorly studied.

The effects of inactivated influenza vaccines on key effectors of innate and acquired immunity are being investigated at the Mechnikov Research Institute of Vaccines and Sera (Moscow). Various types of influenza vaccines were selected for the study. First, their effect on distribution pattern of lymphocyte subpopulations was estimated *in vitro*.

Analysis of the vaccine effect on the immunophenotype of lymphocytes cultured for 72 hours, showed activation of the innate and acquired immunity effectors: NK cells (CD16/56), NKT cells (CD3/CD16/56), B lymphocytes (CD45/CD20), cells with early activation marker (CD45/CD25), T lymphocytes with late activation marker (CD3/HLA-DR), and regulatory T cells (Tregs, CD4/CD25/Foxp3). In view of this, below are characteristics of the cells that most actively responded to influenza vaccines added to PBMC culture.

Natural killer cells are essential to the innate immunity in influenza. Their function is to lyze tumor and virus-infected cells and to regulate innate and adaptive immune responses [19, 20]. Natural killer cells have been reported to identify influenza-infected cells through the NKp44 and NKp46 receptors that bind influenza hemagglutinin. Natural killer cells have also been reported to stimulate cellular immune response, regulate eosinophil maturation, and protect respiratory epithelium [21]. When interacting with peripheral mononuclear cells, PO, a component of the adjuvanted vaccine, significantly increases NK cells' cytotoxic effect on target cells. The phenomenon was observed almost in all donors examined, with the increased effect being especially pronounced in patients with the baseline activity of NK cells at the lower normal limit or decreased [22].

Being phenotypically heterogenous, NKT cells duplicate the functions of NK cells and link innate and acquired immunity [23].

Cytotoxic T lymphocytes identify and kill virus-infected cells. Infected cells present virus core antigens coupled to MHC class I molecules, which ensures their identification and subsequent killing by cytotoxic T lymphocytes [24, 25].

Specific cytotoxic lymphocytes cannot prevent cells from being initially infected with the virus, but they can restrict virus reproduction and enhance virus elimination out of the body. In unvaccinated adults, cytotoxic lymphocytes are crucial for clearing the body from influenza. They release perforin and stimulate apoptosis of virus-infected cells [26, 27].

Efficacy of influenza vaccines is currently assessed from their ability to activate the humoral immune response, as recommended in WHO guidelines. We think that this assessment does not adequately reflect the mechanisms of immune response to viruses. Therefore, it is essential to also study the cellular immunity. Immunodominance, which means that the immune system chooses one or more key epitopes for recognition, is an important factor for the development of vaccines stimulating the cellular immune response [28]. Vaccines aimed at producing cytotoxic T lymphocytes specific for an immunodominant epitope can significantly narrow the cross-reactive range of immune response to various virus strains. The role of antigen delivery route and presentation should also be considered when developing such vaccines. To stimulate a strong cytotoxic immune response, an antigen should be processed and presented by dendritic cells and coupled to MHC class I molecules. These may occur either at the moment dendritic cells are being infected or transduced or when dendritic cells engulf apoptotic bodies from other infected cells. Thus, the induction of cytotoxic immune response varies from strong one (with live attenuated vaccines) to a weaker, lower one (with inactivated whole-virion and subunit vaccines) [21].

B lymphocytes are among the key adaptive immunity effectors in influenza, since they produce anti-hemagglutinin (HA) (mainly against its globular domain) virus-neutralizing antibodies that prevent hemagglutinin from interacting with cellular receptors. Moreover, their Fc portion contributes to virion phagocytosis and to stimulation of antibody-dependent cellular cytotoxicity. HA amino acid sequence homology is about 80% between different strains within one subtype and 40–70% between strains of different subtypes. Besides, anti-neuraminidase antibodies have protective properties. They do not offer virus-neutralizing activity but they can inhibit neuraminidase enzymatic activity, which prevents the virus from spreading. Anti-neuraminidase antibodies also stimulate antibody-dependent cellular cytotoxicity. In addition, anti-neuraminidase antibodies have been shown to protect mice from H5N1 influenza virus [29].

Our study showed high stimulating effect of all studied influenza vaccines on B cell counts in PBMC culture. Adjuvanted vaccine was 1.3-fold more effective than subunit vaccine and 1.1-fold more effective than split vaccine. That means that adjuvanted vaccine activated B cell proliferation more effectively than the inactivated vaccines studied.

B cells were found to produce IgA, IgG, and IgM antibody isotypes in primary infection, while no production of IgM antibodies was observed in secondary infection. IgM antibodies are capable of activating the complement cascade as well as of neutralizing the virus [21, 29]. Secretory immunoglobulins A protect respiratory mucosae, through which influenza enters the body, and are indicative of recent virus exposure. Immunoglobulins G ensure the longest protection against influenza [21, 30].

Comparative analysis of the vaccines studied showed that adjuvanted vaccine is more effective in stimulating NK, NKT cells and Tregs, as well. The vaccine was 1.3- and 1.1-fold more effective than subunit and split vaccines in increasing NK cell count, 2.1- and 1.5-fold for NKT cell count, 1.3- and 1.16-fold for B lymphocyte count, and 1.5- and 1.2-fold for Treg count, respectively. The studied vaccines were not found to activate other cell types.

Natural thymus-derived regulatory cells (nTreg) of CD4 + CD25+ surface phenotype with constitutive expression of Foxp3 transcription factor responsible for their regulatory activity are one of the best documented cell population. Increased Treg number can possibly be explained by the immunoregulatory effect of PO (adjuvant)-containing vaccine. Immunoregulatory function of nTreg is implemented both through cytokine secretion, such as TGF-β and IL-10, and through contact interaction with the effector T lymphocytes and antigen-presenting cells [31, 32].

Innate immune mechanisms are key to protection against pathogens, since they ensure prompt inflammatory reactions including detection of highly conservative structures, which are common to many microorganisms, through special receptors of broad specificity. These are signal PRRs, and TLRs are the most important of them [33–36].

Having recognized a specific pattern, PRRs initiate a series of signal cascades, which make the first line of defense against microorganisms. Besides, these signals initiate maturation of dendritic cells, which prepare the second line of immune response to the infection, known as acquired immunity. Thus, TLRs contribute to the regulation of innate and acquired immunity. Currently known are 11 types of TLRs in humans and 13 types in mice [37, 38]. Four of them (TLR3, TLR7, TLR8, and TLR9) recognize virus RNA and DNA. TLRs have an established role in physiological regulation of pro-inflammatory cytokine production, which are required for immune response to infections caused by bacteria, fungi, and viruses [39]. Inflammation is known to be directly associated primarily with neutrophils, which express almost all identified TLRs, as it has been shown recently. This explains the importance of TLRs in neutrophil activity regulation: LPS-induced TLR4 activation induces the production of pro-inflammatory cytokines and chemokines (IL-1β, IL8, and TNFα); TLR2, TLR4, and TLR9 stimulation is accompanied by respiratory burst and changed expression of adhesion molecules [40, 41].

The study of the effect influenza vaccine has on TLR-positive cell (granulocyte) expression gave the following results.

Patients with initially different anti-influenza AT titers *in vitro* showed statistically significant differences in TLR3, TLR8, and TLR9-expressing cell counts, depending on the type of influenza vaccine added to leukocyte culture.

All the influenza vaccines studied, caused a statistically significant ($p < 0.05$) increase in TLR2-, TLR6-, TLR8-, and TLR9-positive granulocyte counts in PBMC culture, compared to non-stimulated cells.

Subunit vaccine showed statistically significant ($p < 0.001$) stimulating effect on the expression of TLR4-positive granulocytes, compared to control group and split vaccine. TLR4 is known to be an important regulator of neutrophil survival [40–42].

Split vaccine provided better increase in TLR3- ($p = 0.008$) and TLR9- ($p = 0.001$) positive cell counts, compared to subunit vaccine. Both vaccines had similar effect on TLR8+ granulocyte proliferation. TLR3 is an important receptor in recognition of viral double-stranded RNA generated during replication [43]. TLR3 expression by CD4+ и CD8+ lymphocytes is known to be accompanied by their activation, which allows them to get directly involved in various types of immune response [44].

Dendritic cell activation has been reported to occur predominantly with TLR2, TLR3, TLR4, TLR7, and TLR9. TLRs are effective contributors to APC activation, not only because they induce pro-inflammatory cytokine production, but also because they enhance expression of various co-stimulating molecules required for effective antibody recognition [45, 46]. Moreover, TLRs control dendritic cell maturation and antigen-presenting function [47].

Influenza vaccines have been reported to activate innate effectors—the first line of defense to infection—dendritic cells, both myeloid and lymphoid lineages [48]. TLR3 plays an important part in cross-priming of naive CD8 T cells that differentiate to cytotoxic T cells [49, 50]. They are key to killing virus-infected cells. TLR3 expressed on dendritic cells is also essential for NK cell activation via INAM molecule [51].

Adjuvanted vaccine showed high induction potential with respect to TLR9- and TLR8-expressing cells, compared to subunit vaccine ($p = 0.012$ and $p < 0.001$, respectively) and split vaccine ($p = 0.003$ and $p < 0.001$, respectively). TLR8 has been found to recognize viral single-stranded RNA and to be a specific receptor responsible for influenza virus recognition [45, 52]. The increased TLR8-positive cell count in this study can be attributed to the co-stimulating effect of the adjuvant in the adjuvanted vaccine.

TLR9 along with TLR2 and TLR4 are involved in the regulation of B lymphocyte activation, proliferation, differentiation, and survival (this is considered an alternative pathway of B lymphocyte activation) [53]. TLR9 is also supposed to be a PRR key to influenza identification and binding, while recognition of influenza virions by TLR7/8 is significant for the induction of protective immune response to main antigens (hemagglutinin) [54].

Two different intracellular signaling systems are generally recognized at the moment. One of them involves TLR2, TLR4, TLR5, TLR7, TLR9 and intracellular molecules MyD88, IRAK, TRAF, NFkB. This intracellular signaling system usually activates an early pro-inflammatory response. The other intracellular system involves TLR3, TLR4, (might involve TLR7 and TLR8), adaptor protein TRIF and intracellular proteins TRAM, TBK1, and IRF3. This signaling system ensures the activation of anti-virus response. TLR3 is the key component of this signaling pathway, since it interacts with double-stranded viral RNA. TLR4 is equally effective in the activation of both intracellular signaling systems. Thus, there are two important types of innate immune responses. The first type activates antibacterial protection along with the tissue inflammation. The second type provides type I interferon-mediated antiviral response, with interferon being the primary antiviral mediator in innate immunity [55].

5. Conclusion

Thus, the studies have shown that influenza vaccines activate cellular immunity effectors as well as induce humoral immune response. PO-containing adjuvanted vaccine showed the strongest capability of inducing the cellular response, among the three vaccines studied.

Influenza vaccines *in vitro* induced an increase in the number of the innate and acquired immunity effectors: NK cells, NKT cells, B lymphocytes, cells with early activation marker, T lymphocytes with late activation marker, and regulatory T cells.

Despite the fact that influenza vaccines must activate endosomal receptors, they cause nonspecific activation of the surface TLRs. This might be due to the influence exerted by antigen complexes contained in influenza vaccines of various types and due to the presence of an adjuvant in one of the vaccines studied. These vaccines activate TLR signaling cascade and, thus, can probably stimulate key effectors of the innate (DC, NK, and NKT cells) and adaptive

(CTL, B lymphocytes) immunity, which provide antiviral effect and induce body's own defense mechanisms against microbial infection.

6. Vaccination against influenza: the prospect of using adjuvants

The flu is widespread around the world and causes seasonal epidemics, which result in the death of hundreds of thousands of people each year [56]. Complications leading to morbidity and mortality following infection are predominantly observed in high-risk groups: children of early age, people with chronic diseases and pregnant women [57]. According to WHO, globally annual epidemics result in 3,000,000–5,000,000 cases of severe disease and approximately 250,000–500,000 deaths [58].

The vaccination is the most effective tools for preventing of influenza and, as a consequence, reducing the number and severity of post-infectious complications. Inactivated influenza vaccines received the most widely used, due to its high efficiency and low reactogenicity. But, at the same time, inactivated influenza vaccines, including seasonal trivalent vaccines, used for the annual prevention of influenza in the autumn-winter period, are not without some limitations. These vaccines are not enough (effective) immunogenic in vaccinating a number of population groups - small children, pregnant women, the elderly, people with various chronic diseases that are considered to be influenza risk groups. Also, inactivated influenza vaccines are not sufficiently protected against antigenically different strains (drift and heterologous) of the influenza virus that are not contained in the vaccine. In addition, the capacity of all manufacturers may not be sufficient to provide mass vaccine prevention around the world, especially in the event of a pandemic [59–61].

To increase the immunogenicity of inactivated influenza vaccines, adjuvants (immunoadjuvants) have been proposed. With the use of adjuvants, it is possible to increase the immunogenicity of influenza vaccines against a set of antigenically different strains. Adjuvants in the influenza vaccine can also provide efficacy in the immunization of various population groups, including at-risk groups. In addition, a significant increase in the immunogenicity of the vaccine due to the adjuvant will allow the transition to simple (single) immunization regimens, as well as reduce the dose of the antigen (hemagglutinin). This is especially important for pre-pandemic vaccines, because with the same production capacity, more vaccines will be obtained - and as a result, more people are immunized [59, 61].

The action of most adjuvants is based on the prolongation of the AG action, which is provided by the creation of a "depot" of the AG, which slows its absorption. Due to the sorption of AG on certain carriers, the antigen is held in places necessary for exposure of the antigen to antigen presenting cells and lymphocytes. Such an effect occurs when using aluminum alum, immunostimulating complexes, an oil microemulsion [62].

The effect of deposition is also achieved through the use of liposomes [63]. Adjuvants that primarily affect the phagocytic link of the immune system include polyelectrolytes, including PO. Structural association of the AG and polymer-immunostimulant enhances the migration of phagocytes, the functional activity of macrophages in tissues and increases their processing activity [64].

The action of adjuvants depends on the initial immune status of the organism preceding the vaccination. Adjuvants accelerate development and increase the level of immune response, increase the duration of its retention. Long rise and a slow decrease in the intensity of post-vaccination immunity is characteristic of adjuvanted vaccines. At the same time, a reliable immune response is achieved with the help of small doses of AG and a small number of injections of the vaccine [63].

PO possesses expressed immune modulating effects acting first of all on the innate immunity factors such as monocytic-macrophagal system cells, neutrophils and NK-cells and inducing their activation under initially reduced functions. Flow cytochemistry data showed that PO does interact with three lymphocyte subclasses, predominantly binds with monocytes and neutrophils and to a lesser extent with lymphocytes, enhancing intracellular H2O2 production. Hydrogen peroxide being the secondary messenger activates the transcriptional NF-kB factor that is the participant of the cytokines synthesis regulation. The enhancement of the pro-inflammatory cytokines IL-1β, IL6, TNF-α synthesis takes place. Activation by PO cells of monocytic-macrophagal cluster and natural killers promotes mobilization of both cellular and humoral immunity. Finally, all immunity starts up for adequate response development similarly to that as it occurs in natural way [65].

Besides its own clinical application as independent drug, Polyoxidonium is used as immunoadjuvant in new generation vaccines and is a compound in subunit adjuvanted Grippol family vaccines since 1997 when first Grippol® vaccine was registered in Russian market. Due to Polyoxidonium, all Grippol family vaccines contain 3-times lower antigen content in one immunizing dose - 5 mcg per strain, in comparison to 15 mcg per strain in other subunit and split influenza vaccines. This provides Grippol family vaccines with higher safety profile. Today Grippol vaccines are approved and especially recommended for vaccination of cohorts that previously were considered to be not vaccinated (patients with allergic conditions, subjects with chromic somatic diseases, individuals with different immune deficiencies), and children from 6 months of age, and pregnant women. These recommendations were made based on relevant clinical trials results followed by many years practical mass vaccine application experience [66, 67].

Annual vaccination with the "yearly adapted vaccine" is an effective means of prevention and control of influenza in immunocompetent individuals, even in those with a known poor antibody response. In addition to the development of protective antibodies after vaccination, the induction of cell-mediated immunity is considered to be of critical importance [68]. Recent researches concerning the response to influenza vaccination in patients with CVID and unclassified antibody deficiency have shown that while the humoral immune response was strongly impaired, a T cell response against the vaccine was detected in most patients [69].

Seasonal vaccines primarily work through the induction of neutralizing antibodies against the principal surface antigen HA. This important role of HA-specific antibodies explains why previous pandemics have emerged when new HAs have appeared in circulating human viruses. It has long been recognized that influenza virus-specific CD4(+) T cells are important in protection from infection through direct effector mechanisms or by providing help to B cells and CD8(+) T cells. However, the seasonal influenza vaccine is poor at inducing CD4(+) T cell responses and needs to be combined with an adjuvant facilitating this response [70].

Protective immunity induced by SF-10 (synthetic human pulmonary surfactant with a carboxy vinyl polymer as a viscosity improver) against lethal influenza virus infection was partially and predominantly suppressed after depletion of CD8+ and CD4+ T cells (induced by intraperitoneal injection of the corresponding antibodies), respectively, suggesting that CD4+ T cells predominantly and CD8+ T cells partially contribute to the protective immunity in the advanced stage of influenza virus infection [71]. These results suggest that adjuvants can promote effective antigen delivery to antigen presenting cells, activates CD8+ T cells via cross-presentation, and induces cell-mediated immune responses against antigen.

Influenza infection elicits high-affinity IgA in the respiratory tract and virus-specific IgG, which correlates with protection. Long-lived influenza-specific T cells have also been shown to ameliorate disease [72]. Activation of the parameters of innate immunity is critical for the recognition of infection, as well as for the effectiveness of vaccination, which allows not only eliminating pathogens and cells with altered antigenic properties, but also having a significant effect on the formation of adaptive immunity [73].

Development of a universal influenza vaccine currently seems to be quite workable and promising task. Such universal vaccines are expected to contain both antibody production stimulants and inductors of cellular immune response with effectors of innate and adaptive immunity being involved. Adjuvants may play an important part, their functions being aimed both at enhancing immune response to an antigen and at regulating that response [74]. Thus, due to the emergence of a new type of vaccine (adjuvant), in assessing the immunological efficacy is important not only humoral but also cellular immune response.

Conflict of interest

The authors declare no conflict of interest.

Abbreviations

CD	cluster of differentiation
PO	polyoxidonium
TLR's	toll-like receptors
WBCs	leukocytes (white blood cells)
FBS	fetal bovine serum
HAI	hemagglutination inhibition
HAU	hemagglutination unit
RBCs	red blood cells

V	Vaccine
PBMC	peripheral blood mononuclear cell
AB	Antibody
RNA	Ribonucleic acid
MHC	Major histocompatibility complex
HA	hemagglutinin
nTreg	natural thymus-derived regulatory cells
Foxp3	Forkhead box p3
TGF-β	transforming growth factor beta
IL	interleukin
PRRs	pathogen-recognize receptors
LPS	lipopolysaccarides
AG	antigen
DNA	deoxyribonucleic acid
CVID	common variable immunodeficiency
APC	antigen-presenting cell

Author details

Mikhail Petrovich Kostinov[1,2]*, Nelli Kimovna Akhmatova[1], Ekaterina Alexandrovna Khromova[1], Svetlana Anatolyevna Skhodova[1], Vera Nikolaevna Stolpnikova[1], Alexander Petrovich Cherdantsev[3] and Anna Egorovna Vlasenko[4]

*Address all correspondence to: vaccinums@gmail.com

1 I. Mechnikov Research Institute of Vaccines and Sera, Moscow, Russia

2 Federal State-Funded Educational Institution of Higher Education "First Moscow State Medical University named after I.M. Sechenov" of Ministry of Healthcare of Russia, Moscow, Russia

3 Federal State-Funded Educational Institution of Higher Education "Ulyanovsk State University", Ulyanovsk, Russia

4 Novokuznetsk State Institute of Advanced Medical Education, the Branch of Federal State-Funded Educational Institution of Additional Professional Education "Russian Medical Academy of Continuous Professional Education" of the Ministry of Healthcare of Russia, Novokuznetsk, Russia

References

[1] Gross PA, Hermogenes AW, Sacks HS, Lau J, Levandowski RA. The efficacy of influenza vaccine in elderly persons. A meta-analysis and review of the literature. Annals of Internal Medicine. 1995;**123**(7):518-527

[2] Khurana S, Frasca D, Blomberg B, Golding H. AID activity in B cells strongly correlates with polyclonal antibody affinity maturation in-vivo following pandemic 2009-H1N1 vaccination in humans. PLoS Pathogens. 2012 Sep;**8**(9):e1002920. DOI: 10.1371/journal.ppat.1002920

[3] Kositanont U, Assantachai P, Wasi C, Puthavathana P, Praditsuwan R. Kinetics of the antibody response to seasonal influenza vaccination among the elderly. Viral Immunology. 2012 Dec;**25**(6):471-476

[4] Nath KD, Burel JG, Shankar V, Pritchard AL, Towers M, Looke D, Davies JM, Upham JW. Clinical factors associated with the humoral immune response to influenza vaccination in chronic obstructive pulmonary disease. International Journal of Chronic Obstructive Pulmonary Disease. 2014;**9**:51-56

[5] Yerkovich ST, Hales BJ, Carroll ML, Burel JG, Towers MA, Smith DJ, Thomas WR, Upham JW. Reduced rhinovirus-specific antibodies are associated with acute exacerbations of chronic obstructive pulmonary disease requiring hospitalization. BMC 2012;**12**:37

[6] Pera A, Campos C, Lopez N, et al. Immunosenescence: Implications for response to infection and vaccination in older people. Maturitas. 2015;**82**:50-55

[7] Dorrington MG, Bowdish DM. Immunosenescence and novel vaccination strategies for the elderly. Frontiers in Immunology. 2013;**4**:171

[8] Belshe RB, Newman FK, Cannon J, Duane C, Treanor J, Van Hoecke C, Howe BJ, Dubin G. Serum antibody responses after intradermal vaccination against influenza. The New England Journal of Medicine 2004 Nov 25;**351**(22):2286-2294. Epub 2004 Nov 3

[9] Cox F, Roos A, Hafkemeijer N, Baart M, Tolboom J, Dekking L, Stittelaar K, Goudsmit J, Radošević K, Saeland E. Matrix-M adjuvated seasonal virosomal influenza vaccine induces partial protection in mice and ferrets against avian H5 and H7 challenge. PLoS One. 2015 Sep 24;**10**(9):e0135723. DOI: 10.1371/journal.pone.0135723

[10] Smith DJ, Lapedes AS, De Jong JC, Bestebroer TM, Rimmelzwaan GF, Osterhaus AD, Fouchier RA. Mapping the antigenic and genetic evolution of influenza virus. Science. 2004;**305**(5682):371-376. DOI: 10.1126/science.1097211

[11] Krammer F, Palese P. Advances in the development of influenza virus vaccines. Nature Reviews Drug Discovery. 2015;**14**(3):167-182

[12] Altenburg AF, Rimmelzwaan GF, de Vries RD. Virus-specific T cells as correlate of (cross-) protective immunity against influenza. Vaccine. 2015 Jan 15;**33**(4):500-506. DOI: 10.1016/j.vaccine.2014.11.054

[13] Kostinov MP, Zverev VV, editors. Vaccination against Hepatitis B, Influenza and Rubella for Adult Patients with Chronic Diseases. Practice guidelines. Moscow;2009 (in Russian)

[14] Kostinov MP, Solovyova IL. Immunomodulators and Vaccination. Moscow;2013 (in Russian)

[15] Kostinov MP. Immunocorrection of Vaccination in Persons Having Health Problems. Moscow; 2006 (in Russian)

[16] http://www.ema.europa.eu/docs/en_GB/document_library/Scientific_guideline/2009/09/WC500003945.pdf

[17] Mair P, Wilcox R. Robust Statistical Methods in R: Using the WRS2 Package. Technical report, Harvard University; 2016

[18] John H. McDonald. Handbook of Biological Statistics, 2nd edn. Baltimore, Maryland: Sparky House Publishing; 2009

[19] Yokoyama WM. Natural killer cells. In: Paul W, editor. Fundamental Immunology. Philadelphia: Lippincott, Williams & Wilkins; 2013. pp. 395-430

[20] French AR, Yokoyama WM. Natural killer cells and viral infections. Current Opinion in Immunology. 2003;**15**:45-51

[21] Paget C, Ivanov S, Fontaine J, Blanc F, Pichavant M, Renneson J, Bialecki E, Pothlichet J, Vendeville C, Barba-Speath G, Huerre MR, Faveeuw C, Si-Tahar M, Trottein F. Potential role of invariant NKT cells in the control of pulmonary inflammation and CD8+ T cell response during acute influenza A virus H3N2 pneumonia. Journal of Immunology. 2011;**186**(10):5590-5602. DOI: 10.4049/jimmunol.1002348

[22] Ivanova AS, Puchkova NG, Nekrasov AV, Gurkovskaya YaI, Apryatina VA, et al. Mechanisms of adjuvant effects of polyoxidonium. Hematopoiesis Immunology. 2015;**13**(2): 30-92 (in Russian)

[23] Constantinides MG, Bendelac A. Transcriptional regulation of the NKT cell lineage. Current Opinion in Immunology. 2013;**25**:161-167

[24] Slauenwhite D, Johnston B. Regulation of NKT cell localization in homeostasis and infection. Frontiers in Immunology. 2015;**6**:255

[25] Tupin E, Kinjo Y, Kronenberg M. The unique role of natural killer T cells in the response to microorganisms.Nat Rev. Microbiologica. 2007 Jun;**5**(6):405-417

[26] McMichael AJ, Gotch FM, Noble GR, Beare PA. Cytotoxic T-cell immunity to influenza. The New England Journal of Medicine. 1983;**309**(1):13-17. DOI: 10.1056/NEJM 198307073090103

[27] Topham DJ, Tripp RA, Doherty PC. CD8 T cells clear influenza virus by perforin or Fas-dependent processes. Journal of Immunology. 1997;**159**(11):5197-5200

[28] Yewdell JW, Bennink JR. Immunodominance in major histocompatibility complex class I-restricted T lymphocyte responses. Annual Review of Immunology. 1999;**17**:51-88

[29] Sandbulte MR, Jimenez GS, Boon AC, Smith LR, Treanor JJ, Webby RJ. Cross-reactive neuraminidase antibodies afford partial protection against H5N1 in mice and are present in unexposed humans. PLoS Medicine. 2007;**4**(2):e59. DOI: 10.1371/journal.pmed.0040059

[30] Jayasekera JP, Moseman EA, Carroll MC. Natural antibody and complement mediate neutralization of influenza virus in the absence of prior immunity. Journal of Virology. 2007;**81**(7):3487-3494. DOI: 10.1128/JVI.02128-06

[31] Kazimirko NK, Akimova EE, Zavatskiy VYu, Polyakov AS, Tatarenko DP. Immunology of normal pregnancy. Molodoy Ucheny. 2014;**3**(06):132-137 (in Russian)

[32] Kostinov MP, Khromova EA, Savis'ko AA, Kostinova AM. Functional characteristics of the immune system in normal pregnancy and their correlation with vaccination. Consilium Medicum. 2016;**18**(6):59-62 (in Russian)

[33] Willcocks S, Offord V, Seyfert HM, Coffey TJ, Werling D. Species-specific PAMP recognition by TLR2 and evidence for species-restricted interaction with Dectin-1. Journal of Leukocyte Biology. 2013 Sep;**94**(3):449-458. DOI: 10.1189/jlb.0812390

[34] Rakoff-Nahoum S, Medzhitov R. Toll-like receptors and cancer. Nature Reviews Cancer. 2009 Jan; **9**(1):57-63. DOI: 10.1038/nrc2541

[35] Kawai T, Akira S. Toll-like receptors and their crosstalk with other innate receptors in infection and immunity. Immunity. 2011;**34**:637-650

[36] Mahita J, Sowdhamini R. Investigating the effect of key mutations on the conformational dynamics of Toll-like receptor dimers through moleculardynamics simulations and protein structure networks. Proteins. 2018 Jan: 31. DOI: 10.1002/prot.25467

[37] Barreiro LB, Ben-Ali M, Quach H, Laval G, Patin E, Pickrell JK, Bouchier C, Tichit M, Neyrolles O, Gicquel B, Kidd jR, Kidd KK, Alcaïs A, Ragimbeau J, Pellegrini S, Abel L, Casa-nova JL, Quintana-Murci L. Evolutionary dynamics of human Toll-like receptors and their different contributions to host de-fense. PLoS Genetics. 2009;**5**(7):e1000562

[38] Wei T, Gong J, Rössle SC, Jamitzky F, Heckl WM, Stark RW. A leucine-rich repeat assembly approach for homology modeling of the human TLR5-10 and mouse TLR11-13 ectodomains. Journal of Molecular Modeling. 2011;**17**(1):27-36

[39] Engel A, Holt G, Lu H. The pharmacokinetics of Toll-like receptor agonists and the impact on the immune system. Expert Review of Clinical Pharmacology Journal. 2011; **4**(2):275-289

[40] Hyang LT, Paredes CJ, Papoutsakis ET, Miller WM. Gene expression analysis illuminates the transcriptional programs un-derlying the functional activity of ex vivo-expanded granulo-cytes. Physiological Genomics. 2007;**31**(1):114-125

[41] Yoshimura A, Ohishi HM, Aki D, Hanada T. Regulation of TLR signaling and inflammation by SOCS family proteins. Journal of Leukocyte Biology. 2004;**5**(3):422-427

[42] Sabroe LR, Prince EC, Jones et al. Selective roles for Toll-like receptor (TLR)2 and TLR4 in the regulation of neutrophil activation and life span. The Journal of Immunology. 2003; **170**(10):5268-5275

[43] Maitra R, Augustine T, Dayan Y, Chandy C, Coffey M, Goel S. Toll like receptor 3 as an immunotherapeutic target for KRAS mutated colorectal cancer. Oncotarget. 2017 May 23;**8**(21):35138-35135,153. DOI: 10.18632/oncotarget.16812

[44] Asprodites N, Zheng L, Geng D, Velasco-Gonzalez C, Sanchez-Perez L, Davila E. Engagement of Toll-like receptor-2 on cytotoxic T-lymphocytes occurs *in vivo* and augments antitumor activity. FASEB Journal. 2008;**22**(10):3628-3637

[45] Kawai T, Akira S. The role of pattern-recognition receptors in innate immunity: Update on Toll-like receptors. Nature Immunology. 2010 May;**11**(5):373-384

[46] Kumagai Y, Takeuchi O, Kato H, et al. Alveolar macrophages are the primary interferon-alpha producer in pulmonary infection with RNA viruses. Immunity. 2007;**27**:240-252

[47] Manicassamy S, Pulendran B. Modulation of adaptive immunity with Toll-like receptors. Seminars in Immunology. 2009 Aug;**21**(4):185-193

[48] Khromova EA, Akhmatova EA, Skhodova SA, Semochkin IA, Khomenkov VG, Akhmatova NK, Kostinov MP. Effect of influenza vaccines on subpopulations of blood dendritic cells. Journal of Microbiology, Epidemiology and Immunobiology. 2016;(5):23-28 (in Russian)

[49] Schulz O, Diebold SS, Chen M, et al. Toll-like receptor 3 promotes cross-priming to virus-infected cells. Nature. 2005;**433**:887-892

[50] Azuma M, Ebihara T, Oshiumi H, Matsumoto M, Seya T. Cross-priming for antitumor CTL induced by soluble Ag + polyI:C depends on the TICAM-1 pathway in mouse CD11c(+)/CD8α (+) dendritic cells. Oncoimmunology. 2012;**1**:581-592. DOI: 10.4161/onci.19893

[51] Kasamatsu J, Azuma M, Oshiumi H, et al. INAM plays acritical role in IFN-gamma production by NK cells interacting with polyinosinic-polycytidylic acid-stimulated accessory cells. Journal of Immunology. 2014;**193**:5199-5207

[52] Hu T, Suter SR, Mumbleau MM, Beal PA. TLR8 activation and inhibition by guanosine analogs in RNA: Importance of functional groups and chain length. Bioorganic & Medicinal Chemistry. 2018 Jan 1;**26**(1):77-83. DOI: 10.1016/j.bmc.2017.11.020

[53] Jain S, Chodisetti S, Agrewala J. CD40 signaling synergizes with TLR-2 in the BCR independent activation of resting B cells. PLoS One. 2011;**6**(6):e20651

[54] Heer A, Shamshiev A, Donda A, et al. TLR signaling fine-tunes anti-influenza B cell responses. Journal of Immunology. 2007;**178**:2182-2191

[55] Markushin SG. Specifics of innate immunity in viral infections. Epidemiology and Vaccinal Prevention. 2012;**1**(62):72-81 (in Russian)

[56] Kuiken T, Riteau B, Fouchier RA, Rimmelzwaan GF. Pathogenesis of influenza virus infections: the good, the bad and the ugly. Current Opinion in Virology. 2012;**2**(3):276-286. DOI: 10.1016/j.coviro.2012.02.013

[57] Siston AM, Rasmussen SA, Honein MA, et al. Pandemic 2009 influenza A (H1N1) virus illness among pregnant women in the United States. Journal of the American Medical Association. 2010;**303**:1517-1525

[58] WHO: Influenza Fact Sheet. http://www.who.int/mediacentre/factsheets/fs211/en/

[59] WHO. Vaccines against influenza WHO posnion paper ~ November 2012. Weekly Epidemiological Record. 2012;**87**(47):461-476

[60] WHO. Influenza vaccines WHO position paper. Weekly Epidemiological Record. 2005; **80**(33):279-287

[61] Wright P, Neumann G, Kawaoka Y. Orthomyxoviruses. In: Knipe D, Howley P, editors. Fields Virology. 6th ed. Lippincott Williams & Wilkins; 2013

[62] Nikitina TN, Avdeyeva ZhI, Alpatova NA. Study of immune adjyuvant effect of cytokines in experimental models. Cytokines and Inflammation. 2010;**9**(3):19-24 (in Russian)

[63] Medunitsyn NV. Vaccinology M: "Triada-X". 2004. 446 c. (in Russian)

[64] Petrov RV, Khaitov RM. International Journal on Immunorehabilitation. 1999;**11**:C. 13-25. (in Russian)

[65] Dyakonova VA, Dambaeva SV, Pinegin BV, Khaitov RM. Study of interaction between the polyoxidonium immunomodulator and the human immune system cells. International Immunopharmacology. 2004;**4**(13):1615-1623 (in Russian)

[66] Savelyeva GM, Sukhikh GT, Serov VN, Manukhin IB, Radzinsky VE, ediotrs. Gynecology. National Guideline. 2nd edn. Moscow: GEOTAR-Media; 2017. (in Russian)

[67] Boytsov SA, Loukianov MM, Platonova EV, Gorbunov VM, Romanchuk SW, Nazarova OA, Belova OA, Kravtsova EA, Dovgalevsky PYa, Furman NV, Mironova AA, Dolotovskaya PV, Nekrasov AV, Puchkova NG, Abramova MA, Belova EN, Klyashtorny VG, Deev AD. Efficiency of influenza vaccination in patients with circulatory system diseases under dispensary observation in outpatient clinics: prospective follow-up monitoring data. Rational Pharmacotherapy in Cardiology. 2016;**12**(6):703-710. DOI: http://dx.doi.org/10.20996/1819-6446-2016-12-6-703-710 (in Russian)

[68] Principi N, Esposito S. Vaccine use in primary immunodeficiency disorders. Vaccine. 2014;**32**:3725-3731

[69] Hanitsch LG, Lobel M, Mieves JF, Bauer S, Babel N, Schweiger B, Wittke K, Grabowski P,Volk HD, Scheibenbogen C. Cellular and humeral influenza specific immune response upon vaccination in patients with common variable immunodeficiency and unclassified antibody deficiency. Vaccine. 2016 May 5;**34**(21):2417-2423

[70] Christensen D, Christensen JP, Korsholm KS, Isling LK, Erneholm K, Thomsen AR, Andersen P. Seasonal influenza split vaccines confer partial cross-protection against

heterologous influenza virus in ferrets when combined with the CAF01 Adjuvant. Frontiers in Immunology. 2018 Jan 8;**8**:1928. DOI: 10.3389/fimmu.2017.01928 eCollection 2017

[71] Kim H, Kimoto T, Sakai S, Takahashi E, Kido H. Adjuvanting influenza hemagglutinin vaccine with a human pulmonary surfactant-mimicking synthetic compound SF-10 induces local and systemic cell-mediated immunity in mice. PLoS One. 2018 Jan 25; **13**(1):e0191133. DOI: 10.1371/journal.pone.0191133 eCollection 2018

[72] Ascough S, Paterson S, Chiu C. Induction and subversion of human protective immunity: contrasting influenza and respiratory syncytial virus. Frontiers in Immunology. 2018 Mar 2;**9**:323. DOI: 10.3389/fimmu.2018.00323 eCollection 2018

[73] Gasteiger G, D'Osualdo A, Schubert DA, Weber A, Bruscia EM, Hartl D. Cellular innate immunity: An old game with new players. Journal of Innate Immunity 2017;**9**(2):111-125. DOI: 10.1159/000453397. Epub 2016 Dec 23

[74] Esmagambetov IB, Alekseeva SV, Sayadyan Kh.S, Shmarov MM. Modern approach to creation of universal influenza vaccine. Infektsiya i Immunitet. 2016;**6**(2). DOI: http://dx.doi.org/10.15789/2220-7619-2016-2-117-132 (in Russian)

9

Maternal Influenza: Infection, Vaccination, and Compelling Questions

Jill M. Manske

Abstract

Influenza presents a significant risk for increased morbidity and mortality to pregnant women and infants based on evidence from previous influenza pandemics, seasonal epidemics, and the recent H1N1 pandemic. Since 2004, influenza vaccine has been recommended for pregnant women during any trimester of pregnancy to reduce this risk. This chapter presents an overview of influenza risks associated with pregnancy as well as a review of our current understanding of vaccine effectiveness in pregnant women, neonates, and young infants. In addition, some of the current compelling questions related to influenza risk and prevention across all trimesters of pregnancy are explored.

Keywords: influenza vaccine, pregnancy, effectiveness, maternal immunization

1. Introduction

Influenza is a highly contagious, acute respiratory infection (ARI). Each year, it is estimated that 5–10% of adults and 20–30% of children worldwide will become infected with influenza [1]. Pregnant women and infants are at particular risk for influenza. Influenza infection during pregnancy or during the first 6 months of life is a substantial cause of morbidity. Prevention of influenza in these populations is of global health importance.

2. Maternal influenza

Pregnant women are considered a high-risk group for serious illness and complications from influenza. While annual influenza incidence rates in pregnant women are similar to those of nonpregnant women [2–4], influenza infection is associated with increased morbidity and mortality in this subpopulation, with pregnant women having an increased risk of influenza-attributed hospitalizations compared to nonpregnant women [4, 5]. Most likely this is associated with the interaction of the infection with the physiologic and immunologic changes that occur during pregnancy.

Pregnancy-associated changes such as decreased lung capacity, reduced tidal volume, and increased cardiac output likely reduce the capacity of the respiratory and cardiac system to respond to the stress of influenza infection [2, 6]. In addition, during pregnancy there is a progressive suppression of cellular (T-cell mediated) immunity. While this immune suppression serves to protect the developing fetus from maternal cytotoxic T-cell immunity, it can impair the maternal response to viral infections such as influenza [7–11].

The combination of these factors contributes to an increased risk of negative outcomes from influenza infection. If respiratory disease develops, especially during the later stages of pregnancy, it can lead to high morbidity among the pregnant women [6, 12–14]. In a study of hospital admissions records of women admitted between 1994 and 2000 with respiratory conditions during pregnancy, the hospitalization rate was 150/100,000, an admission rate considerably higher than that of nonpregnant women (17/100,000) and corresponding to the rate for people aged 65–69 [5]. Healthy pregnant women ages 20–34 were estimated to be 18 times more likely to be hospitalized for influenza than their nonpregnant peers [5].

While hospitalization rates are increased in all trimesters of pregnancy [4, 15, 16], they are the highest during the third trimester [5, 14, 16–18]. Likewise, there is a strong association of maternal morbidity with this trimester of pregnancy. In a 2003 study, Hartert et al. showed that cardiovascular hospitalization during influenza season increased with each trimester, nearly threefold higher by the third trimester compared to the first trimester [18]. In a study of 8323 healthy pregnant and postpartum women, Lindsay et al. found that the strength of association between influenza exposure and influenza-like illness (ILI) increased as the stage of pregnancy progressed, reporting an odds ratio (OR) of 1.12 (CI, 0.79–1.59) during the first trimester, 1.30 (CI, 0.97–1.73) during the second trimester, and 1.84 (CI, 1.31–2.59) for the third trimester [14]. Other studies have reported that by the third trimester, healthy pregnant women with no comorbidity have the same risk for ILI-associated hospitalization as nonpregnant women with chronic or comorbid conditions [4, 5].

Pregnant women with comorbid conditions such as asthma, diabetes, heart disease, or chronic obstructive pulmonary disease are even more likely to be hospitalized than are pregnant women without chronic conditions [5, 14, 16–18]. Neuzil et al. reported event rates for influenza for low-risk women of 3, 6, and 10 per 10,000 women months in the first, second, and third trimesters, respectively. The event rate in nonpregnant women was 2 per 10,000 women months. Among women with chronic comorbid conditions, rates of 31, 16, and 21 per 10,000 women months were observed during these trimesters, respectively [4].

While considerable data demonstrate increased morbidity and hospitalization from seasonal influenza in pregnant women, mortality appears to be rare in healthy pregnant women during non-pandemic seasons [7, 19, 20]. A study of seasonal influenza among pregnant women over an 8-year period reported an average of five deaths per year and a mean mortality ratio of 2.9 per million live births [21]. However, during pandemics, influenza infection presents a significant increased risk of both morbidity and mortality in pregnant women.

For example, during the pandemic of 1918, pneumonia was reported in 50% of previously healthy pregnant women, leading to case-fatality rates of over 50% [22–26]. In the 1957 pandemic, 50% of the women of childbearing age who died of influenza were pregnant. Furthermore, 10% of all influenza deaths during this pandemic occurred in pregnant women, with the majority occurring during the third trimester [23, 24].

Increased rates of morbidity and mortality in pregnant women also were observed more recently during the 2009 influenza A(H1N1)pdm09 pandemic. In fact, the first reported death of an adult in the United States during this pandemic was a pregnant woman [27]. Of the 45 deaths reported early in the pandemic, 6 (13.3%) were pregnant women, all of whom developed viral pneumonia and respiratory distress syndrome [27–29].

A study of pregnant US women with confirmed or probable influenza during the first month of the outbreak reported 11/34 cases (32.4%) resulted in hospitalization—admissions rates four times higher than those in the general population [30]. Deaths were reported in all three trimesters and were independent of preexisting risk factors. In a California study, pregnant women who were hospitalized with or died from pH1N1 were less likely than nonpregnant women to have a predisposing or comorbid medical condition [31].

A review of published studies following the 2009 pandemic documented that pregnant women were disproportionately represented among hospitalizations, ICU admissions, and deaths. The 120 papers that were included in the review reported 3110 pregnant women from 29 countries with A(H1N1)pdm09 influenza infection, including 1625 (52.3%) who were hospitalized with 2009 H1N1, of whom 378 (23.3%) were admitted to an ICU and 130 (8%) died [32]. Pooling the data from all of the studies included in the review, the authors reported that pregnant women, who represent approximately 1% of the population of United States and Australia, accounted for 6.3% of hospitalizations, 5.9% of ICU admissions, and 5.7% of deaths [32].

Using data from the Centers for Disease Control (CDC) and the Pregnancy Mortality Surveillance System, Callaghan et al. estimated the total burden of pregnancy-related mortality resulting from the 2009 to 2010 pandemic. Confirmed and possible deaths resulting from A(H1N1)pdm09 infection represented the leading cause of pregnancy-related mortality in the United States between the months of April 2009 and June 2010. Of 915 total pregnancy-related deaths during this period, 12% of pregnancy-related deaths were attributed to influenza, 75 (8.2%) classified as confirmed influenza A(H1N1)pdm09 deaths, and 34 (3.7%) classified as possible influenza infection deaths [33]. The authors calculated the pregnancy-related morality ratio for confirmed and possible influenza deaths at 2.2 per 100,000 live births. This represents a significant burden of mortality. The number of deaths (109) during the 2009–2010 influenza season was 20 times greater than the mean number (5) of annual possible influenza deaths reported in a 1998–2005 cohort of pregnancy-related deaths in non-pandemic years [33].

Infants born to influenza-infected women during the pandemic also experienced increased risks of poor clinical outcomes, mostly due to preterm birth. Reports of preterm birth rates ranged from 15 to 30% among infected women [32, 34–36]. Infection with A(H1N1)pdm09 was associated with increased risk of cesarean delivery [32]. In most cases, cesarean delivery was an attempt to improve worsening maternal status rather than out of concern for the infant [32]. Siston et al. reported a cesarean delivery rate of 58% in pregnant women with 2009 H1N1 compared to a baseline cesarean rate of 30.5% [32, 34, 37]. While cesarean deliveries were commonly described, it is likely that this rate was over-reported, since many of the studies reported only severely affected women. Many deliveries were emergencies and performed outside of controlled operating room settings, indicating the urgent nature of these deliveries and the critical status of the women [32].

3. Influenza infection and fetal development

While there is no clear consensus on transplacental transmission of influenza virus or direct viral effects on the fetus [2], the spread of virus beyond the respiratory tract during acute infection is unusual, and vertical transmission, although documented [38–40], appears to be rare [41, 42]. However, even in the absence of vertical transmission, adverse fetal effects can occur, most likely due to the systemic maternal immune response to the infection [43, 44]. Studies have documented inflammatory responses in fetal tissues in response to influenza infection. Such responses could impact the maternal-fetal interface, the placenta, or the fetus directly, leading to pregnancy loss [43]. In addition to direct damage from inflammatory responses, it is hypothesized that maternal hyperthermia can result in adverse fetal outcomes [28, 45]. Maternal hyperthermia during the first trimester of pregnancy, regardless of the cause, has been associated with an increased risk for neural tube defects [46], while fever during labor has been associated with adverse outcomes including neonatal seizures, cerebral palsy, encephalopathy, and death [2, 47–50].

In a large population-based study of influenza infection in over 100,000 women, Hansen et al. observed an increased risk for fetal abnormalities (e.g., central nervous system malfunctions in the fetus, chromosomal abnormalities, suspected damage to the fetus from viral disease) was present in both seasonal (OR 1.53, CI, 1.19–1.95) and pandemic infections (OR 1.48, CI, 1.27–1.73) [51].

A review and meta-analysis of 33 studies published from 1953 to 2013 of first-trimester influenza exposure found that influenza exposure during the first trimester of pregnancy was associated with an increase in congenital abnormalities [adjusted odds ratio (AOR) 2.00, CI, 1.62–4.28]. Anomalies included neural tube defects [odds ratio (OR) 3.33, CI, 2.05–5.40], hydrocephaly (OR 5.74, 1.10–30.00), congenital heart defects (OR 1.56, 1.13–2.14), cleft lip (OR 3.12, CI, 2.20–4.42), digestive system anomalies (OR 1.72, CI, 1.09–2.68), and limb reduction defects (OR 2.03, CI, 1.27–3.27) [52]. A major limitation of this study concerns the fact that it defined influenza exposure as any reported influenza, influenza-like illness, or fever with or without clinical confirmation. The inclusion of wide clinical symptoms without laboratory confirmation of influenza likely resulted in overestimation of the number of infants exposed to influenza during gestation. It therefore cannot be determined whether congenital abnormalities were associated with general, all cause hyperthermia or whether influenza infection poses a unique and specific risk for these outcomes. Nonetheless, these observations suggest that prevention of influenza during the first trimester of pregnancy may reduce risk for congenital abnormalities.

Fetal demise is associated with influenza infection as well. Women with influenza, especially those with pneumonia, had high rates of spontaneous abortion and preterm birth, with 52% of pregnancies ending in spontaneous abortion or preterm delivery during the 1918 pandemic [22, 23, 25].

Using a large nationwide registry, Haberg et al. examined the risk of fetal death after maternal exposure to pandemic influenza infection. The researchers found that pregnant women with a clinical diagnosis of influenza had a nearly twofold increase in the risk of fetal death (adjusted hazard ratio, 1.91; 95% CI, 1.07–3.41) as compared to women who were not exposed to influenza [53].

Pierce et al. assessed perinatal outcomes of maternal A(H1N1)pdm09 infection. The authors found that perinatal mortality was higher in infants born to infected women than in infants of uninfected women (39 per 1000 live births versus 7 per 1000 total births, respectively, $p = 0.001$). This was principally explained by an increase in the rate of stillbirth (27 per 1000 total births versus 6 per 1000 total births, $p = 0.001$) [54].

4. Influenza infection in neonates and young infants

Infants younger than 6 months of age are at a heightened risk for serious illness from influenza, exhibiting the highest rates of severe influenza compared to other pediatric populations [41]. This age group has higher rates of hospitalization, more prolonged ICU stays, and higher fatality rates (0.33 per 100,000 children) than almost any other age group [55–59]. In the United States, estimates of hospitalization rates for young infants (less than 6 months of age) range between 1.8 and 7.2 per 1000 infants, higher than reported rates of hospitalization for children up to 4 years of age (0.14 per 1000) [60] and people 65–80 years of age (0.56–2.13 per 1000) [60–63]. Childhood deaths associated with influenza are most frequent in infants during the first months of life, with mortality rates in infants 0–6 months old more than four times higher than those in older children [59].

Libster et al. [64] documented particularly high mortality rates for infants during the 2009 H1N1 pandemic in Argentina. Of 251 infants and children hospitalized with confirmed A(H1N1)pdm09 infection, 13 (5%) died, for an overall death rate of 1.1 per 100,000 children. Infants were at particularly high risk for fatality, representing the highest death rate at 7.6 per 100,000 children. By comparison, this death rate was 10 times the reported US infant death rate during the relatively serious seasonal influenza season of 2003–2004 [59, 64].

Taken together, these observations highlight the impact of influenza on infants, especially the youngest, and underscore the need for prevention in this vulnerable population.

5. Maternal influenza vaccination

A large body of evidence collected over several decades demonstrates that pregnant women and young infants are at increased risk for complications from influenza, making control of influenza infection in these populations an important public health challenge. Influenza vaccines have been used since 1945 and currently are the primary strategy for preventing influenza infection [65].

Due to the frequent changes of the influenza viral antigens, a vaccine is formatted during the end of the previous season to include the specific antigens of the influenza strains expected to circulate in the following season, with a goal of conferring protection against the upcoming season's strains. Each year, the trivalent inactivated influenza vaccines (IIV3) are formulated to contain three viral components: two influenza A subtypes and one influenza B virus. In 2012, the US Food and Drug Administration (FDA) approved the use of a quadrivalent influenza vaccine (IIV4). The quadrivalent vaccine contains two influenza A subtypes and two influenza B subtypes. In 2009, a monovalent H1N1 vaccine was prepared because the newly recognized strain was identified too late in the season to be included in the trivalent seasonal vaccines [66].

The current inactivated influenza vaccines (IIVs) are composed of inactivated (killed) virus that has been chemically disrupted and purified to form a split-inactivated virus preparation. Such split-virus vaccines contain purified HA and NA antigens and have fewer side effects and reactions than inactivated whole virus vaccines. The IIVs currently available in the United States are split virus or subunit virus similar to the split virus [66].

The other vaccine available in the United States is a live, attenuated influenza vaccine (LAIV). This vaccine is composed of live, attenuated, cold-adapted, temperature-sensitive virus administered directly into the nasal passage. The type A and B strains of influenza in this vaccine can replicate in the nasal passages, stimulating an immune response, but cannot replicate in the lower respiratory tract [67]. While LAIV has been licensed in the United States since 2003, it is not recommended for use in pregnant women [68].

A strategy to increase the effectiveness of IIVs is the addition of adjuvants. Adjuvants are compounds that stimulate the immune system to mount a more robust and protective response to the vaccine. The most commonly used adjuvants in influenza vaccines are the oil-based compounds AS03 and MF59. Adjuvants can allow for the use of lower doses of antigen, resulting in more available doses of vaccine, which may be useful in times of high demand such as during pandemics. While adjuvanted vaccines are not approved for use in pregnant women in the United States, in Canada, and in many European countries, the pandemic vaccine was formulated with adjuvant and administered to pregnant women [69].

Vaccination of pregnant women with IIV has taken place since the 1960s. Universal recommendation for vaccinating woman at all stages of pregnancy has been recommended by the

CDC's Advisory Committee on Immunization Practices (ACIP) since 2004 [65, 70, 71] and by the World Health Organization (WHO) since 2005 [1]. The Advisory Committee on Immunization Practices does not preferentially recommend a specific formulation—trivalent or quadrivalent—of the influenza vaccine [72]. In response to the 2009 H1N1 pandemic, the WHO placed pregnant women, along with caregivers of infants younger than 6 months old, healthcare and emergency services personnel, individuals between 6 months and 24 years, and those aged 25 years or older with chronic medical conditions, in the highest priority group to receive vaccines [73].

The American College of Obstetrics and Gynecology (ACOG) considers prevention of influenza to be an "essential element of prenatal care" [74]. In full support of the ACIP recommendations, ACOG issued new guidelines in September of 2010 stating that all unvaccinated pregnant women at any gestational age be vaccinated against influenza [74].

It is well documented that the antibody (Ab) response to influenza vaccine in pregnant women is similar to that of age-matched, nonpregnant women [75–79]. These observations support a conclusion that influenza vaccination will lead to an effective immune response in pregnant women and thereby provide an important tool in prevention of influenza in this population.

5.1. Effectiveness of maternal influenza vaccines

Pregnant women and neonates are high-risk groups for complications from influenza infection. Control of influenza in this population is an important public health concern. However, due in part to ethical concerns related to enrolling pregnant women in clinical studies, experimental data on influenza vaccination during pregnancy has been scarce, and the quality of the evidence is not consistently high overall [80].

Prior to 2010, there were few well-designed studies specifically addressing vaccine effectiveness in pregnant women. From 1964 to 2008, four studies specifically addressed vaccine effectiveness in pregnant women (**Table 1**). These studies covered eight different influenza seasons and included 51,547 pregnant women.

During a 1962–1963 outbreak of Asian influenza, Hulka measured vaccine effectiveness in pregnant women by asking immunized and nonimmunized patients if they had experienced influenza symptoms during the influenza season. While fewer immunized than unimmunized patients reported respiratory illness with fever (11% versus 20%, respectively), there was no significant difference in reports of respiratory illness between these patients [76].

Black et al. assessed vaccine effectiveness in almost 50,000 pregnant women across five influenza seasons. Vaccine effectiveness was determined by the number of outpatient visits for ILI or hospitalization for influenza or pneumonia. Using these outcomes, the risk of medical visit for respiratory symptoms was no different between vaccinated and unvaccinated women, and hospitalization was rare in both groups [81]. Using the adjusted hazard ratios (AHR = 1.151; CI, 0.979–1.352) from this study, Skowronski and De Serres calculated a vaccine effectiveness of −15% (CI, −35 to 2%) for this study population [7].

In a retrospective case-control study of five influenza seasons (1995–2003), Munoz et al. estimated the potential protective effect of vaccination by recording the occurrence of acute respiratory infection (ARI) in vaccinated and unvaccinated women. The researchers reported a nonsignificant ($p = 0.24$) trend toward lower incidence of medically attended ARI in vaccinated women as compared to unvaccinated women (22.6% of the vaccinated cohort versus 18.9% of the unvaccinated cohort) [82]. Among the women who developed ARI, the number of episodes of ARI was the same, 1.4 illnesses/person in both groups. However, there was a difference in the timing of these episodes, with 9% of the vaccinated cohort reporting ARI episodes during the peak of the influenza season, while 19% of the ARI events in the unvaccinated cohort occurred during the peak ($p = 0.01$, CI, 0.1–0.8) [82]. In this study, only three women were diagnosed with ILI, one vaccinated and two unvaccinated women, all during the peak influenza seasons of 1999–2000 and 2000–2001. These low rates of ILI as well as the small number of vaccinated women in the study population (vaccination rate was 3.5%) are limitations of this study. Using the relative risks reported in the study, vaccine effectiveness was −20% for ARI any time during pregnancy (CI, −59 to 9%) and 39% (CI, −56 to 76%) during the peak of the influenza season [7].

Study	Study period	Participants	Outcomes measured	Influenza vaccine protection
Studies of seasonal IIV during pregnancy				
Hulka [76]	1962–1963	544 pregnant women -363 immunized -181 nonimmunized 176 nonpregnant women -138 immunized -38 nonimmunized	Incidence of influenza-like illness (ILI)	Nonsignificant reduction in incidence of ILI (20% versus 11%)
Black et al. [81]	1997–2002	49,585 pregnant women -3707 immunized -45,878 nonimmunized	Medical visit for respiratory symptoms	No difference in medical visits ($p = 0.088$) Adjusted hazard ratio = 1.151; (CI, 0.979–1.352) Clinical effectiveness: −15% Excluding medical visits for asthma, no difference ($p = 0.988$) Adjusted hazard ratio = 1.001 (CI, 0.838–1.196) Clinical effectiveness: 0%
Munoz et al. [117]	1998–2003	Pregnant women -252 immunized -826 nonimmunized	Medically attended acute respiratory illness (ARI)	Nonsignificant trend toward lower incidence of ARI (22.6% versus 18.9%; $p = 0.24$) Clinical effectiveness: −20% (CI, −59.5 to 9%) any time during pregnancy

Study	Study period	Participants	Outcomes measured	Influenza vaccine protection
				39% (CI, −56 to 76%) during peak of influenza season
Zaman et al. [79]	2004–2005	340 pregnant women -172 immunized with TIV -168 immunized with pneumococcal vaccine	Respiratory illness with fever	Significant reduction of respiratory illness with any fever: Risk difference: −14.2 (CI, −25.5 to 2.9) Clinical effectiveness: 35.8% (CI, 3.7–57.2%) Reduction in respiratory disease with fever over 38 °C: Risk difference: −7.3% (CI, −14.5 to 0.1%) Clinical effectiveness: 43.1% (CI, −9.0 to 70.3%)
Madhi et al. [83]	2011–2012	2116 pregnant women -1062 immunized with IIV3 -1054 received placebo	RT-PCR-confirmed influenza	Clinical effectiveness: 50.4% (CI, 14.5–71.2%)
Thompson et al. [84]	2010–2012	Pregnant women -100 with confirmed influenza -192 with ARI negative for influenza -200 control negative for influenza	RT-PCR-confirmed influenza	Clinical effectiveness: 44% (CI, 5–67%) compared to influenza-negative controls 53% (CI, 24–72%) compared to ARI-negative controls
Studies of PH1N1 vaccine during pregnancy				
Richards et al. [101]	2009–2010	1125 vaccinated 1581 non-vaccinated (unadjuvanted vaccine)	RT-PCR or medical visit during pregnancy with influenza-related ICD-9 diagnosis code	Clinical effectiveness: 61.5% (CI, 15.5–82.5%)
Haberg et al. [53]	2009–2010	117,347 pregnant women (adjuvanted vaccine)		Clinical effectiveness: 70% (AHR, 0.30; (CI), 0.25–0.34)

Table 1. Clinical effectiveness of IIV and A(H1N1)pdm09 influenza vaccine during pregnancy.

The authors of this study speculate that while the receipt of an influenza vaccine may not prevent infection, it is likely to reduce the severity of the disease. However, they provided no data on clinical severity or evidence of such an association with vaccination status. Since there was no confirmation of influenza infection in most patients with ARI, it is impossible to confirm whether clinical symptoms were associated with influenza infection or with other respiratory viruses.

In 2008, Zaman et al. published the first randomized, double-blind, controlled clinical trial (RCT) of influenza vaccine in pregnant women. In this study, 340 pregnant women were randomized to receive either trivalent influenza vaccine (IIV3) or pneumococcal polysaccharide vaccine during the third trimester of pregnancy. This study was part of The Mother's Gift project, a randomized trial with the primary goal of assessing the safety and immunogenicity of pneumococcal vaccines. Therefore, the control arm consisted of mothers who received the pneumococcal vaccine, providing a control for an active, non-influenza vaccine. The authors measured nonspecific respiratory illness with fever and found that vaccinated women were significantly less likely to have respiratory illness, reporting a clinical effectiveness of 35.8% (CI, 3.7–57.2%) for respiratory illness with any fever and 43.1% for fever over 38 °C (CI, −9.0 to 70.3%) [79].

All of these studies share the common weakness that they use clinical symptoms, and not laboratory-confirmed influenza, as the primary outcome. Influenza vaccines are specifically targeted to influenza viruses. Many other respiratory pathogens can cause symptoms similar to influenza, but influenza vaccines are not designed to prevent other causes of influenza-like illness. Hence, clinical symptoms without laboratory confirmation are nonspecific outcomes. Interpretation and quantification of true vaccine effectiveness using only clinical outcomes are problematic, potentially leading to inaccurate estimates of effectiveness. For this reason, laboratory confirmation, either by reverse transcription polymerase chain reaction (RT-PCR) or viral culture, remains the best diagnostic tool for confirming influenza and evaluating vaccine efficacy (VE) and effectiveness.

In 2014, two studies began to address this deficiency in the literature. The research teams estimated influenza vaccine effectiveness in preventing illness among pregnant women using laboratory-confirmed (RT-PCR) influenza as the primary outcome.

Madhi et al. examined maternal and fetal outcomes in 2116 HIV-negative South African women during the 2011–2012 influenza season. 1062 women who received IIV3 were compared to women who received a placebo. Overall vaccine effectiveness at preventing laboratory-confirmed (RT-PCR) influenza in this population was 50.4% (CI, 14.5–71.2) [83].

Using a large health plan database, the Pregnancy and Influenza Project evaluated seasonal vaccine efficacy during the 2010–2011 and 2011–2012 influenza seasons. The authors compared the proportion of vaccinated women among 100 RT-PCR-confirmed influenza cases with the proportion vaccinated among 192 women with ARI who tested negative for influenza, and 200 controls matched by season, site, and trimester [84]. The adjusted vaccine efficacy against influenza was of 44% (CI, 5–67%) using the influenza-negative controls and 53% (CI, 24–72%) for the ARI-negative controls [84].

The 2009 A(H1N1) pandemic provided an opportunity to improve understanding of influenza vaccination during pregnancy. The pandemic allowed an evaluation of the effectiveness of maternal vaccination during an influenza season in which there was a high rate of viral circulation, as well as a close match between the vaccine strain and the circulating viral strain.

Pregnant women were prioritized to receive the vaccine and were strongly advised to be vaccinated [85], resulting in higher than usual vaccination rates [86].

Since the 2009 pandemic, a number of studies have examined monovalent pandemic A(H1N1) vaccination of pregnant women. Synthesizing evidence from this new and expanding database should increase our understanding of maternal influenza vaccination. While most of these studies measured either seroconversion and hemagglutinin inhibition (HAI) titers [87–92] or safety and/or birth outcomes [93–100], two studies specifically examined clinical efficacy of pandemic A(H1N1) vaccine during pregnancy.

In a retrospective cohort study, Richards et al. evaluated influenza infection in 1125 vaccinated and 1581 non-vaccinated women. In this study, influenza infection was defined as testing positive for influenza by RT-PCR or having a medical visit during pregnancy with influenza-related *ICD-9* diagnosis code during the period of 2009 influenza A(H1N1) virus circulation [101]. The researchers reported a vaccine efficacy (VE) of 61.5% (CI, 15.5–82.5%) for 2009 H1N1 influenza vaccine against diagnosed 2009 influenza A(H1N1) infection during the study period among all mothers in the study cohort [101].

A separate population-based study of 117,347 pregnant women in Norway estimated that vaccination during the second or third trimester of pregnancy resulted in a 70% reduction in influenza diagnosis following vaccination with adjuvanted A(H1N1) vaccine (adjusted hazard ratio, 0.30; CI, 0.25–0.34) [53].

While there is significant heterogeneity among these eight clinical studies, presenting wide-ranging estimates of vaccine effectiveness in pregnant women (from −15 to 70%), the evidence of effectiveness data based on laboratory-confirmed influenza is mounting and compelling. The cumulative evidence to date provides three studies showing significant clinical effectiveness during seasonal influenza years, 35.8% against respiratory disease in a RCT [79], 50.4% protection against laboratory-confirmed influenza in a RCT [83], and one large data-base study documenting VE of 44–53% [84]. Two studies of vaccine effectiveness during the 2009 A(H1N1) pandemic estimated VE of 61.5% (unadjuvanted) and 70% (adjuvanted), suggesting that vaccination during a pandemic season may offer more benefit than during non-pandemic years.

These more recent estimates using laboratory-confirmed endpoints are well within the reported vaccine effectiveness for healthy, nonpregnant adults. When combined with the well-documented observation that the antibody response to influenza vaccine in pregnant women is similar to that of nonpregnant women, all current evidence suggests that efficacy of influenza vaccines in pregnant women is similar to the nonpregnant population.

5.2. Maternal vaccination to protect young infants

An important secondary benefit of maternal vaccination appears to be protection of infants from influenza infection during the first months of life, providing an important two-for-one benefit since no influenza vaccine is licensed or recommended for infants younger than 6 months of age.

Maternal vaccination has potential to protect newborns due to the transfer of maternal immunity. Transplacental transfer of antibodies occurs throughout pregnancy, with highest levels during the last 4–6 weeks of gestation [102, 103]. Antibodies (specifically IgG) cross the placenta from mother to fetus during the final weeks of pregnancy, while infants acquire additional immune protection during breastfeeding, when the main class of immunoglobulin transferred in breast milk is IgA [104].

Several studies have demonstrated transplacentally acquired antibodies after natural influenza infection in the mother. One study examined the cord sera of 26 infants who had culture-confirmed influenza when younger than 4 months of age. The authors found a direct correlation between the gestational age at the time of infection and the level of antibody in the cord serum ($p = 0.002$), suggesting a protective effect of transplacentally acquired antibody [105].

During the 1979 influenza epidemic, infants of mothers with serum antibody to influenza (seropositive) were compared to infants of mothers who were seronegative [106]. The infants of seropositive mothers had higher specific serum antibody (IgG) titers against the HA influenza protein than did infants of seronegative mothers. Good correlation was found between maternal antibody titers and titers in infants (correlation, 0.81). No such correlation was found for non-immune mothers and their infants (correlation, 0.24) [106]. However, this study showed no difference in incidence of influenza infection, although infants of immune mothers showed delayed onset of symptoms and shorter duration of illness, suggesting that passive maternal immunization may delay onset and severity.

5.2.1. Serological studies

When evaluating vaccination response to influenza, a serum antibody titer of ≥1:40 against the HA protein is considered to be clinically relevant, resulting in a 50% decrease in symptomatic infection and, therefore, serving as a correlate of protective immunity [107]. Recent analysis of published data indicates an even higher level of clinical protection, estimating that 70% of participants are protected at a titer of 1:40, with protection increasing gradually with higher titers [108].

In the absence of a widely accepted immune correlate of protection for influenza, the analysis of hemagglutinin inhibition (HAI) seroprotection rates is generally considered a useful indicator of protection in vaccinated persons. There are challenges associated with using this antibody titer as a correlate of protection in infants, however, particularly since this correlate was determined in healthy adults [41, 107]. In any event, the US Food and Drug Administration (FDA) uses this HAI antibody titer in evaluation of influenza vaccines, making the HAI antibody titer the standard used by most investigators [40], including those examining vaccine protection in neonates.

In a study examining transplacental transfer of antibody in response to vaccination, Englund et al. studied women during the last trimester of pregnancy who were vaccinated with IIV3 (A/Sichuan/H3N2, A/Taiwan/H1N1, B/Victoria). Maternal immunization resulted in the transfer of influenza-specific IgG to the infants. When measured at the time of delivery, the levels of antibody transferred were high, with between 87 and 99% of antibody detectable in the mother also detectable in the infant [78]. The antibody titers to at least two of the three influenza antigens (influenza H3N2 and influenza B) remained significantly elevated up to 2 months of age [78].

Sumaya and Gibbs vaccinated pregnant women and reported a similar correlation, finding that cord blood HAI antibody in infants correlated with titers of vaccine-stimulated HAI antibody in mothers, with HAI antibody detected in 54% of newborn serum and 73% of maternal serum [75]. This study did not examine infant influenza infection as an outcome, so the study was unable to correlate serum antibody levels with clinical outcome.

While these previous studies demonstrated that maternal antibody appears to be transferred to infants following both natural infection and vaccination, neither study discussed whether the level maternal antibody was high enough to confer protective immunity to the infant [41, 107]. Using HAI titer as a correlate of immunity, Steinhoff et al. did conduct an RCT of maternal influenza vaccine. Serum samples were obtained from 311 mothers before vaccination and at delivery and from 292 infants at birth at 10 weeks and 20–26 weeks later [109]. The proportion of mothers with a protective antibody titer (HAI ≥ 1:40) at the time of delivery was 88% for A/New Caledonia (H1N1), 98% for A/Fujian (H3N2), and 45% for B/Hong Kong. Similar proportions of infants had protective antibody titers at birth [109].

Yamaguchi et al. also examined the immune responses to influenza vaccination during pregnancy by measuring the effect of influenza vaccination (IIV3) in pregnancy, including maintenance of the specific antibody response, and the efficiency of transplacental transfer of the antibody to the fetus. The study included 125 pregnant women, 71 in their second trimester and 54 during the third trimester of pregnancy. The authors reported that vaccination at any time during pregnancy yielded protective levels of antibody in both maternal and fetal blood [110].

In a prospective study examining the immunogenicity and transplacental transmission of antibodies in pregnant women in Asia, Lin et al. enrolled 46 pregnant women who received a single dose of IIV3. Twenty-eight days after vaccination, the seroprotection rate in vaccinated women against H1N1, H3N2, and influenza B was 91.3, 84.8, and 56.5%, respectively [111].

Several additional studies have demonstrated transplacental antibody transfer following maternal vaccination with pandemic H1N1 vaccine. Three studies evaluated adjuvanted A(H1N1) vaccines, and two studied nonadjuvanted A(H1N1)vaccine. All five of the studies documented protective levels of antibody in significant percent of infants (79–95%).

Zuccotti et al. followed 69 mother-infant pairs. The women were vaccinated during their third trimester of pregnancy with MF59-adjuvanted influenza A(H1N1) vaccine. All of the mothers had HAI antibody titers at or above 1:40 at the time of delivery and throughout the 5 months of follow-up. Ninety-five percent of the infants had HAI antibody titers at or about 1:40 at both birth and 2 months of age. By 5 months of age, the proportion of infants with titers of 1:40 dropped to 81.2% [89], suggesting that passively acquired antibody at levels thought to be protective is transferred and persists for at least 5 months.

In a separate study performed at three sites in the UK, researchers followed infants born to mothers who were vaccinated with AS03-adjuvanted H1N1 vaccine during the second or third trimester of pregnancy. This study found that 79% of the infants of vaccinated mothers had serum antibody titers at or higher than 1:40 compared to a background immunity in 19% of infants of unvaccinated women ($p = 0.001$) [112].

Helmig et al. evaluated the serological response of a cohort of women immunized with adjuvanted A(H1N1) vaccine or by natural infection with A(H1N1)pdm09. The authors detected protective antibody levels (>1:40) in a significant number 17/19 (89.5%) of newborns born to vaccinated mothers ($p = 0.001$) [113]. Notably, while natural influenza infection conferred protective antibody levels in mothers, it did not contribute to protective levels in their infants; only 15.8% of infants born to women who had natural influenza infection during pregnancy developed protective levels of antibody at birth.

In a study of nonadjuvanted A(H1N1) vaccine, Tsatsaris et al. measured Ab titers in cord blood of 88 infants born to women vaccinated with a single dose of monovalent A(H1N1) vaccine. The researchers reported 95% (CI, 89–99%) of infants have protective levels of antibody (>1:40) at birth [114], and Fisher et al. also reported protective levels of Ab in cord blood of infants following maternal vaccination with 2009 monovalent A(H1N1) [115].

Taken together, these studies provide an important proof of concept for transplacentally acquired antibody, from either natural infection or vaccination of their mother, to potentially protect young infants from influenza infection and present maternal immunization as a promising strategy for reducing influenza infection in infants.

5.2.2. Clinical studies

Over the past 11 years, nine studies have been published evaluating the effect of maternal immunization on influenza in 97,656 infants across 15 influenza seasons. Six of these studies showed clinical protection; three studies did not (**Table 2**).

Study	Study period	Participants	Outcomes measured	Protection by maternal influenza vaccine
Black et al. [81]	1997–2002	49,585 pregnant women	Hospitalization for pneumonia and influenza	No difference in risk for hospitalization ($p = 0.235$) Adjusted hazard ratio: 0.956 (CI, 0.889–1.029) Clinical effectiveness: 4% (CI, –3 to 11%) No difference in risk including otitis media visit ($p = 0.506$) Adjusted hazard ratio: 0.938 (CI, 0.777–1.132) Clinical effectiveness: 6% (CI, –13 to 22%)
Munoz et al. [117]	1998–2003	225 infants of immunized mothers	Hospitalization or	No difference in hospitalization

Study	Study period	Participants	Outcomes measured	Protection by maternal influenza vaccine
		826 infants of nonimmunized mothers	clinic visits for respiratory conditions	During first month, infants of immunized moms had more clinic visits for bronchitis (p = 0.04) and fewer for respiratory distress (p = 0.04) No other differences
France et al. [116]	1995–2001	3160 infants of immunized mothers 37,969 infants of nonimmunized women	Medically attended acute respiratory illness (ARI)	No reduction in clinic visit rates Incident rate ratio: 0.96 (CI, 0.86–1.07)
Zaman et al. [79]	2004–2005	316 infant-mother pairs followed for 24 weeks	Clinic visits for respiratory illness Laboratory-confirmed influenza before 24 weeks of age (confirmation by rapid test)	63% effective at preventing laboratory-confirmed influenza in infants up to 6 months old (CI, 5–85%) 29% effective in preventing febrile illness (CI, 6.9–45.7%) 42% effective in preventing clinic visit (CI, 18.2–58.8%)
Benowitz et al. [118]	2000–2009	Infants less than 12 months old -220 cases -430 matched controls	Laboratory-confirmed influenza (confirmation by direct fluorescent antibody (DFA) test)	91.5% effective at preventing hospitalization of infants less than 6 months of age (p = 0.001; CI, 61.7–98.1%) No significant effect on infants older than 6 months
Eick et al. [120]	2002–2005	1169 infant-mother pairs	Laboratory-confirmed influenza (confirmation by viral culture, fourfold rise in HAI antibody in cord serum or rapid test)	Laboratory-confirmed influenza decreased among infants born to vaccinated women compared to controls Risk ratio 0.59 (CI, 0.37–0.93) Clinical effectiveness: 41% Hospitalization Risk ratio 0.61 (CI, 0.45–0.84) Clinical effectiveness: 39%
Poehling et al. [126]	2002–2009	Infants less than 6 months old hospitalized with fever or respiratory symptoms -151 cases -1359 controls	Laboratory-confirmed influenza (confirmation by viral culture or PCR)	Hospitalized infants whose mothers were immunized were 45–48% less likely to have laboratory-confirmed influenza Adjusted odds ratio (OR) 0.52 (CI, 0.30–0.91)
Sugimura et al. [127]	2010–2011	200 infants from birth to 6 months of age -106 infants of vaccinated mothers	Laboratory-confirmed influenza (confirmation by rapid test)	Significant difference in incidence of influenza between infants of vaccinated versus unvaccinated mothers (p = 0.019)

Study	Study period	Participants	Outcomes measured	Protection by maternal influenza vaccine
		-90 infants of unvaccinated mothers		
Madhi et al. [83]	2011–2012	2046 infants -1026 infants of vaccinated mothers - 1023 infants of placebo mothers	Laboratory-confirmed influenza RT-PCR	Vaccine efficacy of 48.8% (CI, 11.6–70.4%)

Table 2. Clinical effectiveness of maternal vaccination for protection of infants.

5.2.2.1. *Studies finding no protective effect*

In a retrospective cohort study of 48,639 infants, Black et al. found that infants born to vaccinated women had the same risk of hospitalization for influenza or pneumonia as infants of unvaccinated women (CI, 0.889–1.029). They also reported that maternal vaccination was not a significant determinant of risk for ILI or otitis media [81].

France et al. followed 3160 infants of immunized mothers and 37,969 infants of nonimmunized mothers from 1995–2001 and during four specific seasonal periods: peak influenza, respiratory syncytial virus predominant, periseasonal, and summer weeks [116]. They found no difference in medically attended ARI (incident rate ratio for peak influenza season 0.96, CI, 0.86–1.07), concluding "maternal influenza vaccination did not reduce visit rates during any of the four time periods and did not delay the onset of first respiratory illness" [116].

In a study that included an examination of data over five influenza seasons, Munoz et al. reported similar results, finding no difference in hospitalizations for respiratory illness during the peak of influenza season between infants of vaccinated mothers versus infants of non-vaccinated mothers [117].

5.2.2.2. *Studies finding clinical protection*

While the three earlier studies above found no benefit to infants from maternal vaccination, a more recent matched case-control study of infants less than 12 months old admitted to hospitals for seasonal influenza between 2000 and 2009 reported maternal vaccination to be 91.5% effective (CI, 61.7–98.1%, p = 0.001) in preventing hospitalization of infants younger than 6 months of age [118]. Maternal vaccination was not effective in preventing hospitalization for infants older than 6 months (−41.4% (CI, 0.153–0.918)). In this study, influenza cases from 2007 to 2009 were confirmed by direct fluorescent antibody (DFA) test, which was reported to be 96.2% sensitive and 99% specific for influenza [119]. A limitation to this study is that results from nine influenza seasons were combined, with no information regarding the strain match of vaccine to circulating strain for each influenza season. The researchers did not type the strain of influenza in infected infants, stating that they "did not have adequate power to assess the vaccine's effectiveness by influenza season...and did not type strains to determine whether influenza infections were caused by strains included in the vaccine" [118].

Eick et al. conducted a study in the White Mountain and Navajo reservations over three influenza seasons, November 2002 to September of 2005. In this prospective cohort study, the effect of influenza vaccine during pregnancy on influenza infection in infants was compared between infants of vaccinated women and those born to non-vaccinated women. The authors analyzed 83 confirmed influenza cases. Of these cases, seven (86%) were confirmed by serology, ten (12%) by viral culture, and two (2%) by rapid influenza testing. Using these three measures of influenza infection, the authors reported a 41% reduction in the risk of laboratory-confirmed influenza for infants born to vaccinated women (RR 0.59, CI, 0.37–0.93) and a 39% reduction in the risk of ILI hospitalization (RR 0.61, CI, 0.45–0.84) [120].

The authors of this study pooled the results from three different assay methods, each with different sensitivities, to document influenza infection. Pooling assays with differing diagnostics represents a limitation of this study. Likewise, the use of serology to document influenza in most (86%) of cases represents a weakness of this study. The authors describe serological documentation of influenza infection as a fourfold or greater increase in HAI antibody in serum collected at 2–3 or 6 months compared with previous serum specimen [120]. Significant limitations have been reported regarding the use of serology in diagnosing influenza in adult patients that have been vaccinated with inactivated vaccines [121–123]. Using serology to document influenza infection in young infants presents additional complications.

Infants under 6 months of age have immature, immunologically inexperienced immune systems. Since their ability to produce antibody in response to infection is often delayed or completely absent, many of their serum antibodies are maternally derived. More than 50 years ago, the use of serology for diagnosis of influenza in infancy was questioned. During an influenza outbreak in Glasgow in 1953, fourfold increases in antibody were found in only 20% of infants admitted to pediatric pneumonia wards (as compared to 30% of adult cases) [124]. In two different outbreaks, antibody production was absent or considerably delayed in infected children under 18 months of age, even when virus could be isolated [125]. These observations illustrate the difficulties inherent in using serology to document influenza infection in young infants.

In the only randomized, blinded clinical study to assess infant protection, Zaman et al. reported a vaccine effectiveness of 63% (CI, 5–85%) against laboratory-confirmed influenza in infants up to 6 months of age [79]. Influenza was confirmed by rapid test (Z Stat Flu), which was reported to have a specificity of 80–90% and a sensitivity of 70–72% for type A and type B influenza. When respiratory illness and fever were used as measure of disease, the reported effectiveness was 29% (CI, 7–46%) [79].

A recent study sought to determine whether maternal vaccination during pregnancy was associated with a reduced risk or laboratory-confirmed influenza hospitalizations in 1510 infants over seven consecutive influenza seasons (2002–2003 through 2008–2009) and across three diverse geographic regions of the United States [126]. Of the 1510 infants hospitalized with fever or respiratory symptoms, 151 (10%) had laboratory-confirmed (by viral culture or

RT-PCR) influenza. The proportion of infants who were influenza positive varied significantly across influenza seasons, from 3% in 2006–2007 to 15% in 2003–2004. The percentage of women who were vaccinated also varied by season, from 10% in 2003–2004 to 38% in 2008–2009.

Among influenza-positive infants during all study years, 12% of their mothers reported being vaccinated during pregnancy, while 20% of mothers of influenza-negative infants reported receiving a vaccination [126], yielding an adjusted odds ratio of 0.52 (CI, 0.30–0.91) and suggesting that infants whose mothers received influenza vaccines during pregnancy were 48% less likely to have laboratory-confirmed influenza than infants of unvaccinated women [126].

In a randomized, placebo-controlled trial of influenza vaccination in South Africa, Madhi et al. followed 1026 infants born to women who received IIV3 and 1023 infants born to placebo recipients. The attack rate of influenza was lower among infants of vaccinated mothers (1.9%) than among those whose mothers received placebo vaccine (3.6%), yielding a vaccine effectiveness of 57.5% (CI, 7.6–70.4) in this population [83].

In a prospective study, Sugimura et al. assessed the incidence of fever and laboratory-confirmed influenza in newborns whose mothers were vaccinated during pregnancy with IIV3. Two hundred infants were followed from birth to 6 months of age. Fever was noted in 36 (34%) of the infants in the vaccinated group and 47 (52.2%) of infants born to unvaccinated mothers ($p < 0.007$). The incidence of influenza as diagnosed by rapid test was 0 (0%) and 5 (5.6%), respectively, ($p = 0.019$) [127].

The reviewed studies assessed hospitalization, clinic visits, ARI, or laboratory-confirmed influenza as primary outcomes. Rationale for influenza vaccination often includes additional secondary outcomes such as reduction of absenteeism for household contacts, secondary infections, acute otitis media, or community transmission of influenza. While these outcomes are important in measuring the broad impact of influenza, they do not provide accurate assessment of vaccine efficacy or effectiveness. Such an assessment is essential for evidence-based, reasoned development of public health policy and decision-making about influenza prevention.

In summary, the evidence for newborn protection through maternal vaccination is encouraging, but several studies exhibit methodological limitations. The results of studies measuring rates of ARI, clinic visit, or hospitalization range from no vaccine effect up to 42% effectiveness [81, 116, 117]. The six studies that used some form of laboratory-confirmed influenza (rapid tests, viral culture, or PCR) as the primary outcome are more encouraging, reporting vaccination effectiveness ranging from 41 to 91.5% [79, 83, 118, 120, 126, 127].

While outcomes and study designs differ, in general the data to date suggest that maternal vaccination has the potential to decrease influenza illness in newborns. As such, maternal immunization during pregnancy should continue to be recommended and encouraged for all women.

6. Current challenges

Influenza is a complex disease. For centuries it has eluded complete understanding or control. Constantly evolving and catching us by surprise, influenza is a perpetually emerging disease. The main tool for prevention of influenza is vaccination, the cornerstone for prevention of influenza disease. However, unlike many other vaccines, the effectiveness of influenza vaccines remains moderate to marginal across all populations [128], and in addition, the vaccines need to be administered every year. A universal influenza vaccine providing broad and long-lasting protection continues to be elusive.

These realities—difficult enough in the general population—are even more challenging to understand during pregnancy. Particularly complex is determining how, or if, the changing immune responses over pregnancy vis-a-vis influenza season and vaccination schedules impact vaccine effectiveness and disease outcomes in pregnant women.

A recent critique by Savitz et al. calls into question our most basic understanding of influenza infection during pregnancy, with a particular critique on the quality of the evidence for a benefit of maternal vaccination in prevention of harm from seasonal influenza [129]. Savitz et al. discuss the complications inherent in many current research practices, which serve to limit our understanding of the true picture of maternal influenza. Central to this critique is the notion that both pregnancy and influenza have temporal components; influenza typically is seasonal, with a 2–3-month period of circulation each year. But pregnancy has trimesters, each with distinct fetal developmental stages along with physiological and immunological changes in the expectant mother. To complicate this further, the risk of adverse outcomes from influenza infection is not equal across all trimesters of pregnancy. Therefore, optimizing risk and benefit of vaccination during pregnancy is complicated and likely requires reexamination of influenza risk and benefit across trimesters in association with months of influenza circulation [129].

A recent WHO review of influenza throughout pregnancy found insufficient data from comparable studies to discern which specific weeks, months, or trimesters influenza poses increased risk to pregnant women [130]. Savitz et al. assert that "As with all time dependent states, pregnancies must be followed longitudinally. There needs to be a week-by-week consideration of the pregnancy with regard to vaccination status and circulating influenza viruses" [129].

Aside from complications associated with potential differences in virus exposure across the trimesters of a pregnancy, risks posed to pregnant women also may differ according to the specific strain circulating during a given season, and, likewise, the immune response to vaccination also could differ based on strain [131].

Even when taking yearly strain differences into account, variation in immune responses across trimesters adds yet another complicating variable. It is widely accepted that the immune response to influenza vaccine in pregnant women is indistinguishable from that of nonpregnant women and that gestational age appears to have no effect on antibody response [75, 76, 132, 133].

Findings from more recent studies suggest that we may need to entertain a more nuanced approach to our understanding of the maternal immune response to influenza vaccination—precisely because immunogenicity and seroconversion may not tell the entire story.

In a 2011 study, Ohfuji et al. reported a lower seroprotective antibody response to pandemic A(H1N1) vaccine in pregnant women who had received prior seasonal influenza vaccine and suggested that the potential interference between pH1N1 and seasonal vaccination needed additional investigation [15]. Schlaudecker et al. directly compared immunogenicity of inactivated influenza vaccine in pregnant versus nonpregnant women and found that pregnancy modified antibody responses to the vaccine [134]. They demonstrated a significantly decreased postimmunization HAI geometric mean titer and a nonsignificantly decreased geometric mean ratio (fold increase) to influenza A antigens after influenza vaccine, even though overall seroconversion and seroprotection rates were comparable between the two groups of women. In a 2013 blinded randomized control study, Bischoff et al. found that the immune response to an adjuvanted pandemic A(H1N1) vaccine in pregnant women was decreased compared with nonpregnant women [133]. Sperling et al. examined HAI titers over pregnancy and found that timing of vaccination did not alter response, although there was a trend toward lower responses during the first trimester and six weeks postpartum [135].

A small study of 36 women during the 2012–2014 flu seasons suggests that T-follicular helper (Tfh) cell response to vaccination was highest during the first trimester of pregnancy. Tfh cells are required for the generation of high-quality antibody-producing B cells. Their expansion has been shown to be a predictor of response to influenza vaccination outside of pregnancy suggesting that immunologic changes during pregnancy may impact vaccine response. Notably, there was no significant expansion of Tfh after vaccination during either the second or third trimester [136].

In a study aimed to determine the optimal timing for vaccination within the second or third trimesters of pregnancy, Yamaguchi et al. reported that serum antibody levels in vaccinated women depended not on gestational stage but on the amount of time elapsed, since vaccination antibody titers decreased with time [110]. This observation is supported by other studies documenting that influenza-specific antibodies after vaccination are typically short lived [115].

Two separate studies of vaccine effectiveness in nonpregnant adults during the 2011–2012 influenza season also suggest that vaccine effectiveness wanes with time since vaccination [137, 138]. In both of these studies, vaccination effectiveness waned in people who were vaccinated 93 days—around 3 months—or more before presentation of symptoms. A similar observation was made by Fisher et al. who demonstrated a significant linear decline over time in HAI titers after pH1N1 infection or vaccination ($p = 0.04$ for infected and $p = 0.009$ for vaccinated) [115].

Taken together, these observations support a consensus that pregnant women are capable of mounting a robust immune response to influenza vaccination during the second and third trimester of pregnancy. Experimental evidence during the first trimester is less clear, due in part to a limited number of studies on influenza vaccination during the first trimester.

There is increasing evidence suggesting that—regardless of initial vaccine response—the level of vaccine-mediated anti-influenza-specific antibodies decreases with time. This waning of antibody implies that women vaccinated during the first trimester of pregnancy might be *less* well protected as their pregnancy progresses. It is well documented that serious influenza-related morbidity in healthy pregnant women most often occurs during the second and third trimester of pregnancy. So a reasonable goal appears to be ensuring the highest possible level of protection during the second and third trimesters. Studies on waning immunity suggest that this may be precisely opposite of what occurs in women who are vaccinated early in pregnancy; protection wanes as risk increases.

6.1. Timing maternal vaccination for protection of neonates

Cross-placental transfer of immunity occurs when antibodies cross the placenta via active transport, particularly in the final weeks of pregnancy. It is logical to assume that vaccine-induced maternal antibody transmitted to the fetus will provide protection to the infant during the first months of life, and several studies document increased antibody titers in infants of vaccinated mothers [120].

Comparable to studies of vaccinated mothers, researchers have demonstrated that the titers of influenza-specific antibodies in newborns, while not affected by trimester of maternal vaccination (within second or third trimester), do wane with time and are short lived [75]. Tsatsaris et al. also noted a trend toward lower cord blood antibody titer associated with longer intervals between maternal vaccination and delivery. A similar observation was made by Yamaguchi et al. who reported that transfer rate from the maternal blood to the fetal blood at time of delivery tended to be inversely correlated with duration of gestation postvaccination [110]. Some additional studies have hinted at lower cord blood titers among infants of women vaccinated in the first trimesters, but it is unclear if this is clinically significant [131].

Taken together, these studies serve to highlight the complicated nature of immunity particularly during pregnancy in response to vaccination and invite further virological and epidemiological studies to confirm and fully understand these observations and to correlate changes in antibody titer with clinical outcomes in both mothers and infants. As our understanding evolves, we may need to develop a more nuanced approach—one that takes into consideration the trimester of exposure to both circulating virus and vaccines—to optimize vaccine effectiveness during the period of highest risk of influenza disease.

The recommendation to vaccinate all pregnant women regardless of gestational age is motivated in part by operational concerns. Timing of the influenza vaccine campaigns occurs in the fall in temperate regions. Pregnancy, on the other hand, occurs throughout the year. Since pregnancy presents a period of regularly scheduled and repeat visits, a more tailored approach to influenza vaccine coverage may be appropriate in order to stack the odds in favor of the highest level of protection for both mother and infant.

7. Conclusions

The impact of influenza infection on pregnant women and newborns is well documented. The increased risk for morbidity and mortality has resulted in the universal recommendation that pregnant women be vaccinated for influenza at any stage of pregnancy [65]. Evidence to date suggests that influenza vaccination during pregnancy is similarly effective as in the nonpregnant population. Pregnant women mount robust immune response that correlates with clinical efficacy. This immunity then is transferred to the fetus during gestation, providing clinical benefit to infants less than 6 months of age. And while not a component of this review, there is substantial evidence that influenza vaccines are safe during all stages of pregnancy with no evidence of risk of adverse pregnancy outcome linked to influenza vaccines [3, 65, 131, 139, 140].

Gaps remain in our understanding of influenza risk over all seasons and trimesters, of maternal immunity, and of optimal timing of vaccination. To this end, in January of 2015, the Bill and Melinda Gates Foundation held a meeting of global stakeholders in the maternal influenza field. Participants identified a need for stronger evidence regarding, among other issues, the burden of disease and maternal immunization efficacy [141]. Expanding this evidence base will allow for a deeper understanding of influenza in this population and the development of more robust and efficacious public health approaches toward this disease.

Author details

Jill M. Manske

Address all correspondence to: jmmanske@stthomas.edu

University of St. Thomas, Saint Paul, MN, USA

References

[1] World Health Organization, WHO position paper on influenza vaccines. Wkly Epidemiol Record 2005; 33: 279–287)

[2] Tamma PD, Steinhoff MC, Omer SB. Influenza infection and vaccination in pregnant women. Expert Rev Respir Med 2010;4:321–8.

[3] Mak TK, Mangtani P, Leese J, Watson JM, Pfeifer D. Influenza vaccination in pregnancy: current evidence and selected national policies. Lancet Infect Dis 2008;8:44–52.

[4] Neuzil KM, Reed GW, Mitchel EF, Simonsen L, Griffin MR. Impact of influenza on acute cardiopulmonary hospitalizations in pregnant women. Am J Epidemiol 1998;148:1094–102.

[5] Schanzer DL, Langley JM, Tam TW. Influenza-attributed hospitalization rates among pregnant women in Canada 1994–2000. J Obstet Gynaecol Can 2007;29:622–9.

[6] Jamieson DJ, Theiler RN, Rasmussen SA. Emerging infections and pregnancy. Emerg Infect Dis 2006;12:1638–43.

[7] Skowronski DM, De Serres G. Is routine influenza immunization warranted in early pregnancy? Vaccine 2009;27:4754–70.

[8] Gaunt G, Ramin K. Immunological tolerance of the human fetus. Am J Perinatol 2001;18:299–312.

[9] Szekeres-Bartho J. Immunological relationship between the mother and the fetus. Int Rev Immunol 2002;21:471–95.

[10] Davies M, Browne CM. Pregnancy-associated nonspecific immunosuppression: kinetics of the generation and identification of the active factors. Am J Reprod Immunol Microbiol 1985;9:77–83.

[11] Saleeby E, Chapman J, Morse J, Bryant A. H1N1 influenza in pregnancy: cause for concern. Obstet Gynecol 2009;114:885–91.

[12] Laibl VR, Sheffield JS. Influenza and pneumonia in pregnancy. Clin Perinatol 2005;32:727–38.

[13] Griffiths PD, Ronalds CJ, Heath RB. A prospective study of influenza infections during pregnancy. J Epidemiol Community Health 1980;34:124–8.

[14] Lindsay L, Jackson LA, Savitz DA, Weber DJ, Koch GG, Kong L, et al. Community influenza activity and risk of acute influenza-like illness episodes among healthy unvaccinated pregnant and postpartum women. Am J Epidemiol 2006;163:838–48.

[15] Ohfuji S, Fukushima W, Deguchi M, Kawabata K, Yoshida H, Hatayama H, et al. Immunogenicity of a monovalent 2009 influenza A (H1N1) vaccine among pregnant women: lowered antibody response by prior seasonal vaccination. J Infect Dis 2011;203:1301–8.

[16] Dodds L, McNeil SA, Fell DB, Allen VM, Coombs A, Scott J, et al. Impact of influenza exposure on rates of hospital admissions and physician visits because of respiratory illness among pregnant women. CMAJ 2007;176:463–8.

[17] Cox S, Posner SF, McPheeters M, Jamieson DJ, Kourtis AP, Meikle S. Hospitalizations with respiratory illness among pregnant women during influenza season. Obstet Gynecol 2006;107:1315–22.

[18] Hartert TV, Neuzil KM, Shintani AK, Mitchel EF, Jr., Snowden MS, Wood LB, et al. Maternal morbidity and perinatal outcomes among pregnant women with respiratory hospitalizations during influenza season. Am J Obstet Gynecol 2003;189:1705–12.

[19] Kort BA, Cefalo RC, Baker VV. Fatal influenza A pneumonia in pregnancy. Am J Perinatol 1986;3:179–82.

[20] Housworth J, Langmuir AD. Excess mortality from epidemic influenza, 1957–1966. Am J Epidemiol 1974;100:40–8.

[21] Callaghan WM, Chu SY, Jamieson DJ. Deaths from seasonal influenza among pregnant women in the United States, 1998–2005. Obstet Gynecol 2010;115:919–23.

[22] Nuzum JW, Pilot I, Stangl FH, Bonar BE. 1918 pandemic influenza and pneumonia in a large civil hospital. IMJ Illinois Med J 1976;150:612–6.

[23] Freeman DW, Barno A. Deaths from Asian influenza associated with pregnancy. Am J Obstet Gynecol 1959;78:1172–5.

[24] Greenberg M, Jacobziner H, Pakter J, Weisl BA. Maternal mortality in the epidemic of Asian influenza, New York City, 1957. Am J Obstet Gynecol 1958;76:897–902.

[25] Harris JW. Influenza occurring in pregnant women: a statistical study of thirteen hundred and fifty cases. J Am Med Assoc 1919;72:978–80.

[26] Woolston, W.J., Conley D.O. Epidemic pneumonia (Spanish influenza) in pregnancy: effect in one hundred and one cases. J Am Med Assoc 1918;71:1898–9.

[27] CDC. Novel influenza A (H1N1) virus infection in three pregnant women—United States. MMWR Morb Mortal Wkly Rep 2009;58:497–500.

[28] Panda B, Panda A, Riley LE. Selected viral infections in pregnancy. Obstet Gynecol Clin North Am 2010;37:321–31.

[29] CDC. Hospitalized patients with novel influenza A (H1N1) virus infection-California. MMWR Morb Mortal Wkly Rep 2009;58:536–41.

[30] Jamieson DJ, Honein MA, Rasmussen SA, Williams JL, Swerdlow DL, Biggerstaff MS, et al. H1N1 2009 influenza virus infection during pregnancy in the USA. Lancet 2009;374:451–8.

[31] Louie JK, Acosta M, Jamieson DJ, Honein MA. Severe 2009 H1N1 influenza in pregnant and postpartum women in California. N Engl J Med 2010;362:27–35.

[32] Mosby LG, Rasmussen SA, Jamieson DJ. 2009 Pandemic influenza A (H1N1) in pregnancy: a systematic review of the literature. Am J Obstet Gynecol 2011.

[33] Callaghan WM, Creanga AA, Jamieson DJ. Pregnancy-related mortality resulting from influenza in the United States during the 2009–2010 pandemic. Obstet Gynecol 2015;126:486–90.

[34] Siston AM, Rasmussen SA, Honein MA, Fry AM, Seib K, Callaghan WM, et al. Pandemic 2009 influenza A(H1N1) virus illness among pregnant women in the United States. JAMA 2010;303:1517–25.

[35] Yates L, Pierce M, Stephens S, Mill AC, Spark P, Kurinczuk JJ, et al. Influenza A/H1N1v in pregnancy: an investigation of the characteristics and management of affected women and the relationship to pregnancy outcomes for mother and infant. Health Technol Assess 2010;14:109–82.

[36] Gerardin P, El Amrani R, Cyrille B, Gabriele M, Guillermin P, Boukerrou M, et al. Low clinical burden of 2009 pandemic influenza A (H1N1) infection during pregnancy on the island of La Reunion. PLoS One 2010;5:e10896.

[37] Zhang J, Troendle J, Reddy UM, Laughon SK, Branch DW, Burkman R, et al. Contemporary cesarean delivery practice in the United States. Am J Obstet Gynecol 2010;203:326e1–e10.

[38] Yawn DH, Pyeatte JC, Joseph JM, Eichler SL, Garcia-Bunuel R. Transplacental transfer of influenza virus. JAMA 1971;216:1022–3.

[39] Dulyachai W, Makkoch J, Rianthavorn P, Changpinyo M, Prayangprecha S, Payungporn S, et al. Perinatal pandemic (H1N1) 2009 infection, Thailand. Emerg Infect Dis 2010;16:343–4.

[40] Lieberman RW, Bagdasarian N, Thomas D, Van De Ven C. Seasonal influenza A (H1N1) infection in early pregnancy and second trimester fetal demise. Emerg Infect Dis 2011;17:107–9.

[41] Ortiz JR, Englund JA, Neuzil KM. Influenza vaccine for pregnant women in resource-constrained countries: a review of the evidence to inform policy decisions. Vaccine 2011;29:4439–52.

[42] Hewagama S, Walker SP, Stuart RL, Gordon C, Johnson PD, Friedman ND, et al. 2009 H1N1 influenza A and pregnancy outcomes in Victoria, Australia. Clin Infect Dis 2010;50:686–90.

[43] Uchide N, Ohyama K, Bessho T, Toyoda H. Induction of pro-inflammatory cytokine gene expression and apoptosis in human chorion cells of fetal membranes by influenza virus infection: possible implications for maintenance and interruption of pregnancy during infection. Med Sci Monit 2005;11:RA7–16.

[44] Shi L, Tu N, Patterson PH. Maternal influenza infection is likely to alter fetal brain development indirectly: the virus is not detected in the fetus. Int J Dev Neurosci 2005;23:299–305.

[45] McKinney WP, Volkert P, Kaufman J. Fatal swine influenza pneumonia during late pregnancy. Arch Intern Med 1990;150:213–5.

[46] Moretti ME, Bar-Oz B, Fried S, Koren G. Maternal hyperthermia and the risk for neural tube defects in offspring: systematic review and meta-analysis. Epidemiology 2005;16:216–9.

[47] Coffey VP, Jessop WJ. Maternal influenza and congenital deformities. A follow-up study. Lancet 1963;1:748–51.

[48] Hardy JM, Azarowicz EN, Mannini A, Medearis DN, Jr., Cooke RE. The effect of Asian influenza on the outcome of pregnancy, Baltimore, 1957–1958. Am J Public Health Nations Health 1961;51:1182–8.

[49] Saxen L, Hjelt L, Sjostedt JE, Hakosalo J, Hakosalo H. Asian influenza during pregnancy and congenital malformations. Acta Pathol Microbiol Scand 1960;49:114–26.

[50] Edwards MJ. Review: hyperthermia and fever during pregnancy. Birth Defects Res A Clin Mol Teratol 2006;76:507–16.

[51] Hansen C, Desai S, Bredfeldt C, Cheetham C, Gallagher M, Li D-K, et al. A large, population-based study of 2009 pandemic Influenza A virus subtype H1N1 infection diagnosis during pregnancy and outcomes for mothers and neonates. J Infect Dis 2012;206:1260–8.

[52] Luteijn JM, Brown MJ, Dolk H. Influenza and congenital anomalies: a systematic review and meta-analysis. Hum Reprod 2014;29:809–23.

[53] Haberg SE, Trogstad L, Gunnes N, Wilcox AJ, Gjessing HK, Samuelsen SO, et al. Risk of fetal death after pandemic influenza virus infection or vaccination. N Engl J Med 2013;368:333–40.

[54] Pierce M, Kurinczuk JJ, Spark P, Brocklehurst P, Knight M, Ukoss. Perinatal outcomes after maternal 2009/H1N1 infection: national cohort study. BMJ 2011;342:d3214.

[55] Moore DL, Vaudry W, Scheifele DW, Halperin SA, Dery P, Ford-Jones E, et al. Surveillance for influenza admissions among children hospitalized in Canadian immunization monitoring program active centers, 2003–2004. Pediatrics 2006;118:e610–9.

[56] Izurieta HS, Thompson WW, Kramarz P, Shay DK, Davis RL, DeStefano F, et al. Influenza and the rates of hospitalization for respiratory disease among infants and young children. N Engl J Med 2000;342:232–9.

[57] Neuzil KM, Mellen BG, Wright PF, Mitchel EF, Jr., Griffin MR. The effect of influenza on hospitalizations, outpatient visits, and courses of antibiotics in children. N Engl J Med 2000;342:225–31.

[58] Thompson WW, Shay DK, Weintraub E, Brammer L, Bridges CB, Cox NJ, et al. Influenza-associated hospitalizations in the United States. JAMA 2004;292:1333–40.

[59] Bhat N, Wright JG, Broder KR, Murray EL, Greenberg ME, Glover MJ, et al. Influenza-associated deaths among children in the United States, 2003–2004. N Engl J Med 2005;353:2559–67.

[60] Thompson WW, Weintraub, E., Shay, D.K., Brammer, L., Cox, N., Fukuda, K. Age-specific estimated of US influenza-associated deaths and hospitalizations. Int Congr Ser 2004;1263:316–20.

[61] Iwane MK, Edwards KM, Szilagyi PG, Walker FJ, Griffin MR, Weinberg GA, et al. Population-based surveillance for hospitalizations associated with respiratory syncytial virus, influenza virus, and parainfluenza viruses among young children. Pediatrics 2004;113:1758–64.

[62] Poehling KA, Edwards KM, Weinberg GA, Szilagyi P, Staat MA, Iwane MK, et al. The underrecognized burden of influenza in young children. N Engl J Med 2006;355:31–40.

[63] Centers for Disease Control. Surveillance for laboratory-confirmed, influenza-associated hospitalizations—Colorado, 2004–05 influenza season. MMWR Morb Mortal Wkly Rep 2005;54:535–7.

[64] Libster R, Bugna J, Coviello S, Hijano DR, Dunaiewsky M, Reynoso N, et al. Pediatric hospitalizations associated with 2009 pandemic influenza A (H1N1) in Argentina. N Engl J Med 2010;362:45–55.

[65] Fiore AE, Uyeki TM, Broder K, Finelli L, Euler GL, Singleton JA, et al. Prevention and control of influenza with vaccines: recommendations of the Advisory Committee on Immunization Practices (ACIP), 2010. MMWR Recomm Rep 2010;59:1–62.

[66] Centers For Disease Control. Key facts about 2009 H1N1 flu vaccine. http://www.cdc.gov/h1n1flu/vaccination/vaccine_keyfacts.htm. Published March, 2010. Accessed February 15, 2016.

[67] Ambrose CS, Luke C, Coelingh K. Current status of live attenuated influenza vaccine in the United States for seasonal and pandemic influenza. Influenza Other Respir Viruses 2008;2:193–202.

[68] Centers For Disease Control. General recommendations on immunization: recommendations of the Advisory Committee on Immunization Practices (ACIP). MMWR 2011; 60 (No. 2): 26.

[69] Yudin MH. Risk management of seasonal influenza during pregnancy: current perspectives. Int J Women's Health 2014;6:681–9.

[70] Fiore AE, Shay DK, Broder K, Iskander JK, Uyeki TM, Mootrey G, et al. Prevention and control of seasonal influenza with vaccines: recommendations of the Advisory Committee on Immunization Practices (ACIP), 2009. MMWR Recomm Rep 2009;58:1–52.

[71] Harper SA, Fukuda K, Uyeki TM, Cox NJ, Bridges CB. Prevention and control of influenza: recommendations of the Advisory Committee on Immunization Practices (ACIP). MMWR Recomm Rep 2004;53:1–40.

[72] Centers for Disease Control. Prevention and Control of Influenza: Recommendations of the Immunization Practices Advisory Committee (ACIP). MMWR Morb Mortal Wkly Rep 2013;62:10, 30.

[73] World Health Organization. WHO recommendations on pandemic (H1N1) 2009 vaccines. http://www.who.int/csr/disease/swineflu/notes/h1n1_vaccine_20090713/en/. July 2009. Accessed November 7, 2015.

[74] Centers For Disease Control. Updated interim recommendations for obstetric health care providers related to the use of antiviral medications in the treatment and prevention of influenza for the 2009–2010 season.http://www.cdc.gov/h1n1flu/recommendations.htm. December 2009. Accessed January 12, 2016.

[75] Sumaya CV, Gibbs RS. Immunization of pregnant women with influenza A/New Jersey/76 virus vaccine: reactogenicity and immunogenicity in mother and infant. J Infect Dis 1979;140:141–6.

[76] Hulka JF. Effectiveness of polyvalent influenza vaccine in Pregnancy. Report of a Controlled Study during an Outbreak of Asian Influenza. Obstet Gynecol 1964;23:830–7.

[77] Deinard AS, Ogburn P, Jr. A/NJ/8/76 influenza vaccination program: effects on maternal health and pregnancy outcome. Am J Obstet Gynecol 1981;140:240–5.

[78] Englund JA, Mbawuike IN, Hammill H, Holleman MC, Baxter BD, Glezen WP. Maternal immunization with influenza or tetanus toxoid vaccine for passive antibody protection in young infants. J Infect Dis 1993;168:647–56.

[79] Zaman K, Roy E, Arifeen SE, Rahman M, Raqib R, Wilson E, et al. Effectiveness of maternal influenza immunization in mothers and infants. N Engl J Med 2008;359:1555–64.

[80] Manske JM. Efficacy and effectiveness of maternal influenza vaccination during pregnancy: a review of the evidence. Matern Child Health J 2013;18:1599–609.

[81] Black SB, Shinefield HR, France EK, Fireman BH, Platt ST, Shay D. Effectiveness of influenza vaccine during pregnancy in preventing hospitalizations and outpatient visits for respiratory illness in pregnant women and their infants. Am J Perinatol 2004;21:333–9.

[82] Munoz FM, Englund JA. A step ahead. Infant protection through maternal immunization. Pediatr Clin North Am 2000;47:449–63.

[83] Madhi SA, Cutland CL, Kuwanda L, Weinberg A, Hugo A, Jones S, et al. Influenza vaccination of pregnant women and protection of their infants. N Engl J Med 2014;371:918–31.

[84] Thompson MG, Li D-K, Shifflett P, Sokolow LZ, Ferber JR, Kurosky S, et al. Effectiveness of seasonal trivalent influenza vaccine for preventing influenza virus illness among pregnant women: a population-based case-control study during the 2010–2011 and 2011–2012 influenza seasons. Clin Infect Dis 2014;58:449–57.

[85] Centers for Disease Control. Use of Influenza A (H1N1) 2009 monovalent vaccine: recommendations of the Advisory Committee on Immunization Practices (ACIP). MMWR Morb Mortal Wkly Rep 2009;58:1–8.

[86] Centers for Disease Control. Seasonal Influenza and 2009 H1N1 influenza vaccination coverage among pregnant women–10 states, 2009–2010 influenza season. MMWR Morb Mortal Wkly Rep 2010;59:1541–5.

[87] Horiya M, Hisano M, Iwasaki Y, Hanaoka M, Watanabe N, Ito Y, et al. Efficacy of double vaccination with the 2009 pandemic influenza A (H1N1) vaccine during pregnancy. Obstet Gynecol 2011;118:887–94.

[88] Jackson LA, Patel SM, Swamy GK, Frey SE, Creech CB, Munoz FM, et al. Immunogenicity of an inactivated monovalent 2009 H1N1 influenza vaccine in pregnant women. J Infect Dis 2011;204:854–63.

[89] Zuccotti G, Pogliani L, Pariani E, Amendola A, Zanetti A. Transplacental antibody transfer following maternal immunization with a pandemic 2009 influenza A(H1N1) MF59-adjuvanted vaccine. JAMA 2010;304:2360–1.

[90] Abzug MJ, Nachman SA, Muresan P, Handelsman E, Watts DH, Fenton T, et al. Safety and immunogenicity of 2009 pH1N1 vaccination in HIV-infected pregnant women. Clin Infect Dis 2013;56:1488–97.

[91] Yung CF, Andrews N, Hoschler K, Miller E. Comparing the immunogenicity of AS03-adjuvanted 2009 pandemic H1N1 vaccine with clinical protection in priority risk groups in England. PLoS One 2013;8:e56844.

[92] Puleston R, Bugg G, Hoschler K, Konje J, Thornton J, Stephenson I, et al. Multi-centre observational study of transplacental transmission of influenza antibodies following vaccination with AS03(A)-adjuvanted H1N1 2009 vaccine. PLoS One 2013;8:e47448.

[93] Moro PL, Broder K, Zheteyeva Y, Walton K, Rohan P, Sutherland A, et al. Adverse events in pregnant women following administration of trivalent inactivated influenza vaccine and live attenuated influenza vaccine in the Vaccine Adverse Event Reporting System, 1990–2009. Am J Obstet Gynecol 2011;204:146e1–7.

[94] Kallen B, Olausson PO. Vaccination against H1N1 influenza with Pandemrix((R)) during pregnancy and delivery outcome: a Swedish register study. BJOG 2012;119:1583–90.

[95] Pasternak B, Svanstrom H, Molgaard-Nielsen D, Krause TG, Emborg HD, Melbye M, et al. Risk of adverse fetal outcomes following administration of a pandemic influenza A(H1N1) vaccine during pregnancy. JAMA 2012;308:165–74.

[96] Beau AB, Hurault-Delarue C, Vidal S, Guitard C, Vayssiere C, Petiot D, et al. Pandemic A/H1N1 influenza vaccination during pregnancy: a comparative study using the EFEMERIS database. Vaccine 2014;32:1254–8.

[97] Chambers CD, Johnson D, Xu R, Luo Y, Louik C, Mitchell AA, et al. Risks and safety of pandemic H1N1 influenza vaccine in pregnancy: birth defects, spontaneous abortion, preterm delivery, and small for gestational age infants. Vaccine 2013;31:5026–32.

[98] Heikkinen T, Young J, van Beek E, Franke H, Verstraeten T, Weil JG, et al. Safety of MF59-adjuvanted A/H1N1 influenza vaccine in pregnancy: a comparative cohort study. Am J Obstet Gynecol 2012;207:177.e1–8.

[99] Omon E, Damase-Michel C, Hurault-Delarue C, Lacroix I, Montastruc JL, Oustric S, et al. Non-adjuvanted 2009 influenza A (H1N1)v vaccine in pregnant women: the results of a French prospective descriptive study. Vaccine 2011;29:9649–54.

[100] Tavares F, Nazareth I, Monegal JS, Kolte I, Verstraeten T, Bauchau V. Pregnancy and safety outcomes in women vaccinated with an AS03-adjuvanted split virion H1N1 (2009) pandemic influenza vaccine during pregnancy: a prospective cohort study. Vaccine 2011;29:6358–65.

[101] Richards JL, Hansen C, Bredfeldt C, Bednarczyk RA, Steinhoff MC, Adjaye-Gbewonyo D, et al. Neonatal outcomes after antenatal influenza immunization during the 2009 H1N1 influenza pandemic: impact on preterm birth, birth weight, and small for gestational age birth. Clin Infect Dis 2013.

[102] Simister NE. Placental transport of immunoglobulin G. Vaccine 2003;21:3365–9.

[103] Munoz ET, Deem MW. Epitope analysis for influenza vaccine design. Vaccine 2005;23:1144–8.

[104] Van de Perre P. Transfer of antibody via mother's milk. Vaccine 2003;21:3374–6.

[105] Puck JM, Glezen WP, Frank AL, Six HR. Protection of infants from infection with influenza A virus by transplacentally acquired antibody. J Infect Dis 1980;142:844–9.

[106] Reuman PD, Ayoub EM, Small PA. Effect of passive maternal antibody on influenza illness in children: a prospective study of influenza A in mother-infant pairs. Pediatr Infect Dis J 1987;6:398–403.

[107] Plotkin SA. Correlates of protection induced by vaccination. Clin Vaccine Immunol 2010;17:1055–65.

[108] Coudeville L, Andre P, Bailleux F, Weber F, Plotkin S. A new approach to estimate vaccine efficacy based on immunogenicity data applied to influenza vaccines administered by the intradermal or intramuscular routes. Hum Vaccines 2010;6:841–8.

[109] Steinhoff MC, Omer SB, Roy E, Arifeen SE, Raqib R, Altaye M, et al. Influenza immunization in pregnancy—antibody responses in mothers and infants. N Engl J Med 2010;362:1644–6.

[110] Yamaguchi K, Hisano M, Isojima S, Irie S, Arata N, Watanabe N, et al. Relationship of Th1/Th2 cell balance with the immune response to influenza vaccine during pregnancy. J Med Virol 2009;81:1923–8.

[111] Lin S-Y, Wu E-T, Lin C-H, Shyu M-K, Lee C-N. The safety and immunogenicity of trivalent inactivated influenza vaccination: a study of maternal-cord blood pairs in Taiwan. PLoS One 2013;8:e62983.

[112] Puleston RL, Bugg G, Hoschler K, Konje J, Thornton J, Stephenson I, et al. Observational study to investigate vertically acquired passive immunity in babies of mothers vaccinated against H1N1v during pregnancy. Health Technol Assess 2010;14:1-82.

[113] Helmig RB, Maimburg RD, Erikstrup C, Nielsen HS, Petersen OB, Nielsen LP, et al. Antibody response to influenza A(H1N1)pdm09 in vaccinated, serologically infected and unaffected pregnant women and their newborns. Acta Obstet Gynecol Scand 2015;94:833–9.

[114] Tsatsaris V, Capitant C, Schmitz T, Chazallon C, Bulifon S, Riethmuller D, et al. Maternal immune response and neonatal seroprotection from a single dose of a monovalent nonadjuvanted 2009 influenza A(H1N1) vaccine: a single-group trial. Ann Intern Med 2011;155:733–41.

[115] Fisher BM, Van Bockern J, Hart J, Lynch AM, Winn VD, Gibbs RS, et al. Pandemic influenza A H1N1 2009 infection versus vaccination: a cohort study comparing immune responses in pregnancy. PLoS One 2012;7:e33048.

[116] France EK, Smith-Ray R, McClure D, Hambidge S, Xu S, Yamasaki K, et al. Impact of maternal influenza vaccination during pregnancy on the incidence of acute respiratory illness visits among infants. Arch Pediatr Adolesc Med 2006;160:1277–83.

[117] Munoz FM, Greisinger AJ, Wehmanen OA, Mouzoon ME, Hoyle JC, Smith FA, et al. Safety of influenza vaccination during pregnancy. Am J Obstet Gynecol 2005;192:1098–106.

[118] Benowitz I, Esposito DB, Gracey KD, Shapiro ED, Vazquez M. Influenza vaccine given to pregnant women reduces hospitalization due to influenza in their infants. Clin Infect Dis 2010;51:1355–61.

[119] Landry ML, Cohen S, Ferguson D. Real-time PCR compared to Binax NOW and cytospin-immunofluorescence for detection of influenza in hospitalized patients. J Clin Virol 2008;43:148–51.

[120] Eick AA, Uyeki TM, Klimov A, Hall H, Reid R, Santosham M, et al. Maternal influenza vaccination and effect on influenza virus infection in young infants. Arch Pediatr Adolesc Med 2011;165:104–11.

[121] McDonald JC, Andrews BE. Diagnostic methods in an influenza vaccine trial. Br Med J 1955;2:1232–5.

[122] Petrie JG, Ohmit SE, Johnson E, Cross RT, Monto AS. Efficacy studies of influenza vaccines: effect of end points used and characteristics of vaccine failures. J Infect Dis 2011;203:1309–15.

[123] Rapmund G, Johnson RT, Bankhead AS, Herman YF, Dandridge OW. The diagnosis of Asian influenza virus infection after recent immunization. U S Armed Forces Med J 1959;10:637–49.

[124] Grist NR, Landsman JB. Influenza in Glasgow, 1950–1953. Glasgow Med J 1955;36:69–75.

[125] Anderson SG, Donnelley M, French EL, Kalra SL, White J. Influenza in Victoria, 1950 and 1951. Med JAust 1953;2:44–7.

[126] Poehling KA, Szilagyi PG, Staat MA, Snively BM, Payne DC, Bridges CB, et al. Impact of maternal immunization on influenza hospitalizations in infants. Am J Obstet Gynecol 2011;204:S141–8.

[127] Sugimura T, Nagai T, Kobayashi H, Ozaki Y, Yamakawa R, Hirata R. Effectiveness of maternal influenza immunization in young infants in Japan. Pediatr Int 2015.

[128] Osterholm MT, Kelley NS, Sommer A, Belongia EA. Influenza vaccine efficacy and effectiveness: a new look at the evidence. Lancet Inf Dis, 2012;12:36–44.

[129] Savitz DA, Fell DB, Ortiz JR, Bhat N. Does influenza vaccination improve pregnancy outcome? Methodological issues and research needs. Vaccine 2015;33:6430–5.

[130] World Health Organization. WHO Influenza data taskforce –interim report.2015;1–24.

[131] Kay AW, Blish CA. Immunogenicity and Clinical Efficacy of Influenza Vaccination in Pregnancy. Front Immunol 2015;6:289.

[132] Murray DL, Imagawa DT, Okada DM, St Geme JW, Jr. Antibody response to monovalent A/New Jersey/8/76 influenza vaccine in pregnant women. J Clin Microbiol 1979;10:184–7.

[133] Bischoff AL, Folsgaard NV, Carson CG, Stokholm J, Pedersen L, Holmberg M, et al. Altered response to A(H1N1)pnd09 vaccination in pregnant women: a single blinded randomized controlled trial. PLoS One 2013;8:e56700.

[134] Schlaudecker EP, McNeal MM, Dodd CN, Ranz JB, Steinhoff MC. Pregnancy modifies the antibody response to trivalent influenza immunization. J Infect Dis 2012;206:1670–3.

[135] Sperling RS, Engel SM, Wallenstein S, Kraus TA, Garrido J, Singh T, et al. Immunogenicity of trivalent inactivated influenza vaccination received during pregnancy or postpartum. Obstet Gynecol 2012;119:631–9.

[136] Patel CG, Phillips Heine R, Staats J, Antczak B, Weaver K, Weinhold K, Swamy C. T-follicular helper (Tfh) cell expansion varies by trimester after influenza vaccination in pregnancy. AJOG,2016;214:S57–S58.

[137] Sullivan SG, Komadina N, Grant K, Jelley L, Papadakis G, Kelly H. Influenza vaccine effectiveness during the 2012 influenza season in Victoria, Australia: Influences of waning immunity and vaccine match. J Med Virol 2013;86:1017–1025.

[138] Kissling E, Valenciano M, Larrauri A, Oroszi B, Cohen JM, Nunes B, et al. Low and decreasing vaccine effectiveness against influenza A(H3) in 2011/12 among vaccination target groups in Europe: results from the I-MOVE multicentre case-control study. Euro Surveill 2013;18.

[139] Rasmussen SA, Watson AK, Kennedy ED, Broder KR, Jamieson DJ. Vaccines and pregnancy: past, present, and future. Semin Fetal Neonatal Med 2014;19:161–9.

[140] van der Maas N, Dijs-Elsinga J, Kemmeren J, van Lier A, Knol M, de Melker H. Safety of vaccination against influenza A (H1N1) during pregnancy in the Netherlands: results on pregnancy outcomes and infant's health: cross-sectional linkage study. BJOG 2015.

[141] Sobanjo-Ter Meulen A, Abramson J, Mason E, Rees H, Schwalbe N, Bergquist S, et al. Path to impact: A report from the Bill and Melinda Gates Foundation convening on maternal immunization in resource-limited settings; Berlin—January 29–30, 2015. Vaccine 2015;33:6388–95.

10

Cholesteryl Pullulan Nanoparticles-Encapsulated TNF-α: An Effective Mucosal Vaccine Adjuvant Against Influenza

Tsunetaka Ohta

Abstract

We encapsulated tumor necrosis factor-α (TNF-α), a major proinflammatory cytokine, into cholesteryl pullulan (CHP) to prepare TNF/CHP nanoparticles. In this chapter, the immune response-enhancing capability of the nanoparticles to act as a vaccine adjuvant against influenza is described. TNF/CHP nanoparticles showed excellent storage stability, and they enhanced host immune responses to external immunogens. We applied the nanoparticles in a mouse model of influenza virus infection to investigate their adjuvant ability. Nasal administration of TNF/CHP nanoparticles combined with a conventional split vaccine was effective at inducing systemic IgG_1 as well as mucosal IgA, and it protected mice against a lethal challenge of A/PR/8/34 (H1N1) influenza virus. Mechanistic studies showed that the nanoparticles enhanced antigen uptake by dendritic cells (DCs) and moderately induced the expression of inflammation-related genes in nasal-associated lymphoid tissue (NALT), leading to the activation of both B and T cells. A preliminary safety study revealed no severe toxicity to TNF/CHP nanoparticles. Slight-to-moderate influences in nasal mucosa were observed only after repeated administration and they were reversible. Our data show that TNF/CHP nanoparticles effectively enhance both humoral and cellular immunity via nasal administration and could be a potential adjuvant for vaccines against infectious diseases like influenza.

Keywords: adjuvant, mucosal, nanoparticle, CHP, TNF-α

1. Introduction

Vaccines are the most effective interventions against infectious diseases such as influenza. Many vaccines, however, are only effective at preventing onset and aggravation of symptoms, and less effective at preventing infection, particularly with respiratory infections. One reason for this is that the major administration routes of conventional vaccines, including subcutaneous (*s.c.*) and intramuscular (*i.m.*), induce neutralizing IgG antibody in blood but not mucosal IgA antibody, which is more effective at preventing infection. The efficacy of IgG antibody against variant or mutated viruses is very limited because it has highly restricted cross-protective capabilities. Conversely, IgA antibody on mucosa shows wide cross-protection and can block infection [1, 2]. When immunizations are delivered at the mucosa, IgA antibody is induced on mucosal surfaces throughout the body and IgG antibody is produced in the blood. Since mucosal vaccination induces immunity in both the systemic and mucosal compartments [3, 4], enhanced antigen-specific mucosal immunity is a clear goal for next-generation vaccines. Mucosal, especially nasal, vaccines are ideal because of their effectiveness in preventing infection via the respiratory tract. Nasal vaccines have the additional benefit of improved patient compliance and greater clinical convenience as well.

One significant drawback of mucosal vaccines is that they generally do not induce strong enough immune responses. The recent component-split vaccines, while avoiding many negative patient reactions, tend to be less immunogenic by themselves even in the case of intravenous (*i.v.*) or *i.m.* administration. Generally, children and the elderly tend to respond less to vaccinations, which may lower the preventive power of the population [5]. Therefore, adjuvants must be administered simultaneously with the vaccine in order to enhance vaccine-specific immune responses. Alum salts are the most commonly used adjuvant, but they are neither suitable for all vaccines nor always capable of eliciting the desired immune responses. Other types of adjuvants are being tested, such as liposomes, emulsions, and their combinations [6, 7]. The development of safe, effective, and suitable adjuvants is an important component in the future of mucosal vaccines.

Several groups have examined the use of cytokines (proteinaceous bioactive substances) as a new type of vaccine adjuvant due to their potent effects on the immune system [8–10]. Although some encouraging results have been reported, cytokines are not yet in the practical use as adjuvants. One of the important points to consider is the type of drug delivery system (DDS). Recently, our group tried to generate a new type of vaccine adjuvant by combining cytokines and biocompatible saccharide materials. This chapter describes the creation of human tumor necrosis factor-α (TNF-α) encapsulated by cholesteryl pullulan (CHP) resulting in TNF/CHP nanoparticles. We investigated the potential of the nanoparticles as a nasal vaccine adjuvant by examining its ability to protect against lethal influenza infection in a mouse model and conducting further mechanistic analyses on innate and acquired immunity.

2. Tumor necrosis factor-α (TNF-α)

TNF-α is a major proinflammatory cytokine primarily produced by T cells and macrophages, and it is bioactive in a homotrimeric form [11]. It was first described as a potent anti-tumor factor, but it is now known to play an integral role in host defense. It activates innate and adaptive immunity by stimulating dendritic cell (DC) maturation and subsequent T cell activation as well as contributing to inflammatory responses [12, 13] (**Figure 1**).

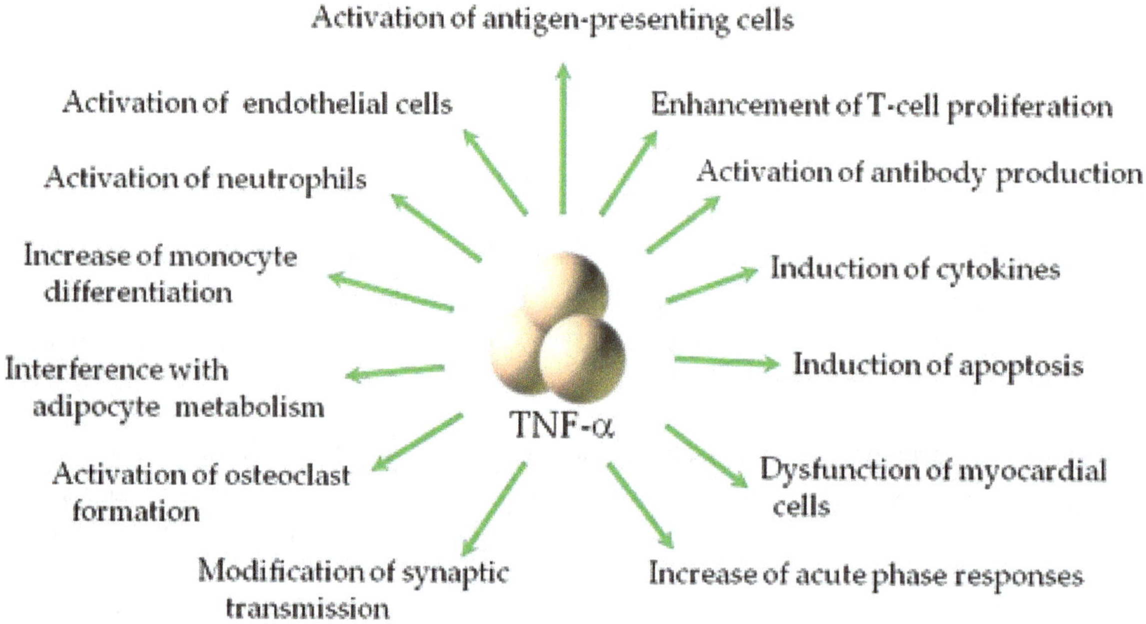

Figure 1. Various actions of TNF-α.

Interestingly, it was recently shown that TNF-α exerted adjuvant activities against pathogenic infections [14, 15]. Although there were some attempts to develop TNF-α (as well as other cytokines) as a vaccine adjuvant, successful practical results have not been reported. This is probably because TNF-α causes unfavorable biological reactions when administered systemically, and it is rapidly degraded when delivered at the mucosal surface. To overcome these obstacles, some investigators have attempted to generate protease-resistant mutant TNF-α molecules and have reported some potential as a vaccine adjuvant at the experimental level [16, 17].

3. Pullulan and cholesteryl pullulan (CHP)

One method of establishing a safer and more effective way to administer bioactive substances that is gaining popularity is a nanoparticle DDS. For nanoparticle materials, polysaccharides have been shown to possess several favorable characteristics in comparison with synthetic polymers currently used. Unlike synthetic polymers that could accumulate in the body to levels beyond the renal clearance, saccharides are biocompatible, meaning they are degraded by intrinsic enzymes inside the body [18, 19]. In this study, we used pullulan to create DDS nanoparticles.

Pullulan is a natural and chemically neutral homopolysaccharide consisting of α-1, 6-linked maltotriose units (maltotriose is three glucose molecules linked with α-1, 4 glycosidic bonds). It is produced primarily by fermentation of starch by strains of the fungus *Aureobasidium pullulans* [20]. By introducing hydrophobic moieties onto the hydrophilic pullulan molecule, amphiphilic coploymers can be generated. A representative is cholesteryl pullulan (CHP) [21, 22] (**Figure 2**).

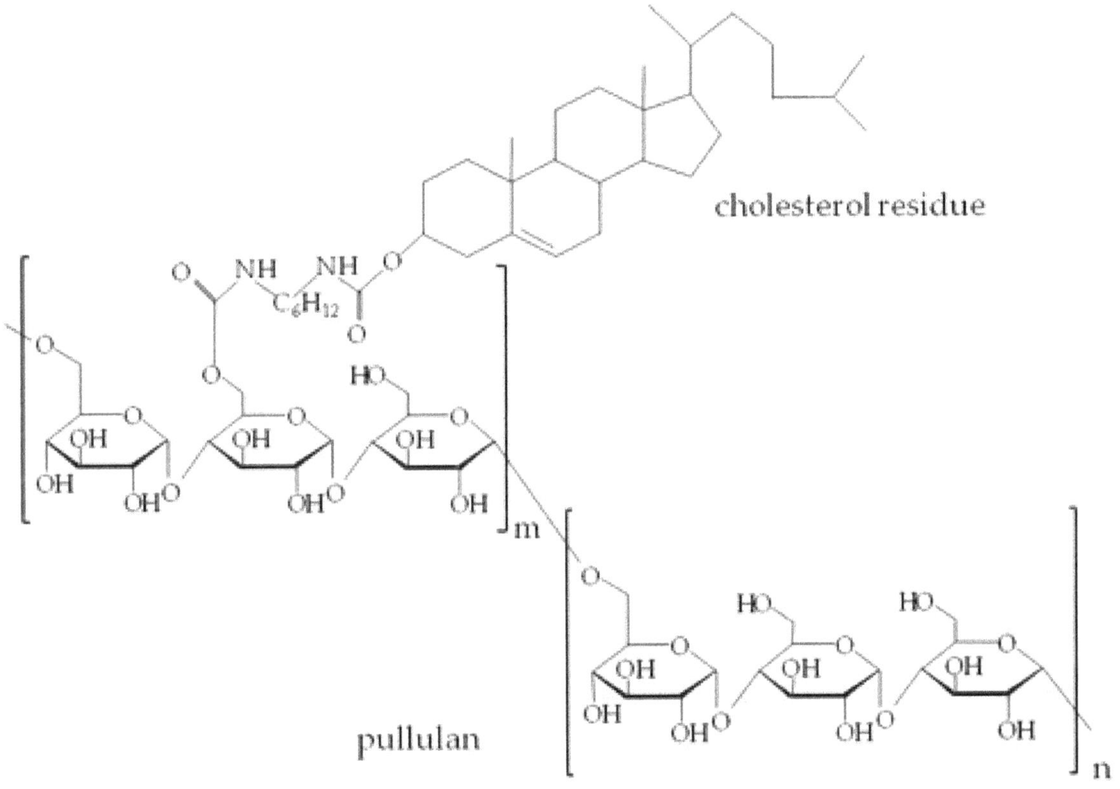

Figure 2. Chemical structure of CHP. m, n; integer values. In PUREBRIGHT CP-100T (NOF Co., Tokyo, Japan), 1–3% of glucose units are modified with cholesterol residues.

CHP self-assembles into nanoparticles in aqueous solution and entraps various molecules in its internal space through hydrophobic interactions. The hydrophilic shell serves as a stabilizing interface between the hydrophobic core and the external aqueous environment. It also protects the entrapped molecule from mechanical, chemical, or enzymatic attacks from outside the particle, and it acts as a superior carrier for delivery. It also allows slow release of the encapsulated materials [23–25]. Furthermore, the CHP nanoparticles showed prolonged circulation and thermodynamic stability in animal models [26].

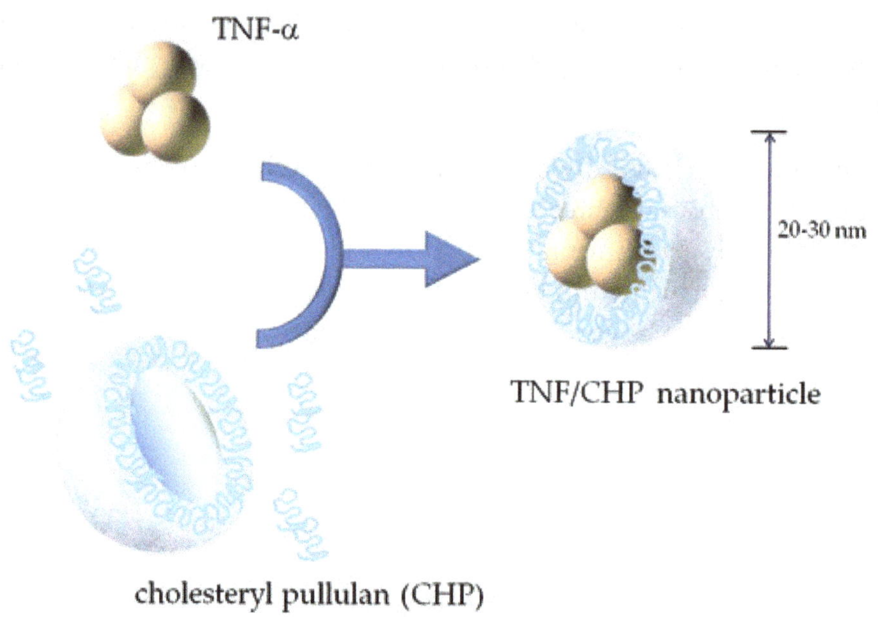

Figure 3. Schematic model of self-assembling of TNF/CHP nanoparticles. TNF-α is shown in the trimeric, bioactive form. The diameter of the particle is approximately 20–30 nm.

Pullulan-based nanoparticles have been used for the delivery of proteins, anticancer drugs, imaging agents, and nucleotides. CHP nanoparticles are efficiently transferred to antigen-presenting cells such as macrophages and/or DCs, and they elicit strong immune responses [27, 28]. CHP is under vigorous investigation for establishing novel vaccine therapies against several types of cancers [29–31]. We created CHP nanoparticles containing TNF-α, which are described in the following sections (**Figure 3**).

4. TNF/CHP nanoparticles

4.1. Preparation of TNF/CHP nanoparticles

In this study, we used TNF-α derived from a human lymphoblastoid cell line, BALL-1 [32], and CHP (PUREBRIGHT CP-100T) from NOF Corporation. CHP encapsulated active trimeric TNF-α to form stable nanoparticles as schematically shown in **Figure 3**. The encapsulating process was time- and temperature-dependent; at 37°C, more than 95% of the TNF-α was encapsulated into CHP complexes after 5 days of incubation; at 4°C, very few, if any, TNF/CHP nanoparticles were formed.

The resulting nanoparticles were relatively uniform. The mode and average sizes of the particles were 27.2 and 42.4 nm based on dynamic light scattering (DLS) results. This was not very different from the size of the blank CHP particles with a mode of 27.6 nm and an average of 42.8 nm (**Figure 4**). Stoichiometric analyses showed that a TNF/CHP nanoparticle consisted of a TNF-α active trimer (ca. 50 kDa) in a CHP tetrameric complex (ca. 400 kDa).

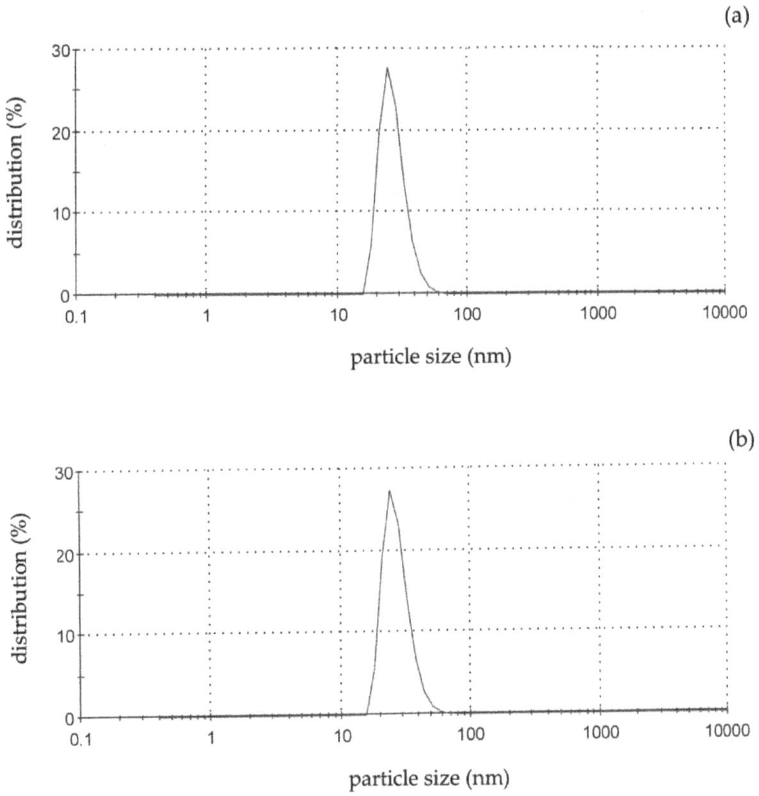

Figure 4. Size distribution of TNF/CHP nanoparticles. Two hundred fifty μg/mL TNF-α and 12 mg/mL CHP were mixed, sterilized by filtration, and incubated at 37°C for 5 days. CHP self-assembled with TNF-α molecules to form nanoparticles. The particle size was determined by DLS with a Zetasizer Nano ZS (Malvern Instruments Ltd., Malvern, UK). (a) TNF/CHP nanoparticles, (b) blank CHP particles. Reproduced with permission from Nagatomo D. et al., [33].

4.2. Storage stability of TNF/CHP nanoparticles

Stability of the nanoparticles was evaluated after various treatments by measuring the level of TNF-α. To estimate the amount of encapsulated TNF-α, methyl-β-cyclodextrin (Me-β-CD) was used to disrupt the CHP complex and release the TNF-α as previously described [26]. The results showed that the nanoparticle retained its integrity and kept TNF-α molecules active inside the complex in aqueous solution at room temperature for at least 21 days (**Figure 5a**). Furthermore, even after five cycles of freezing and thawing, 80% of the particles remained intact (**Figure 5b**). These results show that the TNF/CHP nanoparticles have excellent storage stability. However, upon contact with high concentrations of dissolved proteins, such as serum albumin, the nanoparticles rapidly released the encapsulated TNF-α (data not shown), probably replaced by proteins from the external environment as reported [34]. This calls an attention to the usage of the nanoparticles, such as *i.v.* injection.

Me-β-CD is known to interact with cholesteryl groups and disrupt CHP complexes to release the substance inside the particles [26]. The amount of Me-β-CD required to disrupt the TNF/CHP nanoparticles was approximately 100 mg/mL, much higher than the 0.3 mg/mL reported for Interleukin-12 (IL-12)/CHP nanoparticles [35], suggesting that the affinity between TNF-α and CHP was much stronger than that of IL-12 and CHP. The molecular interaction of TNF-α and CHP that creates this strength is an interesting area for further study.

Many medical formulations, especially biologicals, require storage at low temperatures or freezing. On the contrary, the TNF/CHP nanoparticles could be stored in solution and without refrigeration. Our formulation offers improved convenience of handling and transportation.

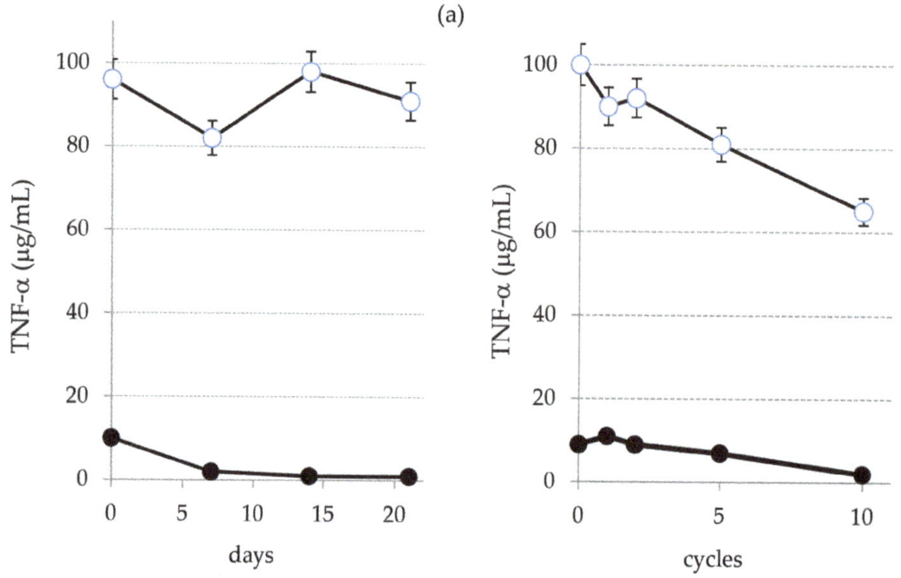

Figure 5. Stability of TNF/CHP nanoparticles *in vitro*. TNF/CHP nanoparticles were incubated in Dulbecco's phosphate buffer at 25°C or repeatedly freeze-thawed (−80°C/25°C). An aliquot was examined for the amount of active TNF-α. Samples were treated with 100 mg/mL Me-β-CD at 37°C for 2 h to release TNF-α from the particles. The amount of TNF-α was determined by an enzyme-linked immunosorbent assay (ELISA) system. (a) storage stability at 25°C; (b) stability through freeze-thaw cycles. Open circle, treated with Me-β-CD; closed circle, without Me-β-CD. (mean ± SD, n = 3).

5. Immune responses induced by TNF/CHP nanoparticles administered nasally

Although TNF-α is known to have immune-enhancing activity [14], severe and unfavorable effects have hampered its practical use. Based on the stability described in the previous section, we hypothesized that delayed release of TNF-α from TNF/CHP nanoparticles would promote the beneficial effects of TNF-α while avoiding harmful events. We examined the adjuvant activity of the TNF/CHP nanoparticles, for example, enhanced induction of antigen-specific antibodies in mice, particularly in the case of nasal administration. We used a commercial influenza virus hemagglutinin vaccine (IVV), which is a component-split and trivalent vaccine for seasonal influenza. It consists of the inactivated hemagglutinin (HA) antigens from A/Brisbane/59/2007 (H1N1), A/Uruguay/716/2007 (H3N2), and B/Brisbane/60/2008. The nasally administered TNF/CHP nanoparticles combined with the IVV induced significant levels of

IgA in the nasal wash, as well as IgG_1 in blood plasma (**Figure 6a, b**). These are comparable to those of the positive control cholera toxin B subunit (CTB), the most powerful adjuvant in experimental settings [35]. Furthermore, IVV with CHP alone (without TNF-α) or with free TNF-α failed to induce significant levels of antibodies when compared to IVV with no adjuvant. The TNF/CHP nanoparticles alone did not induce a measurable antibody response against IVV. To further examine antigen specificity, we performed hemagglutinin (HA)-specific hemagglutination inhibition (HI) assay for the different types of influenza virus included in the vaccine. The TNF/CHP nanoparticles with IVV induced significant HI activity against all types of HA used (A/H1N1, A/H3N2, and B) (**Figure 6c**).

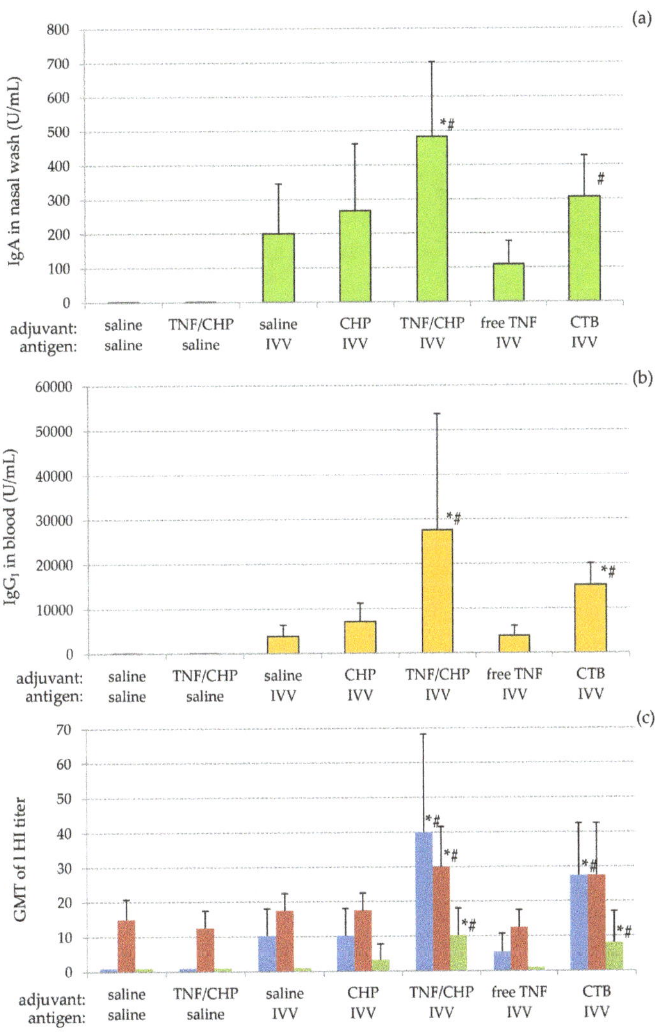

Figure 6. Adjuvant effects of TNF/CHP nanoparticles administered nasally. BALB/c mice were nasally given IVV (SEIKEN, Denka Seiken Co., Ltd., Japan) (0.3 μg/mouse) and TNF/CHP nanoparticles (5 μg/mouse of TNF-α) or CTB (0.8 μg/mouse) once a week for 4 weeks. The nasal wash and blood plasma were prepared from the mice, and the levels of IVV-specific IgA and IgG_1 were determined by ELISA. (a) IgA levels in nasal wash, (b) IgG_1 levels in blood plasma, (c) HI titer in blood plasma against different HA types of influenza virus expressed in GMT (geometric mean titer). Blue column, type A/H1N1; red column, type A/H3N2; green column, type B. (mean ± SEM, n = 8). *, $P < 0.05$ vs. saline/IVV; #, $P < 0.05$ vs. free TNF/IVV. Adapted with permission from Nagatomo D. et al., [33].

These data indicate that TNF/CHP nanoparticles administered nasally can induce not only mucosal but also systemic immunity significantly and efficiently, comparable to the effects of CTB. In addition, the nasal vaccination covers a broad range of antigenicity as previous reports suggested [1, 2]. Also, just for reference, the induction of specific antibodies was seen for other antigens, such as Hepatitis virus type A vaccine, diphtheria toxoid, and cedar pollen allergen (data not shown). Those suggest that TNF/CHP nanoparticles have the potential as a vaccine adjuvant with a broad range of applications, as well as influenza.

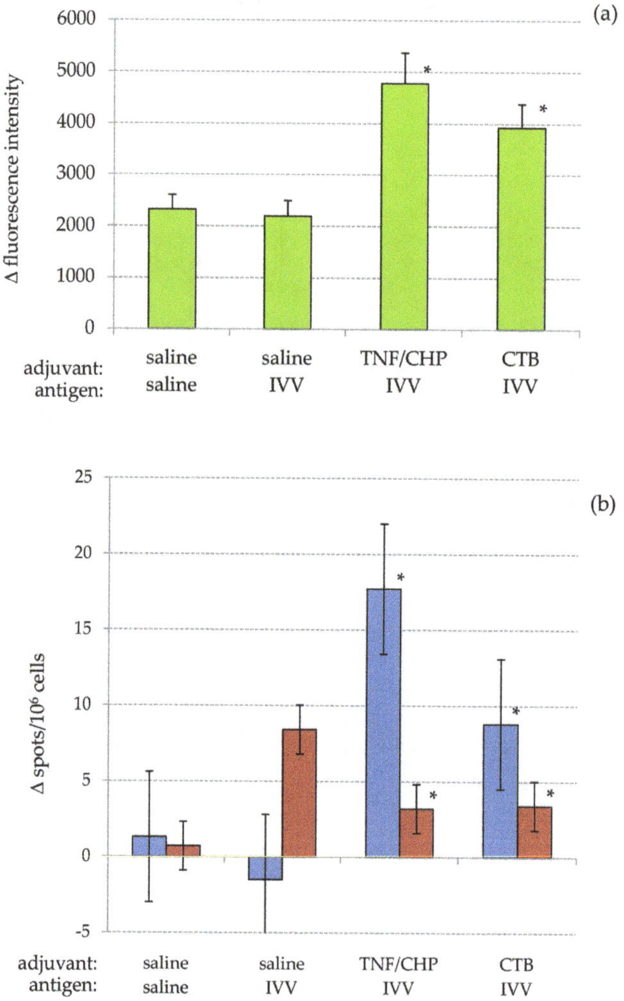

Figure 7. Proliferation and cytokine production by splenocytes from mice nasally administered TNF/CHP nanoparticles and IVV. BALB/c mice were given IVV (0.3 μg/mouse) and TNF/CHP nanoparticles (5 μg/mouse as TNF-α) or CTB (0.8 μg/mouse) by the nasal route as previously described. Splenocytes were prepared from the mice. Then, IVV-specific proliferation and IL-4/IFN-γ-producing cells were examined with alamarBlue and ELISpot, respectively. The results represent the difference (Δ) between data from experiments with and without IVV antigen stimulation. (a) proliferation response. (b) cytokine production. Blue column, IL-4 production; red column, IFN-γ production (mean ± SEM, n = 8). *, $P < 0.05$ vs. saline/IVV. Adapted with permission from Nagatomo D. et al. [33].

The antigen-specific T cell responses of the vaccinated animals were examined by challenging their isolated splenocytes with IVV. IVV-specific proliferation in the TNF/CHP nanoparticle group was comparable to that of CTB (**Figure 7a**). We also measured cytokine production to understand what kind of T cell response occurred. IVV alone increased IFN-γ production, while the addition of either adjuvant (TNF/CHP nanoparticle or CTB) suppressed IVV-induced Interferon-γ(IFN-γ) production. The TNF/CHP nanoparticles combined with IVV also produced IL-4 cytokine to a higher level than IVV with CTB (**Figure 7b**). These experiments suggest that the nasally administered adjuvant shifted the Th1/Th2 balance to a Th2-dominant state, which confirms previous results obtained with a mutant TNF-α [17].

6. Protective effect of TNF/CHP nanoparticles in lethal challenge of influenza virus on mice

To directly address the stimulatory effect of the TNF/CHP nanoparticle adjuvant on protective immunity, we challenged immunized mice with a lethal dose of influenza virus. Mice were nasally immunized with IVV with or without TNF/CHP nanoparticles once a week for 3 weeks. Then, they were challenged with the antigenically distinct influenza virus A/Puerto Rico/8/34 strain at a lethal dose (**Figure 8**). The mice that received only IVV died by 8 days post challenge, which was comparable to mice without IVV immunization. The TNF/CHP nanoparticles without the IVV slightly delayed the time to death, but all of the animals eventually died. On the contrary, combined administration of IVV and TNF/CHP nanoparticles showed a highly protective effect with 90% of the mice surviving lethal challenge. The effect was comparable to that of the CTB adjuvant. Free TNF also showed a somewhat protective effect. Interestingly,

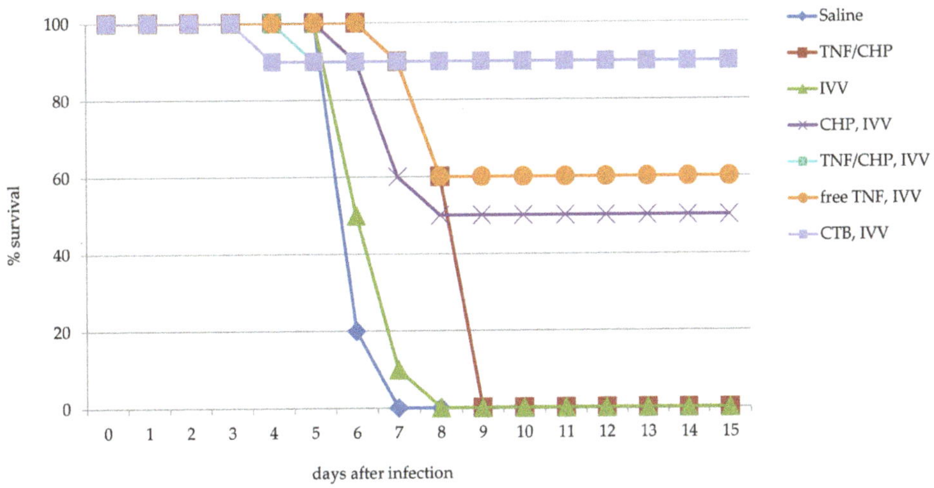

Figure 8. Protective effect of TNF/CHP nanoparticles adjuvant against lethal influenza virus challenge in mice. BALB/c mice were nasally administered with IVV with or without an adjuvant once a week for 3 weeks. Seven days after the final immunization, mice were challenged nasally with influenza virus (Puerto Rico/8/34, 10 LD_{50}) and then monitored daily. Mice that were moribund or that had lost more than 20% of their body weight were considered to have reached an experimental endpoint and were humanely euthanized by anesthetization. Blue diamond, saline only; red square, TNF/CHP nanoparticles only (5 μg/mouse of TNF-α); green triangle, IVV only (0.3 μg/mouse); purple cross, IVV with blank CHP nanoparticles (240 μg/mouse); blue square, IVV with TNF/CHP nanoparticles (5 μg/mouse of TNF-α); orange circle, IVV with free TNF (5 μg/mouse); purple dot, IVV with CTB (0.8 μg/mouse) (n = 10). Reproduced with permission from Nagatomo D. et al. [33].

CHP only (without TNF-α) provided a certain level of protection as an adjuvant, as we observed 50% survival. Importantly, the nasally administered TNF/CHP nanoparticles induced significant protective immunity in spite of the distinct antigenicities [36], suggesting that they have a potential for inducing broad cross-protection.

Antibodies became detectable after the second or third vaccination and reached plateau levels thereafter in mice vaccinated with TNF/CHP nanoparticles. The surviving animals immunized with IVV and TNF/CHP nanoparticles had immunological memory, including IgG_1 in plasma, and IgA in nasal/vaginal wash and feces. This memory was maintained at high levels for more than 90 days, and these mice responded to a boosting challenge of the IVV to further elevate the antibody levels (**Table 1**). These data indicate that the nanoparticles induced systemic immunity and long-lived memory, a critical feature for successful vaccine adjuvants. Overall, our data demonstrate that TNF/CHP nanoparticles are effective as a vaccine adjuvant for nasally delivered IVV.

TNF/CHP nanoparticles enhanced an IgA response not only at the site of application (e.g., in the nasal wash) but also at distant mucosal sites, such as the intestine (feces), vaginal, and salivary glands (data not shown). IgA antibody elicited at the mucosa is of vital importance as the natural route of infection for influenza is via the respiratory mucosa. Hence, local mucosal protection against pharyngeal carriage is likely to be decisive for preventing disease [37]. Conventional parenteral vaccines are not able to stimulate mucosal immune responses, thus restricting their efficacy in infections of mucosal surfaces such as the respiratory tract [1]. Our nasal vaccine/adjuvant formulation consisting of the IVV and TNF/CHP nanoparticles effectively induced both systemic and mucosal protective immunity.

	IgG_1 titer in plasma (U/mL)				**IgA titer in feces extract (U/mL)**			
Adjuvant	**Unimmunized**	**None**	**TNF/CHP nanoparticles**	**CTB**	**Unimmunized**	**None**	**TNF/CHP nanoparticles**	**CTB**
1 day before boost								
Day 90	n.d.	21,338 ± 2,438.9	16,917 ± 9,392.0	8,700 ± 5,510.3	n.d.	4.2 ± 3.5	14.4 ± 16.7	13.1 ± 10.8
12 days after boost								
Day 112	36.6 ± 43.2	19,764 ± 13,601.2	53,769 ± 29,893.7	37,729 ± 29,281.3	34.6 ± 33.3	19.8 ± 8.3	64.4 ± 63.4	58.2 ± 37.1

BALB/c mice were nasally administered with IVV (0.3 μg/mouse), with or without TNF/CHP nanoparticles (5 μg/mouse of TNF-α) or CTB (0.8 μg/mouse) once a week for 4 weeks. Ninety-one days after the immunization, the mice were boosted with IVV (0.9 μg/mouse). Twenty-one days after the boosting challenge, the blood plasma was prepared and the feces were extracted with 10 volumes of water. The IgG_1 in blood plasma and IgA in feces extract were examined (mean ± SEM, $n = 8$).
n.d., not detected.

Table 1. Induction of immunological memory by TNF/CHP nanoparticles.

Muraoka et al. proposed that CHP-based nanoparticles preferentially deliver antigen to antigen-presenting cells in the lymph nodes, which potentiates effective immune responses [38]. This might be the reason why the TNF/CHP nanoparticles induced excellent protective immunity. They, however, reported that CHP itself did not show an adjuvant effect in the context of a tumor vaccine [31]. Interestingly, CHP only (without TNF-α) showed a certain level of protective efficacy in our study. The reason for the discrepancy between their results and ours is not clear. It is unlikely, given the short time frame, that TNF-α was replaced *in vivo* by IVV antigens to form IVV/CHP nanoparticles that were then delivered to the lymph node. Another factor that is critical for adjuvant activity is particle size [39]; however, size is not an issue in our case since the DLS analyses showed no difference in particle size between the TNF/CHP nanoparticles and empty CHP particles (**Figure 4**). Most probably, the difference has to do with varying mechanisms to elicit protection against external pathogens, such as influenza virus, and internal antigens, such as tumor antigen.

7. Mechanistic analyses of effects of TNF/CHP nanoparticles

7.1. Activation of immune cells in NALT

Being focused on the nasal route of vaccination, we examined immune cells in nasal tissues after immunization. The mucosal surfaces contain abundant B cells, T cells, and plasma (or DC) cells. After repeated immunization of animals for 3 weeks, cells from the nasal-associated lymphoid tissues (NALT) were prepared from mice, and expression of a surface marker for DCs (CD11c) and activation markers for B cells (CD80 and CD86) were examined by flow cytometry. The ratios of $CD80^+/CD11c^+$ cells; $CD86^+/CD11c^+$ cells were 0.20; 0.33, 0.30; 0.44, and 0.33; 0.50% for saline, IVV, and IVV with TNF/CHP nanoparticles, respectively (data not shown). Even though the degree was small, IVV vaccination with or without TNF/CHP nanoparticles activated DCs and B cells. Also, TNF/CHP nanoparticles did not have a prominent effect on DC or B cell activation.

7.2. Antigen uptake and activation of NALT and nasal passage cells

We next focused on the early immune response of nasal mucosal tissues. Uptake of antigen by the mucosal tissues is essential for the induction of immune responses [40]. Therefore, we examined antigen uptake by NALT-resident and nasal passage DCs, the inductive sites of the common mucosal immune system [41]. In these experiments, we used ovalbumin (OVA) as a model antigen and assessed antigen uptake by DCs in the NALT and nasal passage cells by flow cytometry at 6 h after immunization. Immunization of mice with OVA combined with TNF/CHP nanoparticle activated antigen uptake by both NALT and nasal passage DCs. TNF/CHP nanoparticles stimulated DCs most in the nasal passage mucosal immune tissue (**Figure 9**). We also found that TNF/CHP nanoparticles enhanced expression of DC and B cell activation markers (CD40, 80, and 86) in a bone marrow-derived immature DC preparation *in vitro* (data not shown).

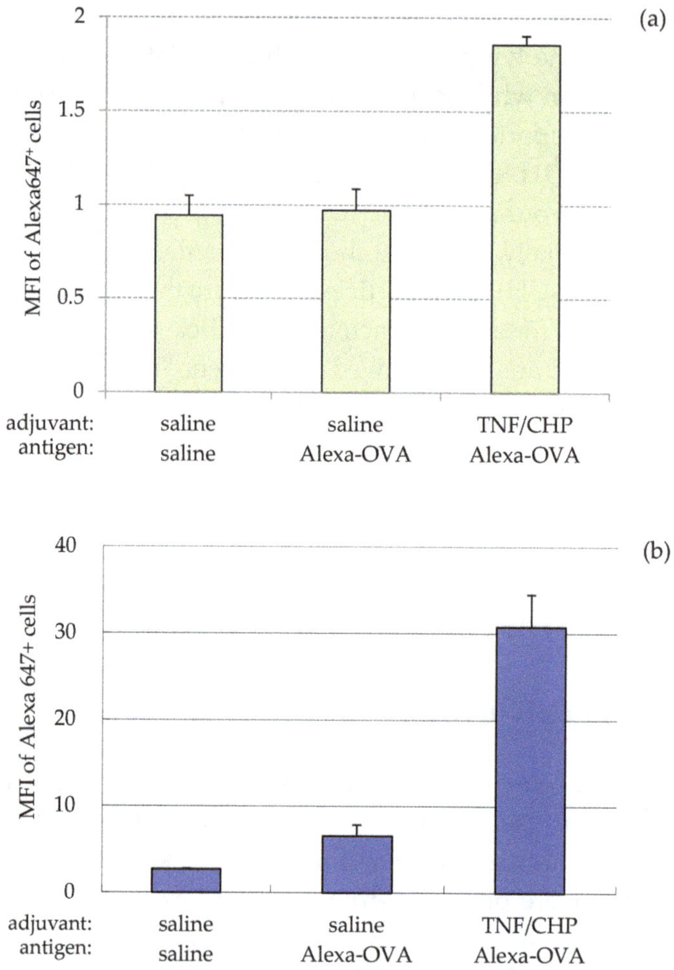

Figure 9. Antigen uptake of NALT and nasal passage DCs after TNF/CHP nanoparticles administration. BALB/c mice were nasally immunized with 10 μg of Alexa 647-labeled OVA antigen with or without TNF/CHP nanoparticles as an adjuvant. Six hours after the immunization the NALT and the nasal passage cells were prepared [42] and subjected to flow cytometric analysis. Antigen uptake was determined by detecting the Alexa 647 florescence intensity and the DC marker ($CD11c^+$ cells) in parallel, for example, ratio of Alexa 647^+/$CD11c^+$. (a) NALT DCs, (b) nasal passage DCs. MFI, mean fluorescence intensity (mean ± SD, n = 4). Adapted with permission from Nagatomo D. et al. [33].

7.3. Expression of inflammatory signals in NALT

Vaccine adjuvants trigger the innate immune system allowing enhanced humoral and cellular responses against the co-administered vaccine antigens. To understand innate immune system activation caused by the TNF/CHP nanoparticles after immunization, we conducted gene expression profiling in NALT cells 2, 6, and 26 h after nasal administration of IVV antigen with or without the nanoparticles. By scattering analyses, the gene expression of inflammation- and immunity-related molecules was found to be significantly upregulated (data not shown). These included the triggering receptor expressed on myeloid cells 1, fibronectin 1, CD14, Toll-like receptor (TLR) 2, TLR3, IL-1β, IL-1 family 9, and IL-6. We confirmed the level of inflammation-related molecules in activated NALT cells by quantitative polymerase chain reaction (PCR) analysis. Expression of the inflammatory markers was enhanced when an adjuvant was included (TNF/CHP nanoparticles, free TNF, or CTB), while CHP itself did not show significant enhancing activity. Among the molecules tested, significant increases in expression occurred for IFN-γ, IL-1α, IL-1β, IL-6, CXCL2, IL-12β, CD14, and lipopolysaccharide (LPS)-binding protein (**Figure 10**). The degree of enhancement varied from gene to gene, but the greatest increase of expression was observed for IL-6 and IL-12β.

Overall, free exogenous TNF-α elicited the strongest increase in expression of inflammatory markers, and the enhancement tended to be highest at 2 h post-immunization. TNF/CHP nanoparticles elicited a moderate increase in gene expression by comparison, but the pattern over time was similar to that of free TNF-α. One reason for the discrepancy in gene expression between free TNF and the nanoparticles could be that the nanoparticles cause a slow release of TNF-α, prolonging the immune-stimulatory effect. The pattern of expression over time was very different for most genes when stimulated with CTB adjuvant. For example, although the expression of IL-12β was prominent at 6 h post-immunization when CTB was used as an adjuvant, the IL-12β response was much lower with TNF/CHP nanoparticles at the same time point.

Taken together, TNF/CHP nanoparticles delayed activation of innate immunity. By prolonging and dampening the stimulatory effect of TNF-α CHP seemed to minimize the unfavorable effects of TNF-α while promoting its beneficial activities. One important safety issue related to the development of nasal vaccines is the potential dissemination of vaccine antigens to the central nervous system (CNS). Past reports suggested that nasal administration of CTB allowed it to reach the CNS and accumulate in olfactory tissues. It caused Bell's Palsy in clinical studies, probably due to IL-12β production, and the use of CTB in humans was prohibited [43, 44]. In this context, the lower expression level of IL-12β seen in our experiments with TNF/CHP nanoparticles could be a beneficial safety feature.

Regarding CHP itself, a shell of the nanoparticles did not show immune-enhancing activity, such as increasing IgG_1 and IgA or the expression of inflammation-related genes (**Figure 10**). However, CHP did confer a certain level of protection in a lethal influenza virus challenge (**Figure 8**). We cannot easily account for these conflicting observations; there are other pathways and mechanisms likely involved and waiting to be clarified.

8. Safety study of TNF/CHP nanoparticles

General safety was preliminarily examined according to the OECD guidelines for testing chemicals [45]. Mice nasally administered with a combination of TNF/CHP nanoparticles and IVV either once or four times were subjected to an acute or a repeated toxicity study, respectively.

8.1. General symptoms, ophthalmic examination, body weight, and body temperature

No general symptoms or behavioral anomalies in either male or female animals were correlated with the IVV with TNF/CHP nanoparticles treatment during the study period. In ophthalmic examinations, there were no test material-related ocular findings observed. Body

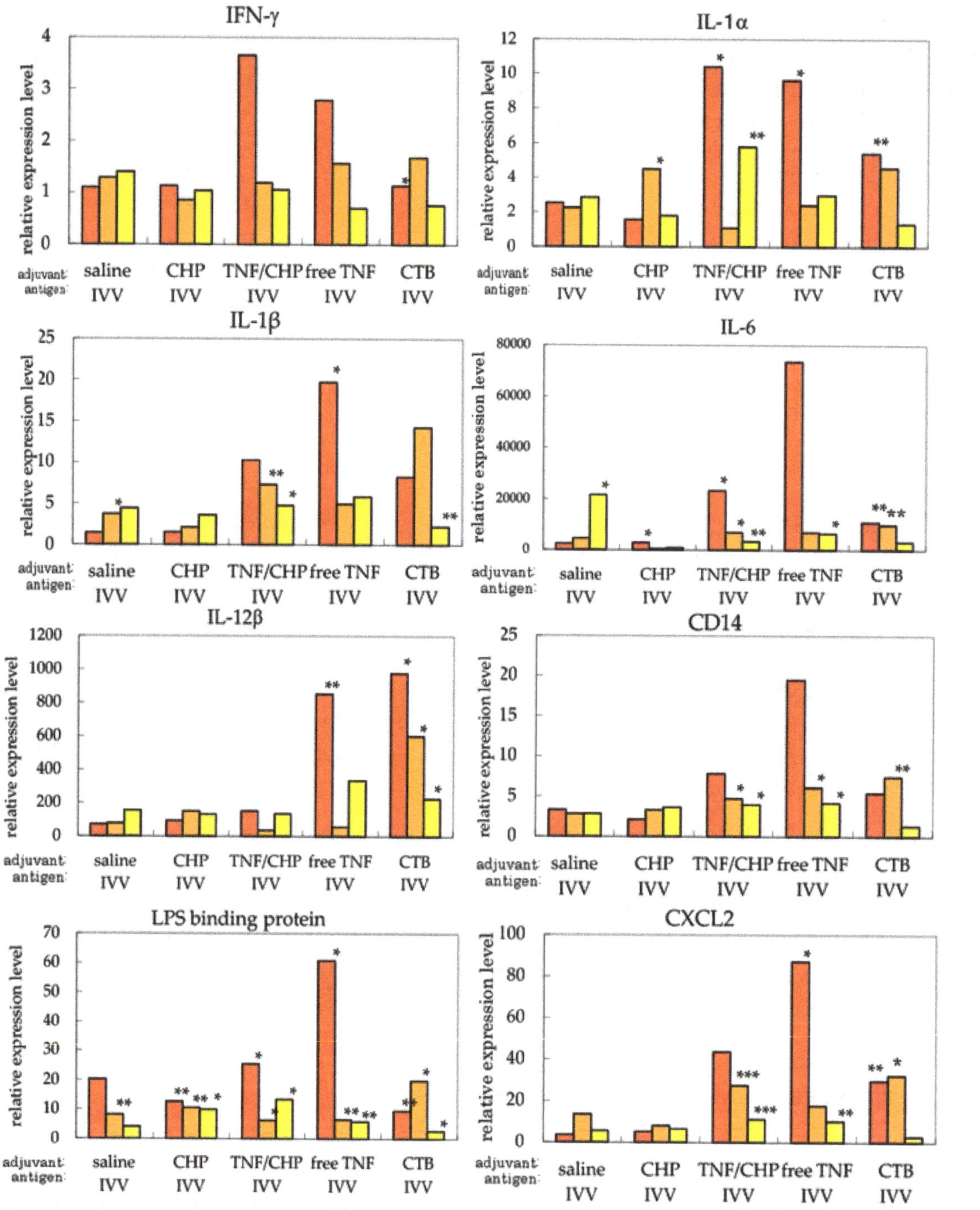

Figure 10. Gene expression in NALT after TNF/CHP nanoparticles administration. mRNA was prepared from NALT cells of BALB/c mice 2, 6, and 26 h after administration of TNF/CHP nanoparticles and IVV. Gene expression related to innate and adaptive immune responses was analyzed by quantitative PCR and normalized to glyceraldehyde 3-phosphate dehydrogenase (GAPDH) expression. Data are shown as relative level vs. control (means of quadruple experiments). Red column, 2 h; orange column, 6 h; yellow column, 26 h post treatment. *, $P < 0.05$; **, $P < 0.01$; ***, $P < 0.001$ vs. saline control. Adapted with permission from Nagatomo D. et al. [33].

weight and body temperature were not statistically different among the treatment groups (data not shown).

8.2. Hematology, blood biochemistry, and urinalysis

Hematology evaluations were performed during and at the end of study. There were no differences in any of the tested parameters (white blood cell, red blood cell, hematocrit, lymphocyte, neutrophil, eosinophil, basophil, and monocyte) between controls and TNF/CHP nanoparticles with the IVV treatment. For blood biochemistry, we examined total protein, albumin, urea nitrogen, creatinine, Na^+, K^+, Cl^-, Ca^{2+}, inorganic phosphate, aspartate aminotransferase (AST), alanine aminotransferase (ALT), lactate dehydrogenase (LDH), amylase (AMY), γ-glutamyl transpeptidase (γ-GT), total cholesterol, triglyceride, high density lipoprotein (HDL)-cholesterol, total bilirubin, and glucose. Urobilinogen, bilirubin, ketone body, glucose, protein, pH, specific gravity, nitrite salt, and leucocytes were examined during the study period. All differences found during the study fell within historical control value ranges and were not considered test material-related (data not shown).

8.3. Pathology and major organ weights

Gross pathology of all the animals was examined at the end of the study. The major organs (brain, heart, lung, kidney, liver, ovary, testis, spleen, adrenal, and thymus) were weighed at the end of the study in all of the animals. No change was noted as test material-related (data not shown).

8.4. Histopathology

The histopathology of tissues from animals in each group was examined. As discussed in Section 7.3, there were some concerns of possible harmful effects on the CNS. However, no abnormalities in the brain, especially olfactory bulb, were noted in any animals after histological examination. There were some effects observed at the administration site (nasal mucosal tissue). While single administration showed no effect, repeated administration with IVV alone showed a slight infusion and TNF/CHP nanoparticles combined with IVV induced slight-to-moderate infusion and infiltration of inflammatory cells (lymphocytes, neutrophils, eosinophils, and mast cells). However, the response was reversed with time since the infusion diminished to trace proportions after the 2-week cessation period. No excessive inflammatory symptoms, such as formation of edema or fibrosis, were noted (data not shown).

Overall, no obvious immunotoxicity was detected. Although further evaluation is required, our results demonstrate that the toxicity of TNF/CHP nanoparticles is relatively low and safe as a nasal vaccine adjuvant against influenza.

Very recently, Onishi et al. reported that hydroxypropyl-β-cyclodextrin (HP-β-CD), another type of saccharide-based material that can form nanoparticles, exhibited adjuvant activity and elicited a strong protective effect against influenza virus in mice and cynomolgus macaques [46]. They suggested the involvement of follicular helper T cells via myeloid differentiation primary gene 88 (MyD88)- and TANK-binding kinase (TBK)-dependent pathways. Their findings may shed some light on additional mechanisms at play with nanoparticles as vaccine adjuvants. However, they mentioned the cytotoxicity of HP-β-CD at more than 0.5% *in vitro*, probably because of β-CD's ability to extract cholesterol out of cell membranes [47]. TNF/CHP nanoparticles might represent a preferable alternative.

A probable precaution for the practical use of TNF/CHP nanoparticles is avoiding contact with high concentrations of dissolved proteins as mentioned in Section 4.2. Unless, encapsulated TNF-α would be released from the nanoparticles and the adjuvant activity would be diminished. This means that the nanoparticles is not suitable for *i.v.* administration and premixed formulation with vaccine antigen. For the best performance, we recommend to administer the TNF/CHP nanoparticles on mucosa, such as nasal surface, after mixing with the vaccine antigen just before use.

9. Conclusions

The results of this study demonstrate that TNF/CHP nanoparticles are effective as a vaccine adjuvant against influenza when administered via the nasal mucosal route. Moreover, the ability of TNF/CHP nanoparticles to stimulate comparatively balanced systemic and mucosal immune responses makes them a potentially promising vaccine adjuvant for inducing immunity against infectious pathogens. In the short term, TNF/CHP nanoparticles may aid the development of new nasal influenza vaccines. Looking further ahead, we propose that combining TNF/CHP nanoparticles with next-generation vaccine platforms that do not rely on the cold chain will offer valuable alternatives for vaccination in a variety of settings.

Acknowledgements

The author is very grateful to Dr. Ayato Takada of Research Center for Zoonosis Control, Hokkaido University for his expertise with influenza challenge of mice. The author is also thankful to the staff of R&D Center, Hayashibara Co., Ltd. for their excellent technical assistance, especially Mr. Daiki Nagatomo and Ms. Madoka Taniai for the mechanistic analyses of action, and Dr. Shigeyuki Arai for the histopathological examination.

Author details

Tsunetaka Ohta

Address all correspondence to: tsunetaka.ota@hb.nagase.co.jp

R&D Center, Hayashibara Co. Ltd., Okayama, Japan

References

[1] Kikuta K, Hirabayashi Y, Nagamine T, Aizawa C, Ueno Y, Oya A, Kurata T, and Tamura S. Cross-protection against influenza B type virus infection by intranasal inoculation of the HA vaccines combined with cholera toxin B subunit. Vaccine. 1990;8:595–599.

[2] Ichinohe T, Kawaguchi A, Tamura S, Takahashi H, Sawa H, Ninomiya A, Imai M, Itamura S, Odagiri T, Tashiro M, Chiba J, Sata T, Kurata T, and Hasegawa H. Intranasal immunization with H5N1 vaccine plus Poly I:Poly C12U, a Toll-like receptor agonist, protects mice against homologous and heterologous virus challenge. Microbes Infect. 2007;9:1333–1400.

[3] Holmgren J and Czerkinsky C. Mucosal immunity and vaccines. Nat. Med. 2005;11:S45–S53.

[4] Kiyono H and Fukuyama S. NALT-versus Peyer's-patch-mediated mucosal immunity. Nat. Rev. Immunol. 2004;4:699–710.

[5] Goodwin K, Viboud C, and Simonsen L. Antibody response to influenza vaccination in the elderly: a quantitative review. Vaccine. 2006;24:1159–1169.

[6] Garcon N, Leroux-Roels G, and Cheng WF. Chapter 4, Vaccine adjuvants. In: Garçon N, Stern PL, Anthony L. Cunningham AL, edited. Understanding Modern Vaccines: Perspectives in Vaccinology. Amsterdam: Elsevier; 2011;1: pp. 89–113. ISSN 2210–7630.

[7] De Gregorio E, Caproni E, and Ulmer JB. Vaccine adjuvants: mode of action. Front. Immunol. 2013;4:214. doi:10.3389/fimmu.2013.00214.

[8] Boyaka PN, Lillard JW, and McGhee J. Interleukin 12 and innate molecules for enhanced mucosal immunity. Immunol. Res. 1999;20:207–217.

[9] Tovey MG and Lallemand C. Adjuvant acitivity of cytokines. Methods Mol. Biol. 2010;626:287–309.

[10] Boyaka PN and McGhee JR. Cytokines as adjuvants for the induction of mucosal immunity. Adv. Drug Deliv. Rev. 2001;51:71–79.

[11] Aggarwal BB, Kohr WJ, Hass PE, Moffat B, Spencer SA, Henzel WJ, Bringman TS, Nedwin GE, Goeddel DV, and Harkins RN. Human tumor necrosis factor, production, purification, and characterization. J. Biol. Chem. 1985;260:2345–2354.

[12] Wajant H, Pfizenmaier K, and Scheurich P. Tumor necrosis factor signaling. Cell Death Differ. 2003;10:45–65.

[13] Calzascia T, Pellegrini M, Hall H, Sabbagh L, Ono N, Elford AR, Mak TW, and Ohashi PS. TNF-alpha is critical for antitumor but not antiviral T cell immunity in mice. J. Clin. Invest. 2007;117:3833–3845.

[14] Brunner C, Seiderer J, Schlamp A, Bidlingmaier M, Eigler A, Haimerl W, Lehr HA, Krieg AM, Hartmann G, and Endres S. Enhanced dendritic cell maturation by TNF-alpha or

cytidine-phosphate-guanosine DNA drives T cell activation *in vitro* and therapeutic anti-tumor immune responses *in vivo*. J. Immunol. 2000;165:6278–6286.

[15] Chen Z, Huang H, Chang T, Carlsen S, Saxena A, Marr R, Xing Z, and Xiang J. Enhanced HER-2/neu-specific antitumor immunity by cotransduction of mouse dendritic cells with two genes encoding HER-2/neu and alpha tumor necrosis factor. Cancer Gene Ther. 2002;9:778–786.

[16] Kayamuro H, Abe Y, Yoshioka Y, Katayama K, Nomura T, Yoshida T, Yamashita K, Yoshikawa T, Kawai Y, Mayumi T, Hiroi T, Itoh N, Nagano K, Kamada H, Tsunoda S, and Tsutsumi Y. The use of a mutant TNF-α as a vaccine adjuvant for the induction of mucosal immune responses. Biomaterials. 2009;30:5869–5876. doi:10.1016/j.biomaterials.2009.07.009.

[17] Kayamuro H, Abe Y, Yoshioka Y, Katayama K, Yoshida T, Yamashita K, Yoshikawa T, Kawai Y, Mayumi T, Hiroi T, Itoh N, Nagano K, Kamada H, Tsunoda S, and Tsutsumi Y. Mutant TNF-alpha, mTNF-K90R, is a novel candidate adjuvant for a mucosal vaccine against HIV. Pharmazie. 2010;65:254–256.

[18] Kean T and Thanou M. Biodegradation, biodistribution and toxicity of chitosan. Adv. Drug Deliv. Rev. 2010;62:3–11. doi:10.1016/j.addr.2009.09.004.

[19] Toole TB. Hyaluronan: from extracellular glue to pericellular cue. Nat. Rev. Cancer. 2004;4:528–539.

[20] Lethers TD. Biotechnological production and applications of pullulan. Appl. Microbiol. Biotechnol. 2003;62:468–473.

[21] Prajapati VD, Jani GK, and Khanda SM. Pullulan: an exopolysaccharide and its various applications. Carbohydr. Polym. 2013;95:540–549. doi:10.1016/j.carbpol.2013.02.082.

[22] Akiyama E, Morimoto N, Kujawa P, Ozawa Y, Winnik FM, and Akiyoshi K. Self-assembled nanogels of cholesteryl-modified polysaccharides: effect of the polysaccharide structure on their association characteristics in the dilute and semidilute regimes. Biomacromolecules. 2007;8:2366–2373.

[23] Akiyoshi K, Kobayashi S, Shichibe S, Mix D, Baudys M, Kim SW, and Sunamoto J. Self-assembled hydrogel nanoparticle of cholesterol-bearing pullulan as a carrier of protein drugs: complexation and stabilization of insulin. J. Control. Release. 1998;54:313–320.

[24] Akiyoshi K, Sasaki Y, and Sunamoto J. Molecular chaperone-like activity of hydrogel nanoparticles of hydrophobized pullulan: thermal stabilization with refolding of carbonic anhydrase B. Bioconj. Chem. 1999;10:321–324.

[25] Shimizu T, Kishida T, Hasegawa U, Ueda Y, Imanishi J, Yamagishi H, Akiyoshi K, Otsuji E, and Mazda O. Nanogel DDS enables sustained release of IL-12 for tumor immunotherapy. Biochem. Biophys. Res. Commun. 2008;367:330–335.

[26] Letchford K and Burt H. A review of the formation and classification of amphiphilic block copolymer nanoparticulate structures: micelles, nanospheres, nanocapsules and polymersomes. Eur. J. Pharm. Biopharm. 2007;65:259–269.

[27] Kobiyama K, Aoshi T, Narita H, Kuroda E, Hayashi M, Tetsutani K, Koyama S, Mochizuki S, Sakurai K, Katakai Y, Yasutomi Y, Saijo S, Iwakura Y, Akira S, Coban C, and Ishii KJ. Nonagonistic Dectin-1 ligand transforms CpG into a multitask nanoparticlate TLR9 agonist. Proc. Natl. Acad. Sci. U.S.A. 2014;111:3086–3092. doi:10.1073/pnas.1319268111.

[28] Mody KT, Popat A, Mahony D, Cavallaro AS, Yu C, and Mitter N. Mesoporous silica nanoparticles as antigen carriers and adjuvants for vaccine delivery. Nanoscale. 2013;5:5167–5179. doi:10.1039/c3nr00357d.

[29] Shiku H, Wang L, Ikuta Y, Okugawa T, Schmitt M, Gu X, Akiyoshi K, Sunamoto J, and Nakamura H. Development of a cancer vaccine: peptides, proteins, and DNA. Cancer Chemother. Pharmacol. 2000;46:S77–S82.

[30] Kageyama S, Wada H, Muro K, Niwa Y, Ueda S, Miyata H, Taniguchi S, Sugino SH, Miyahara Y, Ikeda H, Imai N, Sato E, Yamada T, Osakao M, Ohnishi M, Harada N, Hishida T, Doki Y, and Shiku H. Dose-dependent effects of NY-ESO-1 protein vaccine complexed with cholesteryl pullulan (CHP-NY-ESO-1) on immune responses and survival benefits of esophageal cancer patients. J. Transl. Med. 2013;11:246. doi: 10.1186/1479-5876-11-246.

[31] Kageyama S, Kitano S, Hirayama M, Nagata M, Imai H, Shiraishi T, Akiyoshi K, Scott AM, Murphy R, Hoffman EW, Old LJ, Katayama N, and Shiku H. Humoral immune responses in patients vaccinated with 1-146 HER2 protein complexed with cholesteryl pullulan nanogel. Cancer Sci. 2008;99:601–607.

[32] Fukuda S, Ando S, Sanou O, Taniai M, Fujii M, Masaki N, Nakamura K, Ando O, Torigoe K, Sugimoto T, and Kurimoto M. Simultaneous production of natural human tumor necrosis factor-α, -β and interferon-α from BALL-1 cells stimulated by HVJ. Lymphokine Res. 1988;7:175–185.

[33] Nagatomo D, Taniai M, Ariyasu H, Taniguchi M, Aga M, Ariyasu T, Ohta T, and Fukuda S. Cholesteryl pullulan encapsulated TNF-α nanoparticles are an effective mucosal vaccine adjuvant against influenza virus. BioMed Res. Int. 2015;2015:471468. doi: 10.1155/2015/471468.

[34] Ayame H, Morimoto N, and Akiyoshi K. Self-assembled cationic nanogels for intracellular protein delivery. Bioconjug. Chem. 2008;19:882–890. doi:10.1021/bc700422s.

[35] Wu HY, and Russell M. Induction of mucosal and systemic immune responses by intranasal immunization using recombinant cholera toxin B subunit as an adjuvant. Vaccine. 1998;16:286–292.

[36] Ichinohe T, Watanabe I. Ito S, Fujii H, Moriyama M, Tamura S, Takahashi H, Sawada H, Chiba J, Kurata T, Sata T, and Hasegawa H. Synthetic double-stranded RNA

poly(I:C) combined with mucosal vaccine protects against influenza virus infection. J. Virol. 2005;79:2910–2919.

[37] Patel H, Yewale C, Rathi MN, and Misra A. Mucosal immunization: a review of strategies and challenges. Crit. Rev. Ther. Drug Carrier Syst. 2014;31:273–303.

[38] Muraoka D, Harada N, Hayashi T, Tahara Y, Momose F, Sawada SI, Mukai SA, Akiyoshi K, and Shiku H. Nanogel-based immunologically stealth vaccine targets macrophages in the medulla of lymph node and induces potent antitumor immunity. ACS Nano. 2014;8:9209–9218. doi:10.1021/nn502975r.

[39] Oyewumi MO, Kumar A, and Cui Z. Nano-microparticles as immune adjuvants: correlating particle sizes and the resultant immune responses. Expert Rev. Vaccines. 2010;9:1095–1107. doi:10.1586/erv.10.89.

[40] Yuki K and Kiyono H. New generation of mucosa adjuvants for the induction of protective immunity. Rev. Med. Virol. 2003;13:293–310.

[41] Mestecky J and McGhee JR. Immunoglobulin A (IgA): molecular and cellular interactions involved in IgA biosynthesis and immune response. Adv. Immunol. 1987;40:153–245.

[42] Rodriguez-Monroy MA, Rojas-Hernandez S, and Morefno-Fierros L. Phenotypic and functional differences between lymphocytes from NALT and nasal passages of mice. Scand. J. Immunol. 2007;65:276–288.

[43] Mutsch M, Zhou W, Rhodes P, Bopp M, Chen RT, Linder T, Spyr C, and Steffen R. Use of the inactivated intranasal influenza vaccine and the risk of Bell's palsy in Switzerland. N. Engl. J. Med. 2004;350:896–903.

[44] van Ginkel FW, Jackson RJ, Yuki Y, and McGhee JR. Cutting edge: The mucosal adjuvant cholera toxin redirects vaccine proteins into olfactory tissues. J. Immunol. 2000;165:4778–4782.

[45] OECD. OECD Guidelines for the testing of chemicals and related documents [Internet]. Available from: http://www.oecd.org/chemicalsafety/testing/oecdguidelinesforthetestingofchemicals.htm. [Accessed: 2016-03-18].

[46] Onishi M, Ozasa K, Kobiyama K, Ohata K, Kitano M, Taniguchi K, Homma T, Kobayashi M, Sato A, Katakai Y, Yasutomi Y, Wijaya E, Igarashi Y, Nakatsu N, Ise W, Inoue T, Yamada H, Vandenbon A, Standley DM, Kurosaki T, Coban C, Aoshi T, Kuroda E, and Ishii KJ. Hydroxypropyl-β-cyclodextrin spikes local inflammation that induces Th2 cell and T follicular helper cell responses to the coadministered antigen. J. Immunol. 2015;194:2673–2682. doi:10.4049/jimmunol.1402027.

[47] Atger VM, de la Llera Moya M, Stoudt GW, Rodrigueza WV, Phillips MC, and Rothblat GH. Cyclodextrins as catalysts for the removal of cholesterol from macrophage foam cells. J. Clin. Invest. 1997;99:773–780.

Permissions

All chapters in this book were first published in SFDCI, by InTech Open; hereby published with permission under the Creative Commons Attribution License or equivalent. Every chapter published in this book has been scrutinized by our experts. Their significance has been extensively debated. The topics covered herein carry significant findings which will fuel the growth of the discipline. They may even be implemented as practical applications or may be referred to as a beginning point for another development.

The contributors of this book come from diverse backgrounds, making this book a truly international effort. This book will bring forth new frontiers with its revolutionizing research information and detailed analysis of the nascent developments around the world.

We would like to thank all the contributing authors for lending their expertise to make the book truly unique. They have played a crucial role in the development of this book. Without their invaluable contributions this book wouldn't have been possible. They have made vital efforts to compile up to date information on the varied aspects of this subject to make this book a valuable addition to the collection of many professionals and students.

This book was conceptualized with the vision of imparting up-to-date information and advanced data in this field. To ensure the same, a matchless editorial board was set up. Every individual on the board went through rigorous rounds of assessment to prove their worth. After which they invested a large part of their time researching and compiling the most relevant data for our readers.

The editorial board has been involved in producing this book since its inception. They have spent rigorous hours researching and exploring the diverse topics which have resulted in the successful publishing of this book. They have passed on their knowledge of decades through this book. To expedite this challenging task, the publisher supported the team at every step. A small team of assistant editors was also appointed to further simplify the editing procedure and attain best results for the readers.

Apart from the editorial board, the designing team has also invested a significant amount of their time in understanding the subject and creating the most relevant covers. They scrutinized every image to scout for the most suitable representation of the subject and create an appropriate cover for the book.

The publishing team has been an ardent support to the editorial, designing and production team. Their endless efforts to recruit the best for this project, has resulted in the accomplishment of this book. They are a veteran in the field of academics and their pool of knowledge is as vast as their experience in printing. Their expertise and guidance has proved useful at every step. Their uncompromising quality standards have made this book an exceptional effort. Their encouragement from time to time has been an inspiration for everyone.

The publisher and the editorial board hope that this book will prove to be a valuable piece of knowledge for researchers, students, practitioners and scholars across the globe.

List of Contributors

Kostinov Mikhail Petrovich
Federal State-Funded Research Institution "Scientific Research Institute of Vaccines and Sera named after I.I. Mechnikov", Moscow, Russia Federal State-Funded Educational Institution of Higher Education "First Moscow State Medical University named after I.M. Sechenov" of Ministry of Healthcare of Russia, Moscow, Russia

Cherdantsev Alexander Petrovich
Federal State-Funded Educational Institution of Higher Education "Ulyanovsk State University", Ulyanovsk, Russia

Shmitko Anna Dmitrievna, Akhmatova Nelly Kimovna and Polyschuk Valentina Borisovna
Federal State-Funded Research Institution "Scientific Research Institute of Vaccines and Sera named after I.I. Mechnikov", Moscow, Russia

Kostinova Aristitsa Mikhailovna
National Research Center–Institute of Immunology Federal Medical-Biological Agency of Russia, Moscow, Russia

Praulova Darya Alexandrovna
Dmitriy Rogachev Federal Research Center of Pediatric Hematology, Oncology and Immunology of the Ministry of Health of Russian Federation, Moscow, Russia

Protasov Andrey Dmitrievich and Zhestkov Alexander Victorovich
Federal State-Funded Educational Institution of Higher Education "Samara State Medical University" of Ministry of Healthcare of Russia, Samara, Russia

Tezikov Yuriy Vladimirovich
Department of Obstetrics and Gynecology №1, Samara State Medical University, Samara, Russia

Andrey Dmitrievich Protasov, Mikhail Petrovich Kostinov, Alexander Victorovich Zhestkov, Mikhail L'vovich Shteiner, Svetlana Vyacheslavovna Kazharova, Yuriy Vladimirovich Tezikov and Igor Stanislavovich Lipatov
Samara State Medical University, Samara, Russian Federation Mechnikov Research Institute of Vaccines and Sera, Moscow, Russian Federation

Yasemin Budama-Kilinc and Rabia Cakir-Koc
Department of Bioengineering, Chemical and Metallurgical Engineering Faculty, Yildiz Technical University, Esenler, Istanbul, Turkey

Chen Wang, Chengshui Liao and Wufan Zhang
Key Laboratory of Veterinary Oncological Immunology, Henan University of Science and Technology, Luoyang, China

Deyuan Li and Puyan Chen
Key Laboratory of Animal Bacteriology of China's Department of Agriculture, Nanjing Agricultural University, Nanjing, China

Ewan Peter Plant, Tatiana Zagorodnyaya, Elvira Rodionova, Alin Voskanian-Kordi, Vahan Simonyan, Zhiping Ye and Majid Laassri
Center for Biologics Evaluation and Research, US Food and Drug Administration, Silver Spring, MD, USA

Atsushi Yasuda and Motoyuki Esaki
Ceva Animal Health, Yokohama, Japan

Kristi Moore Dorsey
Ceva Animal Health, Lenexa, Kansas, USA

Zoltan Penzes and Vilmos Palya
Ceva Animal Health, Budapest, Hungary

Darrell R. Kapczynski
Exotic and Emerging Avian Viral Disease Research Unit, Southeast Poultry Research Laboratory, U.S. National Poultry Research Center, Athens, Georgia, USA

Yannick Gardin
Ceva Animal Health, Libourne, France

Ronghui Wang
College of Biosystems Engineering and Food Science, Zhejiang University, Hangzhou, China Department of Biological and Agricultural Engineering, University of Arkansas, Fayetteville, AR, USA

Yanbin Li
College of Biosystems Engineering and Food Science, Zhejiang University, Hangzhou, China Department of Biological and Agricultural Engineering, University of Arkansas, Fayetteville, AR, USA Center of Excellence for Poultry Science, University of Arkansas, Fayetteville, AR, USA

Mikhail Petrovich Kostinov
I. Mechnikov Research Institute of Vaccines and Sera,

Moscow, Russia Federal State-Funded Educational Institution of Higher Education "First Moscow State Medical University named after I.M. Sechenov" of Ministry of Healthcare of Russia, Moscow, Russia

Nelli Kimovna Akhmatova, Ekaterina Alexandrovna Khromova, Svetlana Anatolyevna Skhodova and Vera Nikolaevna Stolpnikova
I. Mechnikov Research Institute of Vaccines and Sera, Moscow, Russia

Alexander Petrovich Cherdantsev
Federal State-Funded Educational Institution of Higher Education "Ulyanovsk State University", Ulyanovsk, Russia

Anna Egorovna Vlasenko
Novokuznetsk State Institute of Advanced Medical Education, the Branch of Federal State-Funded Educational Institution of Additional Professional Education "Russian Medical Academy of Continuous Professional Education" of the Ministry of Healthcare of Russia, Novokuznetsk, Russia

Jill M. Manske
University of St. Thomas, Saint Paul, MN, USA

Tsunetaka Ohta
R&D Center, Hayashibara Co. Ltd., Okayama, Japan

Index

www.ingramcontent.com/pod-product-compliance
Lightning Source LLC
LaVergne TN
LVHW060542210926
848485LV00005B/1240

* 9 7 8 1 6 3 9 8 7 3 2 2 7 *